She Was An... During World War II

I loved this book. Jeane has captured these two nurses so well they became real to me as did the other characters. Using the genre of historical fiction, I got a complete picture of the time and experiences of nurses and the worlds they worked in.

My niece had not heard of the Bataan Death March, and she is 41! I know from speaking to others that a lot of the history of WWII is being lost, and especially the part nurses played in ensuring that our military personnel were well cared for was largely forgotten. As a veteran and a nurse, I could relate to this both personally and professionally. Jeane Slone's work is so good, all students and the general public need to and must read her books.

— Donna Cambra BSN (retired Army Nurse), MFT

I was very moved by the story even though I knew from Jeane's other four books that the women were strong. But it was a surprise to see how strong, dedicated and skilled they were here in the face of combat danger, human suffering, and discrimination. I wouldn't be surprised if the book becomes a movie.

—Bob Matreci, Pacific Coast Museum staff member, Santa Rosa, CA, Vietnam Veteran, World War II history buff

Jeane Slone shines a powerful spotlight on the immense courage, extreme fortitude, and personal resilience of World War II nurses serving our country while enduring intensely difficult and potentially lethal combat conditions. The story is insightful with its keen historical depictions of this critical era, and deftly conveys the experience and impact of segregation in the Armed Forces. Certainly, the strength and dedication of her characters will leave an indelible impression on readers.

Anita Rowell, co-author with her father, Dr. Granville Coggs, of his biography, *Soaring Inspiration: The Journey of an Original Tuskegee Airman*

She Was An American Combat Nurse During World War II

A Historical Novel

Jeane Slone

SHE WAS AN AMERICAN COMBAT NURSE
DURING WORLD WAR II

ISBN: 978-1-7320741-3-2

Printed in the United States of America
First Printing, 2023

Table of Contents

Author's Note

The terms "Negro" and "Colored" have been used when appropriate to maintain the historical perspective of the resources used. Note that the term "Black" was first popularly used in 1966 by Stokely Carmichael, political activist. Political activist Jesse Jackson later popularized the term "African American" in 1990. The terms "Jap" and "Nip" were used commonly during WW II and while considered offensive today, are historically accurate.

Any questionable language usage in this text is drawn directly from the author's historical sources, and has been left intact for the sake of authenticity of the verbiage of the time. Such usage should not be considered a reflection on the author's personal principles and ethics.

Acknowledgments

I could not have produced this five-year project without my incredible, patient, knowledgeable, and perfectionist editor, Cris Wanzer, www.ManuscriptsToGo.com. She has always expressed such a sincere love of my historical novels.

Thanks to my four beta readers, who reviewed the draft manuscript and had super "hawk-eye" abilities in finding errors and making suggestions in their fields of expertise.

Thank you to **Donna R. Cambra**, Army Nurse Corps, retired, BSN, MFT, mother and grandmother.

Donna joined the Army in 1974 after graduating from high school. She won a four-year prestigious scholarship from the University of Maryland to the Walter Reed Army Institute of Nursing Medical Center, which was approved by Congress. The Army needed nurses for the Vietnam War, so this program was created, and accepted male and female students as officer candidates. In 1978, Ms. Cambra graduated as a 1st Lieutenant and attended officers' basic training at Ft. Sam Huston, San Antonio, Texas. She was given orders for Letterman Army Medical Center at the Presidio, San Francisco, CA and spent six years as a medical-surgical nurse working with Korean and Vietnam veterans. She was also head nurse in the metabolic research unit. As a veteran, Donna has volunteered for the American Legion Post 293 in Cloverdale, CA.

Donna began reading the manuscript right before her kidney transplant and went right on to proofreading it during her recovery. Her comment about changing the ending of the last chapter of Nurse Dottie was implemented. It was very helpful to consult Ms. Cambra about the ranks, titles, and status of the nurses, physicians, and U.S. Army personnel in the book.

I wish to also thank Donna for telling me about the official anthem of the 1944 Army Nurse Corps, which was added to the book. Ms. Cambra said that her graduating class from nursing school in 1978 sang the same 1944 song.

Bob Matreci spent the Vietnam era working on electronics for nuclear weapons and B-52 Stratofortress Bomber modifications for low-level missions. He had a 32-year career in the R&D Lab at Hewlett-Packard designing spectrum analyzers. He is a member of the Pacific Coast Air Museum staff specializing in its Air Show Safety Post and the restoration of a WW II remote-controlled machine gun from the B-29 and A-26 bombers. Bob lives in Santa Rosa, CA and is a WW II buff. Thank you, Bob, for your helpful comment about changing the ending of Nurse Dottie's last chapter. Mr. Matreci's suggestion to place a timeline with dates and places in the book plus more maps was well received and implemented. I was quite surprised when Bob contacted me to buy my historical novels again because he had lost his home in the horrific fires in Sonoma County.

Mrs. Shirley Rowell was born in 1927 and birthed her daughter at Grady Hospital in 1951. She was born and raised in Atlanta, Georgia and grew up in a neighborhood near Grady Hospital. Mrs. Rowell resides in Lucas Valley, CA. I wish to thank Shirley for her keen eye regarding accurate Negro vernacular in the 1940s.

Anita Coggs Rowell was born and raised in the San Francisco Bay Area. She is co-author with her father, Dr. Granville Coggs, of his biography, *Soaring Inspiration: The Journey of an Original Tuskegee Airman*. Anita attended the ceremonies at the U.S. Capitol in Washington, DC when the Tuskegee Airmen received the Congressional Gold Medal in 2007. She also attended the January 20, 2009 Presidential Inauguration of Barrack Obama with her father in Washington, DC, where Dr. Coggs was invited to sit near the front of the stage with many other Tuskegee Airmen. Anita lives in Northern California with her husband, and they have two adult daughters. She is a graduate of the University of California,

Berkeley, and received her MBA from San Francisco State University.

I wish to thank Anita for her many interesting comments. She was surprised that Negroes were banned from the Red Cross donor program and that the segregation of blood was required during WW II. It was quite funny when Anita wrote this after reading about how to remove leeches: *"Now that I know how to remove leeches from someone's body, I hope I never have to use this information!"* Anita also suggested that Dottie not be so concerned about being able to "prove the worth of her race" and suggested writing instead, "I want to make my family proud."

I wish to thank **Walter M. Macdougall**, author of *Angel of Bataan – The Life of a World War II Army Nurse in The War Zone and At Home.* Mr. Macdougall put me in contact with Rodney Tenney for permission to use the lovely photograph of his Aunt Alice on the cover of my historical novel. Mr. Macdougall taught middle grade and high school to many of Alice Zwicker's nieces and nephews and met her when she attended evening programs for his students.

Walter read in the local newspaper that Alice was one of the 68 nurses interned at Santo Tomas Internment Camp. He became interested in writing about Alice and began his research by contacting Rod Tenney, the oldest of Alice's nieces and nephews and the genealogist for the family.

Mr. Macdougall and Mr. Tenney collaborated on three years of research for the book *Angel of Bataan*. Both Macdougall and Tenney paid a researcher at the National Archives to acquire the zip files of Alice Zwicker's interrogation from the War Department, a transcription of which appears at the end of this book.

I also wish to thank **Rod Tenney**, nephew of Alice M. Zwicker, 1st Lt., ANC, N-720222, who kindly sent me 26 zip files and granted permission to publish them. The files contained the interrogation from the War Department testimonies about the Japanese internment of his Aunt Alice. Rob told me when he visited his Aunt Alice in her Maine cottage that she would say to him, "You play the cards you are dealt."

Thank you, **Mary Robertson,** who kindly gave me permission to use the beautiful photograph of her Aunt Olive Lucas on the cover of my book. Olive was in the Army Nurse Corps and served at the 335th Station Hospital in Tagap, Burma.

Mary Robertson's writing project began in 1998, when her father asked if she could find anything about her Aunt Olive's service in the Army Nurse Corps. Ms. Robertson wrote a five-part series for the *Talbot Spy, Nonpartisan Education-based News for Talbot County Community* in Maryland titled "The Story of Olive Lucas." Her aunt had just had a stroke and did recover; however, she lost all memory of her time in the Army Nurse Corps. Olive's family did not have letters or diaries but did have many photographs. Ms. Robertson, in researching Olive Lucas, discovered that most of her records were lost in the 1973 fire at the National Personnel Records Center in St. Louis, MO. Eighty percent of the Army service records for those discharged between November 1912 and January 1960 were lost. Mary Robertson found information from US Army records, books, websites, newspapers, interviews, and personal narratives about various nurses who were in the Army Nurse Corps at the same time as Olive, which was 1942 to 1945.

Thank you to the Healdsburg Library, Healdsburg, CA reference department where many of the intelligent, helpful staff were able to find newspaper articles and books that I couldn't locate for my research.

Finally, thank you to my history-buff husband, Dennis Ness, for his support and for sharing his military knowledge in excellent detail for all of my historical novels.

She Was An American Combat Nurse During World War II

Chapter One
Nurse Beatrice Harrington

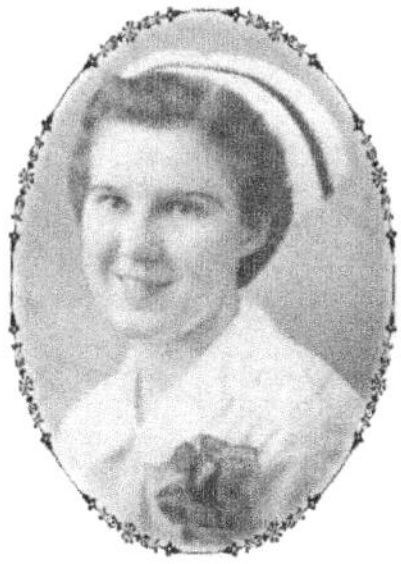

The year was 1942, and I found myself lying in a grave-like hole in the ground covered in dirt and jungle debris. Tree rats scurried up and down the sides of the foxhole and insects crawled all over me. The sharp, high-pitched whizzing sound of a bomb zoomed over my head. Oh my god, it sounded so close! I scrambled to arrange jungle foliage and branches around my foxhole for camouflage from the enemy while I waited for the bombing to end.

Another bomb dropped nearby with a flash of fire. I opened my mouth to keep my eardrums from bursting and tightened the leather chinstrap on my helmet. The entire area around me was showered with incendiary particles. I ducked my head and prayed it would be the last bomb. I had to get back to work to help patch up the casualties.

The explosions continued, shooting flames in every direction and shaking the jungle floor. To fight off the fear of the Japanese airplanes overhead, I closed my eyes and forced myself to think back to why I had become a nurse…

Years earlier, my dad became sick with influenza. With the help of a nurse, I tended to him the best I could at his bedside. After he passed away, as an only child, I continued to live at home and tried to comfort my grief-stricken mother. Later, and against her wishes, I decided to choose nursing as a career.

Mother ranted, "Beatrice, it's one thing that you took care of your father, but with total strangers, you'll be exposed to indecent male genitalia as well as infectious venereal diseases. Southern women of good character *do not* become nurses! Besides, why would you want to empty disgusting bedpans and change bloody bandages?"

I kept my head down and waited for the tirade to end, but in my mind, I plotted an escape.

Mother continued, "This is *not* a proper vocation and it is *not* a way to meet a respectable Southern beau for marriage. You should have settled on a husband after we paid for your coming-out cotillion ball when you were 16."

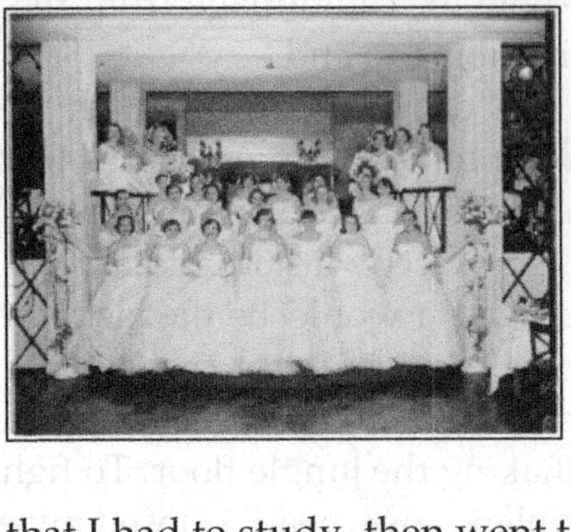

I mumbled that I had to study, then went to my bedroom and closed the door. Mother did not understand my shyness when it came to boys. After all, I was taller and slightly heavier than most of them, and had to wear glasses to boot, all of which made me stick out like a homely young girl.

I adjusted my wire-rimmed eyeglasses and escaped into

another world with a nice thick book titled *Gone with the Wind* – a story from a different time.

In 1937, I attended Grady Memorial Hospital School of Nursing in Atlanta, Georgia. I excelled in my studies, and that, paired with the extra hours I worked at the hospital, came to fruition when I received my Registered Nurse diploma. I felt the crisp official document between my fingers and hugged it to my chest, then beamed with pride as I sat alone in my bedroom once again.

My mother continued to be oblivious to the pride my nursing career gave me. "Beatrice," she lectured one day, "you don't even need to work. Your father left us plenty of money."

I learned to ignore her comments and followed my dreams. After another year went by, I earned the title of Chief of Nursing at Grady. My tall stature commanded the obedience of the nurses working under me as well as the respect necessary to run a hospital.

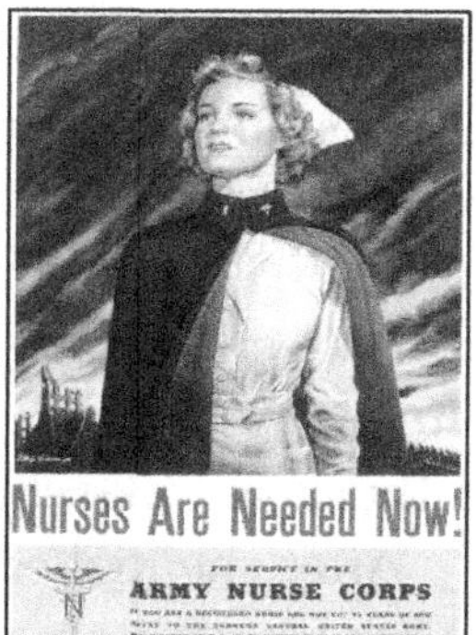

One day at the hospital, during a much-needed break, I flipped through a nursing magazine and came upon a poster of a nurse with the headline, "Join the United States Army Nurse Corps." My heart raced as I pictured myself in my nurse's uniform, and I could almost feel the wind in my hair like the image of the nurse in the magazine conveyed. I was ready to show my patriotism, especially after reading the slogan under the photograph that exclaimed, "Serve your country and travel the world to see exotic lands!"

That's the ticket! I thought. This was how I could continue my nursing career, travel, and get out from under my mother's oppressive thumb.

On my day off, I put on my white, starched nurse's uniform with my badge that read *Grady Hospital, Chief Beatrice Harrington,* and wrapped my blue, red-lined cape around my shoulders. I pushed my dull brown hair into my nurse's cap as best I could, then walked to the Red Cross Recruitment Center, my shoulders back and my head held high.

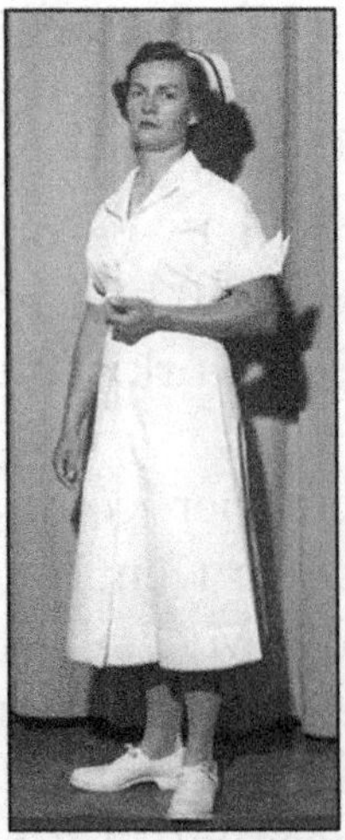

I pulled open the heavy door and walked inside with confidence. With a slight twitch in my hands, I presented my credentials to a serious woman in a Red Cross uniform and introduced myself. When she heard me say "Chief of Nursing," her eyebrows rose and her face glowed with enthusiasm, like she was about to catch a big fish.

After she looked over my papers, she presented her hand. "Miss Harrington, welcome to the United States Army Nurse Corps. Please read these forms and sign below." She handed me a pen.

I slid my finger down the pages as I read the forms line by

line, then held the pen tight to produce a proper signature.

Officer Clark rose from behind her desk. With a shiny, red-lipstick smile, she placed her hand over her heart and said, "Repeat after me..."

She recited the Nightingale Pledge, and I repeated each line after her.

> *I solemnly pledge myself before God and in the presence of this assembly, to pass my life in purity and to practice my profession faithfully. I will abstain from whatever is deleterious and mischievous and will not take or knowingly administer any harmful drug.*
>
> *I will do all in my power to maintain and elevate the standard of my profession and will hold in confidence all personal matters committed to my keeping and all family affairs coming to my knowledge in the practice of my calling. With loyalty will I endeavor to aid the physician in his work and devote myself to the welfare of those committed to my care.*

That finished, she shook my hand once more and said, "Thank you for joining the Army Nurse Corps. Your service is needed as we have fewer than 1,000 nurses in the United States who have enlisted. And as you know, there is a war going on in Europe and we might need more. You'll receive your assignment for basic training within two weeks in the mail."

I floated home, trying to hide my immense smile. I hoped my eyes weren't too full of sparkles as I opened the front door. Mother was in her sitting room. I waved a quick hello and slipped past her to my bedroom.

Over dinner that night, Mother's voice rose to a high pitch as she again brought up the subject of my nursing career. "Beatrice, how can you continue to empty bedpans and be around all those illnesses?"

I sighed. "Mom, I've told you this before. I'm chief of

nursing, which means I'm a supervisor and don't do those jobs anymore." I gripped my fork as my cheeks flushed.

"But how can you meet a husband at such a place? What about the doctors? Are they all married?" Her tired, grayish eyes bored into mine.

I set my fork down and leaned forward. "Mother, I've joined the Army Nurse Corps," I announced.

"You *what?*" She stopped eating and crossed her arms. "Now you'll be with only girls, for heaven's sake!"

I shoved a big bite of mashed potatoes into my mouth.

Mother's eyes filled with tears. She whispered, "Can you change your mind?"

"I cannot and will not." I pushed my chair back from the dining room table, cleared my plate to the kitchen, then stormed off to my room to read a chapter from my thick, enticing novel.

Two weeks later, Mother drove me to the train station. From there, I would leave for Fort Huachuca, Arizona for basic training.

"Darling, I have a present for you." She held out a small, thin white box. She took the lid off and said, "This was your grandmother's. Wear it for good luck and take care of the diamonds on it." She handed me an ornate, dainty watch and dabbed her teary eyes. "Make sure you don't lose it."

"Thank you, Mom. I will treasure it and think of you and Grandma when I wear it. Don't worry, I'll write to you as much as possible."

She kept crying as I got out of the car.

"Have fun playing bridge at Mrs. Wilson's tonight," I said cheerfully as I closed the car door.

A short time later, my mother seemed frail and small as I looked at her out of the train window by my seat. I wiped a tear from my eye, then turned the diamond-studded watch around on my wrist and admired how it glittered in the sunshine beaming through the window.

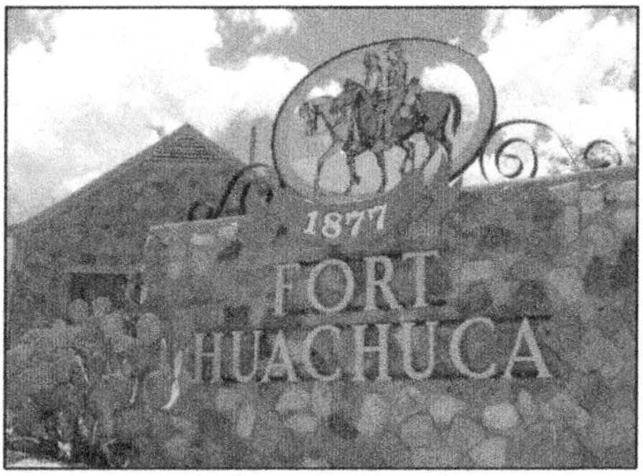

Full of excitement, I arrived at Fort Huachuca in July of 1941 for four weeks of basic training. The summer desert heat was different from the heat I was used to in the South. It was an extremely dry heat, not sticky like at home. I hauled my suitcase through the immense base, which was set on a vast number of acres, and looked around for a sign to guide me.

One of the officers noticed I was lost and said, "Welcome to Fort Huachuca. Are you looking for your barracks?" He puffed his cigar, then put it out in the dirt with his boot.

"Yes," I answered.

"I'm Sgt. McDonald. Follow me." He grabbed my suitcase. "By the way, remember to always salute all officers on the base."

"Thank you, sir. I'm Chief Harrington."

The sergeant brought me to a long, wooden, freshly painted barracks with a sign on it that read *Whites Only*. He pulled open the door and set my suitcase inside. "Here's your new home."

I introduced myself and the group of 30 nurses in the barracks greeted me warmly. It seemed to be a lively, social environment filled with laughter. Everyone was dressed either in nursing uniforms or casual outfits. Each of the women introduced themselves and said where they were from.

"What are those?" I asked, pointing to a stack of boxes near the wall.

"They must be our uniforms," Veronica said as she retrieved a box and tore it open.

Cute, red-headed Molly grabbed one as well. She peered inside and said, "These are some kind of overalls, not uniforms."

Susie pulled out a set of coveralls and inspected the label. "Jeepers, size men's 42 large! No way am I wearing that!" She threw them down. "These coveralls are not designed for our curves. They're too big and will make me look fat!"

I took control of the situation. "Girls, I think these are what we'll have to wear for the rigors of basic training. They must be men's surplus. Here, Agnes, you and I are bigger women. Let's take the 44 large coveralls. The smaller nurses can try the 42 size." I shuffled through another box. "Look, here's a bunch of men's khaki shirts and pants. At least we can roll them up better. Help yourself, gals, this is all we seem to have."

Molly put on a pair of pants. "Look, Chief, they have attached belts." She handed out pants to the others.

"Thanks, Molly." I grabbed a pair of size 44s and stepped into them, then pulled the pants up over my full figure. My nursing shoes were a size 13 so I had no trouble fitting into the provided soldier boots. The socks were also for large men.

Everyone stripped down to their underwear and donned either coveralls or shirts and pants. The belts cinched up the waists and when we rolled up the sleeves and legs, the outfits fit better. Some of the nurses had safety pins, which helped tuck in the excess fabric as well. Everyone tried on the men's boots. Most of the women found size five too big, but they stuffed the toes with extra socks, which helped.

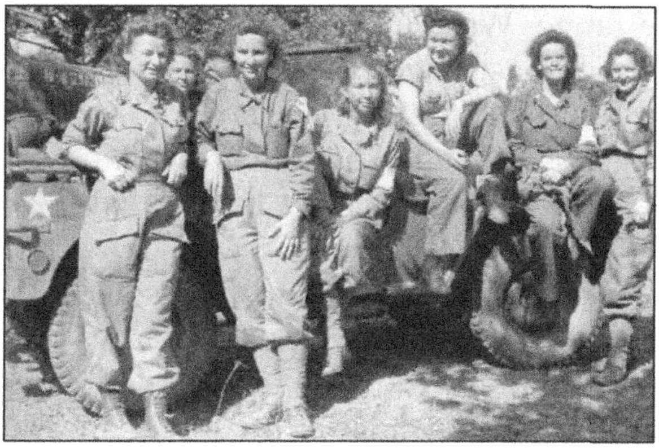

In the morning, we woke to the sound of a bugle and dashed outside to find the dining room for breakfast. We passed by a group of medical corpsmen, who blew wolf whistles at us and admired our new "uniforms."

Sgt. McDonald came to the mess hall and told us to meet him outside after chow for calisthenics. I was a bit worried about calisthenics since I was slightly overweight and had never been one to participate in high school sports. Nonetheless, I put on my happy face and said to my nurses, "It will be fun to exercise with everyone outside."

Agnes protested, "I don't think I can do those—doesn't that mean push-ups also?"

Veronica, who wore lipstick, bragged, "Oh, goody! I was a cheerleader. We'll have a wonderful time!"

A short time later, we were outside in the hot desert sun. Sgt. McDonald had us stand in several lines. He stood in front of us, and in a flash did two push-ups, then two jumping jacks followed by trunk twists, two sit-ups, and one lunge.

"Chief," he said to me. "Make sure everyone does 10 sets of these exercises. I have a meeting to attend." He rushed off.

I was taken by surprise to be left in charge but made sure everyone did the exercise sets, including myself. We took our time and it wasn't too bad.

A smaller sergeant came by and ordered us to follow him

to the rifle range. We trailed after him, then stood in lines again waiting for instruction.

Sgt. Boyd said, "Girls, I'm going to teach you how to fire a rifle at a target." He handed out the firearms.

Susie said, "This is too heavy for me. Don't you have a lighter one?"

Sgt. Boyd chuckled. "No, one size fits all. I'll show you how to use it. Lay prostrate and put your arms on a sandbag like this..." He got down on the ground and demonstrated. "Then look through the sight at the target and squeeze the trigger. Your semi-automatic gun has an eight-shot clip in it, and you have eight tries to shoot the bullseye on the target."

He fired his rifle and hit the bullseye eight times. The nurses clapped.

The sergeant asked, "Who wants to go first?"

When no one stepped forward, I volunteered. I tried but didn't hit the target. None of the nurses did but the sergeant didn't seem concerned.

"Nice try. It's a good thing we're not at war and it's not part of your job as nurses. But because it's in your basic training curriculum, everyone must at least try."

We were drenched with sweat during most of our basic training days in the desert climate of Fort Huachuca. As chief, I found that the constant exercise was not an easy task and I had no experience with athletics, but I had to set an example for the nurses and kept my attitude positive to keep my staff's morale up.

I became pals with Molly and after a couple of weeks of training, we each got a pass for day leave, so we decided to explore Huachuca. I wore my casual shirtwaist two-tone print dress with a matching belt and my black, low pumps, which were great for practical walking. My new hat covered my ordinary brown hair. I watched Molly fashion her light-red hair into a series of rolls in the front, then she tied a big red bow that gathered the rest in the back.

"You have gorgeous hair, Molly, and your plaid dress shows off your nice figure."

"Thanks, Chief. My hair, of course, I got because I'm Irish. My older sister handed down the dress to me and I'm lucky she kept it clean. I like your bonnet—it suits your dress." Molly put on her dainty pumps, which had open toes and higher heels than mine, though I was still taller than her.

We took the bus into town. When we disembarked at the bus stop, a group of boys hooted and whistled at Molly.

She giggled and remarked, "Did you see the one with the wavy blond hair and blue eyes? He was a hot dish."

I laughed. "I'm glad we decided not to wear our nurses' uniforms. You wouldn't have gotten as many whistles. Let's go into that gift shop. I'd like to find something to take home to my mother."

"I'd like to get a cigarette lighter for my brother, who's away at college," Molly added.

After our purchases, we walked down the sidewalk with the Arizona heat beating down on us.

"There's an ice cream sign in that department store window. Let's go in there to get out of the sun," I suggested. I got my lace hanky out of my purse and dabbed the sweat off my forehead before we went in.

We both ordered ice cream sodas piled high with whipped cream and sprinkles. The soda jerk flirted with Molly the entire time.

A short time later, on the bus back to the base, Molly and I chatted nonstop about our little escape from the grind of basic training.

Time passed and our final day of training arrived. We met Sgt. Boyd outside, and he handed out canteens, helmets, and gas masks.

"This is your last day. You are required to go on a 10-mile hike in the mountains while carrying all your gear," he said.

Annie whined, "Ten miles? Yikes! I can't do that."

Before I could reprimand her, Sgt. Boyd said, "Don't worry, I'll follow behind you in a jeep. Take your time. We have all day."

As we climbed up the mountain, I spied a deer grazing in a nearby patch of grass. I announced in a whisper, "Look, there's a deer."

Susie, who was from Chicago, said, "I've never seen a deer. I love its puffy white tail."

The group was silent as the reddish-brown, slender animal stared back at us in wonder with big brown eyes, then disappeared back into the woods.

Toward the last part of the hike, we all longed for flat land, which would be a sure sign that we were near the base. As we walked along, we heard a strange gobble noise that frightened some of the nurses. Agnes, who was from a rural state, laughed and assured us that it was just a harmless wild turkey.

We trudged on and I hoped we were close to the end of our hike. It became hotter by the minute. Upon hearing the monotonous groans from our group, I announced, "Water break!"

The nurses emitted deep sighs as we all sat down, and everyone gulped water from their canteens.

"Only drink half, we need it to last," I said.

After a few more complaints, everyone got up.

"Let's keep our thoughts on the fact that tomorrow, we get to go to the hospital and learn about nursing overseas. And this, girls, means *sitting!* Something I'm sure you'll all enjoy."

We were on our way down the mountain as the sun began to set. *Surely, we must be close to the end by now,* I thought hopefully. Though I kept up a brave front, I would definitely be happy when this part of basic training was over.

Chapter Two
Nurse Dora Mae Williams

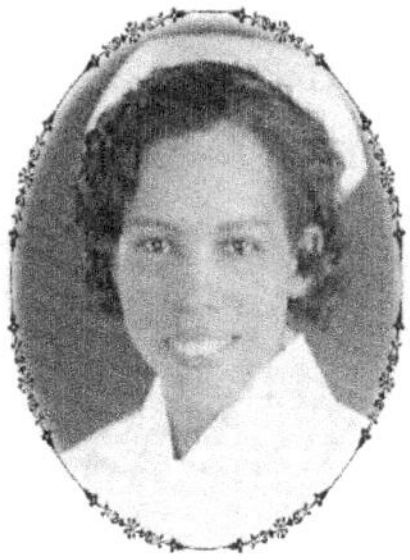

At 21 years of age, I was ready to see the world, and my acceptance into the Army Nurse Corps would be my financial ticket to do so. Although I was on the short side of the height scale, I made up for it with my feistiness and appeared tall and confident. Or so I thought. Daddy always called me small but mighty. He was a Buffalo Soldier in World War I, and the first Negro colonel in the U.S. Army. I was the oldest child in my family and wanted to follow in his footsteps and join the Army as a nurse. So, I applied. And when the letter arrived from the Army, I tore it open with anticipation.

> *To Dora Mae Williams, June 1941*
>
> *Your application to the Army Nurse Corps cannot be given favorable consideration as there are no provisions in Army regulations for the appointment of colored nurses in the Corps.*
>
> *Surgeon General, James C. Magee*
> *US Army Medical Corps*

I threw the letter down on the table and mumbled, "Segregation is as prominent in the military as it is in the South."

I was furious. After all, it took three-and-a-half years to obtain my Registered Nurse degree while I worked at the hospital and studied for school. With much pride, I had graduated at the top of my class from the Grady Hospital Municipal Training School for Colored Nurses in Atlanta, Georgia. I assumed that since I had proven my worth, I would be accepted into the Army Nurse Corps without question. My application was rejected solely because of my race! I shouted, "I shall persevere!"

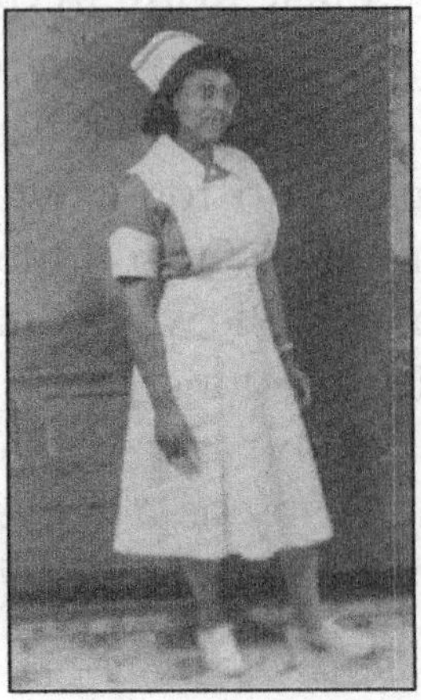

I wrote a letter of complaint to the National Nursing Council for War Service and much to my surprise, received a letter back a few weeks later.

Dear Miss Williams,

You may be assured that we are doing everything we can to remove the present discrimination which Negro nurses are facing in the Army.

Our Advisory Council, and the National Nursing

Council for War Service, are working on the matter, and we hope very soon that you will be called for service.

I am turning your letter over to the National Association of Colored Graduate Nursing as another evidence of discrimination.

Kind personal regards,
Mabel K. Staupers, R.N. Executive Secretary

A few days after the horrific bombing of Pearl Harbor, I heard soul-stirring appeals from the Red Cross on the radio asking for blood donations, so I took it upon myself to go to the local Red Cross to donate blood. But when I arrived at the office, the supervisor frowned at me.

"I'm sorry, the National Offices have barred Negro blood donors at this time," she said.

I left in tears, shocked again at the rejection. I wanted to say to her, "Did you know that most of my Negro nurse colleagues buy defense bonds?" But I didn't have the nerve.

During a break at work the next day, I shared with my fellow nurses what had happened at the Red Cross office. Martha showed me a poem she had cut out of our local newspaper, written by Geraldyne Ghess, a high school student.

Had I wealth, I'd burn it all;
Not one cent for the Red Cross call.
Our money is good ... our blood is bad.
But, still that shouldn't make us mad.
Are they afraid they'll all turn black?
Is that why our blood they lack?

Undeterred, I continued to do an outstanding job at the hospital but yearned for something more. Georgia was the only state I had ever been in, and I wanted to travel the world and support myself at the same time. But I was not a quitter and was taught to never give up. Mama called it "stick-to-itiveness." Both of my parents expected everyone in the family to emulate this trait. And so, with a lot of hard work and determination, I earned the title of Chief of Nursing at the segregated C&D wing of the colored section of the hospital.

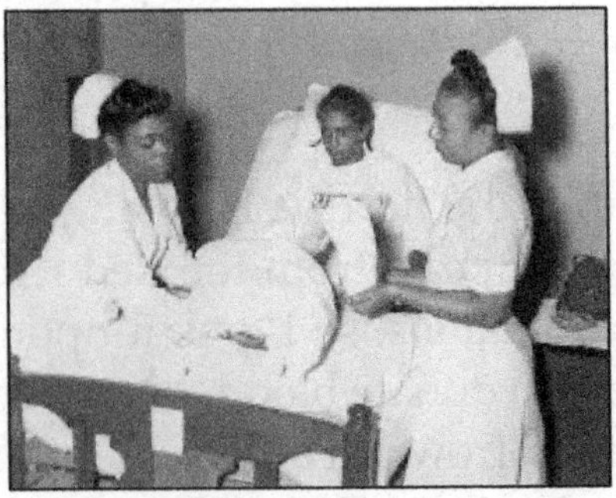

The field of nursing came naturally to me after I had cared for my five brothers and two sisters when the influenza virus struck the family. It hit everyone except my mama and me. God must have known we needed to be spared to help the rest of the family get better. When Daddy became incapacitated by the virus and passed away, that's when I heard my calling to be a nurse.

I received a decent public school education provided by no-nonsense Georgia Negro teachers who wanted to produce productive citizens despite the Jim Crow laws of that time, which made Negro and White races separate. I knew the White schools were better funded, so our education was lower quality. My teachers would say, "Make do and learn. Use it up and wear it out."

Mama had to cook and clean for a well-to-do White family to earn the needed income to support us. I helped earn a second income in housekeeping at the hospital but still managed to graduate from high school at the same time. I loved having my own money, which allowed me to contribute income to the family and buy a Coca-Cola whenever I wanted to.

After high school, I was accepted into nursing school and learned basic skills, like how to bathe patients, take vital signs, and empty bedpans. I was fascinated by the nursing laboratory, which expanded my limited knowledge as a student nurse. We practiced taking each other's blood pressure, temperature, and learned how to use a stethoscope. We learned proper techniques to prevent bed sores by turning each other over without causing injury. My friend, Martha, tickled me when she rolled me over and I giggled the entire time.

Our "fun" escapades ended after our chief of nursing became ill, went on leave, and was replaced by old Chief Graft. We all wondered where they had dug her up from. My first encounter with her was when I was assigned to the surgery ward. I had to bathe an obese, middle-aged woman who had just had abdominal surgery. It took me an hour to give her a bath because she was so large, and I had to be careful of her wounds the entire time.

Old Chief Graft, full of fire, chastised me. "Miss Williams, it took you an entire hour to bathe your patient. I timed you. It should have taken 15 minutes. You will never advance in this career if you don't speed it up!"

I bit my lip, glanced down at my nursing shoes with flushed cheeks, and mumbled, "Yes, ma'am."

The next day, I spied the chief with a scowl on her wrinkled face as she inspected a new nursing student. "Ellie, your nursing pin is crooked."

After Ellie straightened her pin, Chief Graft declared, "You need to do something with that unruly hair of yours. Pull your cap on tighter."

Ellie tried to pull more of her curly strands under her nursing cap without success. The aged chief just clucked her tongue and left to go after her next victim.

I began to worry whether I would make it to graduation with this boss, who seemed to be on the lookout for any little mistake. But I was determined not to be one of the nurses in training who let their emotions take over, which would mean certain failure.

The next week, Irene, who was ready to graduate, ended up quitting and walked out on her shift. It was hard to stand Chief Graft's drive for perfection. Her authoritative rule made for constant conflict and resulted in poor performance from all of the student nurses.

One of the hardest parts of nursing for me was the sound of patients vomiting or coughing up phlegm. It was the noise of it that made me gag. Sometimes I would hear a patient throw up and I'd have to look around to see whether the chief was nearby, then I'd turn my head and swallow hard while I took deep breaths, got a pan, and went to attend to the patient.

Our own Negro physicians were not permitted to work in the hospital. This meant we were under the rule of the White attending doctors. On one of my shifts, I had to care for Mr. Johnson, who had liver cancer. A White doctor, Doctor Miller, gave him oxygen, but the patient still passed away right before my eyes. The doctor looked at his watch, stated the time, then gave me a hard stare.

I looked at him in wonder as he demanded, "What are you waiting for? Write down the time of death on the chart and prepare the body." He rushed out of the room.

I stared at poor Mr. Johnson, the dead man, and shivered as I thought about my father's death.

Head nurse Alma walked in. "Dottie, why are you standing around doing nothing?"

"I don't know how to prepare a dead body...can you help me?" I stammered.

After she heard the word "dead," she averted her eyes and looked out the window. "After a man dies, you must prepare the body for the mortuary and cover all the orifices—the mouth, nostrils, penis, and anus – with bandages. This is done so the body fluids don't drain out prematurely. Go and get the bandages and an ID tag. Write the patient's name on the tag, then tie it to his big toe."

She turned to walk out of the room but I stopped her.

"Please, help me…"

Alma raised her voice, "No, I will not."

I pleaded, "Please just watch me to make sure I do it right. I've never done this before."

She said louder, "No, I don't deal with dead bodies, and I never will!" Then she bolted out of the room.

I looked after her with amazement. This nurse was about to graduate, and I wondered, would the hospital pass her? I looked back at Mr. Johnson, pulled myself together, and resolved to finish the job. If I let every death affect me, then how could I save lives?

Praise the Lord, the next year, I replaced Chief Graft who, much to the staff's relief, retired.

Even though the students at the school for Negro nurses followed the same curriculum as the White nurses, segregation continued and the two programs did not mix. Rumor had it that the White doctors viewed Negro patients as expendable, which made a perfect opportunity for experimentation. As chief, I kept a secret eye on these young new White physicians to make sure they did a proper job. It peeved me to think that colored people could not receive medical care from their own race at the hospital. The Negro physicians in Atlanta were not allowed to admit their own patients or even visit them in the colored ward at Grady.

The hospital provided segregated dormitories for out-of-state nurses of both races. After I heard constant complaints from my student nurses about their housing, one night I went to visit their dorms. I went to the basement of the hospital and left the door just slightly ajar so I could see inside but not disturb the 20 nurses, who were sound asleep. The dismal beds were only two feet apart. There were no lamps or tables, and the air was fetid due to the nearby toilet facilities. Under every bed was an open suitcase being used as a dresser. As I peered around the dim basement, a huge rat brushed past me. I clamped my surprised mouth shut, then spun on my heels and left, glad I lived with my family in the country. We were crowded at home but at least we had windows, pictures on the wall, and space to go outside for fresh air.

One night during an uneventful shift, I decided to explore the White hospital wing. It was quite new, renovated by a recent fundraising campaign. So, I slipped into the A&B White dormitory, which was separated by a single hallway from the Negro C&D wing.

I crept down the hall as if sneaking into a church service late. It sparked a memory…

When I was a young girl, on a hot July day, I had the urge to sip from the "Whites Only" water fountain in my hometown. I wanted to see if that water tasted better than the water from the substandard "colored only" fountain. Besides, no one was around. I took a long drink.

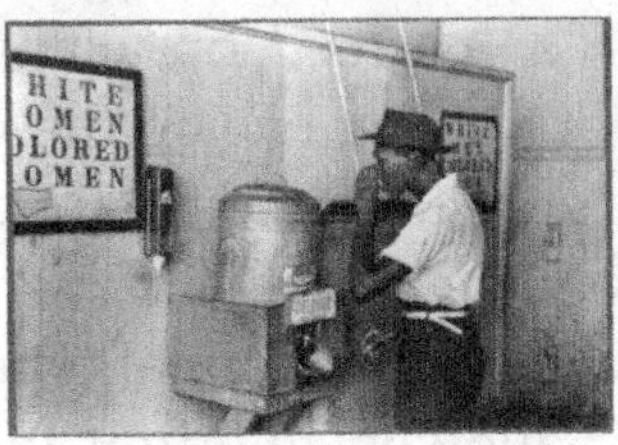

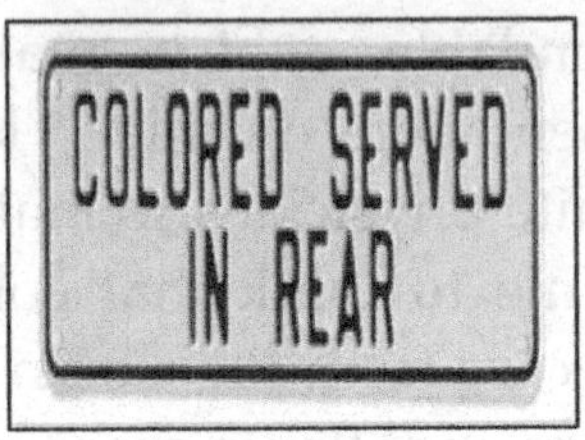

A gang of White boys snuck up behind me, and a tall blond boy pushed the back of my head into the spigot, causing the water to spray me in the face. He yelled out to impress his buddies, "Don't cha know, girl, that niggers aren't allowed to drink from our fountains?" He flipped his finger toward the "Whites Only" sign.

"I can't read," I fibbed and inched away from them, then

ran like the dickens back home.

It turned out, the water tasted the same. It was just from a much fancier fountain.

Mama was outside hanging the wash when I raced into the yard. "Dora, what are you runnin' from?"

Not able to fib to my mother, I said, "I wanted to taste the water from the White fountain…to see if it tasted better than ours."

She frowned. "Don't you ever break any Jim Crow laws. You could get killed!" After she saw the fear in my eyes, her voice softened. "Honey, White folks rule. Someday we'll be equal but until that day comes, promise me you will not defy any laws."

I broke out in tears. Mama put down the laundry basket and held me in her arms.

When I calmed down, I asked, "Why do we have different toilets and water fountains?"

"Well, baby, it's like this. The White folks think we are dirty people and don't want us to use the same fountains or let our butts touch the same toilets."

"But Mama, it's not true! We are clean people. And we clean the White folks' houses! Mama, who is Jim Crow?"

"It's not a person. It means that colored people and White people, by law, have to stay separate."

"But…why, Mama?"

"White people made the laws, and we can only hope that someday our people will rise up and be treated the same. I am blessed to work for the Sanborn family, who make me feel like a family member rather than a servant. Someday, honey, maybe we'll have the same rights as White people. Come inside now and help me make supper."

Both of my parents were proud people and gave all of us the confidence to not fear our White neighbors or hold them in awe. But they did not tolerate fibs or mischief.

My insatiable curiosity flamed as I snapped out of my reverie and peered into the dim light of the new, spacious White dormitory. Each private room had two beds, dressers, and tables with cute little lamps on them. Beyond that area was a library and a science lab. There were 16 private rooms and 40 double-occupancy rooms, several parlors, recreation rooms, a large auditorium, and a dining room.

I tiptoed toward the dining room but was interrupted when a White nurse walked up behind me.

"What are you doing in this section?" She scanned my face.

"I'm the new housekeeper," popped out of my mouth.

"Then where are your supplies?" Her voice was loud and woke up one of the other nurses.

"I'd better go get them." I scampered out of there like a caught thief.

On my way home, I weaved my way to the back of the crowded bus where colored people were required to sit. I once again pondered the separate and not-so-equal segregation laws, and things like the dormitories at Grady. It was a well-known fact that White nurses were paid more than Negro nurses, even though Grady was a public hospital funded by city taxes. I shook my head, thinking about the refusal of my application in June. I was heartbroken that the Army Nurse Corps would not take Negro nurses. I wondered if my letter of complaint to the National Nursing Council for War Service would do any good. It was so unfair.

As chief, I found myself involved with several tricky racial segregation situations. I checked in a young Negro man who'd had a kitchen accident and needed a blood transfusion, but had a rare blood type. He was the cook for a White family and his employer, Mrs. Sadler, brought him in. It was hospital policy to never mix blood from two different races and the glass bottles were required to be labeled with the bold letter "N" for Negro. As precious time was lost in an attempt to find the correct racial blood type for the hemorrhaging patient, Mrs. Sadler insisted that we take her blood to determine what type she had.

A short time later, when I told her she had the same blood type as our patient, she pleaded with me, "My cook is valuable and has been with our family for many years. I beg you, take my blood to save him."

I relented but worried about losing my job. I decided to bend the rules, and had the Negro cook and his White employer lie side by side in the hospital corridor between the White and Negro wings of Grady.

One young White nursing student walked by and asked, "Will this make him White?"

I rolled my eyes. "I don't think so," I replied. "But at least he won't be dead."

The procedure was successful, the cook survived, and thank goodness, I didn't get caught breaking the rules and terminated.

Another incident occurred at Grady when a woman was struck by a car while crossing a city street in Atlanta, and was taken into the hospital, unconscious. Mrs. Wilson was light-skinned and was checked into the White section for care by mistake. A colored man who said he was her husband came into the Negro section to inquire about her.

I looked at the intake records and told him, "No, she's not here."

"I know she is," Mr. Wilson said as he gripped the counter.

"Is she White or Negro?"

It felt like a stupid question, but I was relieved when he answered, "My wife is a light Negro."

I called over to the White section. Chief Beatrice Harrington answered and said Mrs. Wilson was indeed registered there. Chief Harrington had her transferred to our Negro section immediately and Mrs. Wilson received a needed "N" blood transfusion. Indeed, Mrs. Wilson did look quite White, but I was obligated to follow the law. The definition of a Negro was that even if a person had only 1/16 Negro blood, they were still considered Negro.

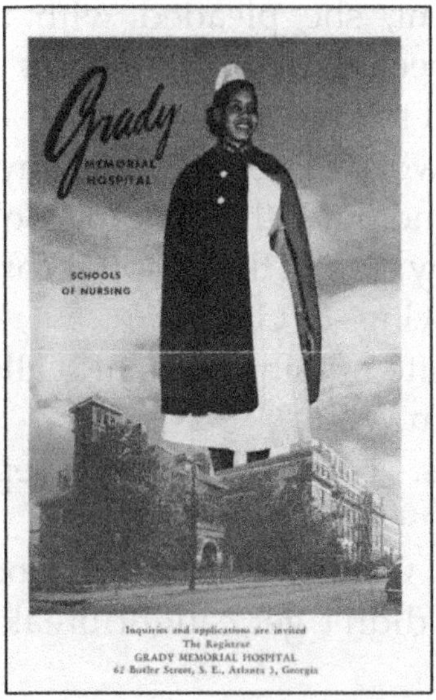

Our hospital was abuzz with talk about the war as it continued to escalate and spread into many countries. I heard that Chief Bea Harrington of the White Grady Hospital left to join the Nurses Corps overseas on the island of the Philippines. After the surprise attack from the Japanese on our territory of Hawaii, I read that the Philippines had been continuously bombed. I hoped Chief Harrington was OK.

I read in the May 1942 *American Journal of Nursing* that Negroes were to be accepted into the Army Nurse Corps. This meant that I might have a chance to join! They must need Negro nurses now that America had declared war.

As I flipped through the journal, I saw a poster that read, "Nurses are needed now for the war effort! You can save many lives! If you are a registered nurse and are between the ages of 21–40 years old, sign up at your local Red Cross Department."

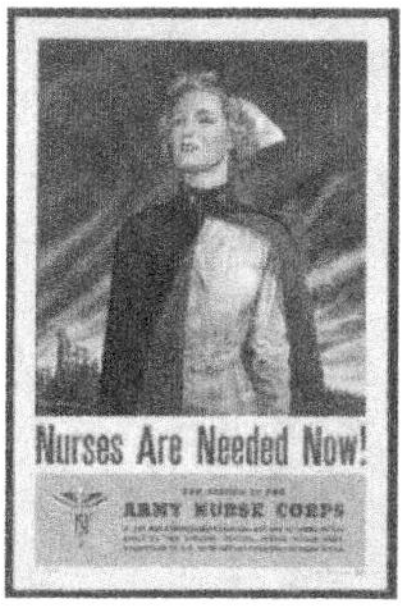
Nurses Are Needed Now!
ARMY NURSE CORPS

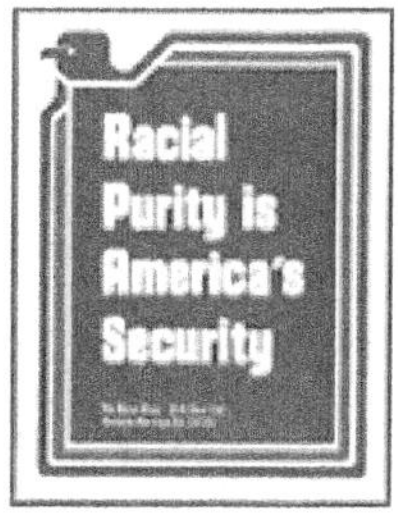
Racial
Purity is
America's
Security

I put my finger on the poster of the nurse. I couldn't identify with her blond, wavy hair, but our uniform was the same. What sparked my interest was that the pay was higher than the pay at the hospital, and the words "serve your country and see the world" inspired me. I felt a rush of excitement at the prospect of a big change in my life. So, on my day off, I marched myself down to the American Red Cross to enlist in the Army Nurse Corps.

The wrinkle-faced lady behind the desk looked up at me, then down at her paperwork.

"Good morning. I'm here to join the Army Nurse Corps," I said.

She stared at me. "We do not accept Negroes."

"I am chief of nursing at Grady Hospital." I showed her my badge.

The woman continued to ignore me and shuffled through her papers. I left the Red Cross office in a cloud of depression but continued to perform my duties at Grady Hospital.

On my break, I read the newly arrived June 1942 *American Nursing Journal* and found a hope-filled article that stated: *The Army Nurse Corps is accepting applications for a quota of 56 Negro nurses at three segregated Army bases – Camp Livingston, Louisiana; Camp Huachuca, Arizona; and Camp Florence, Arizona.*

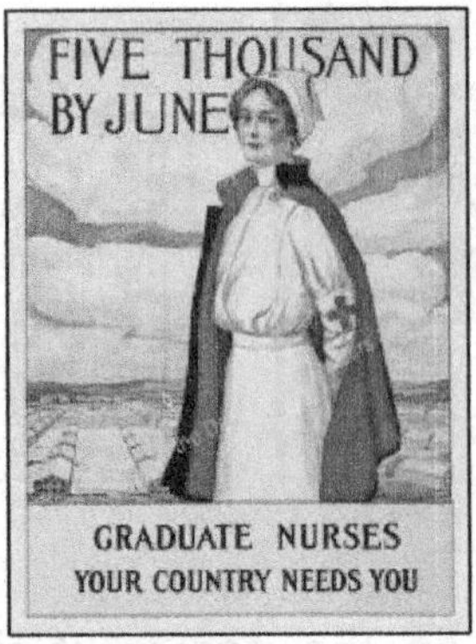
FIVE THOUSAND BY JUNE
GRADUATE NURSES
YOUR COUNTRY NEEDS YOU

Once again, I proceeded to the American Red Cross office and showed the tight-lipped woman behind the desk the article.

She drummed her fingers on her papers, then handed me an application. "Mail this to the surgeon general. Now, if you'll excuse me, I have a lot of work to do."

I sent the application to the surgeon general with a recommendation from a Grady physician. Since I was chief of nursing, I was certain I would be accepted this time; however, the low number of 56 applicants made me bite a nail off.

When I received a letter from the Army Nurse Corps, I bowed my head and said a prayer before I opened it.

> *By command of Surgeon General James C. Magee, US Army Medical Corps*
>
> *Dora Mae Williams is accepted into the Army Nurse Corps and can hereby report on July 12, 1942 to Fort Huachuca, Arizona to complete your basic training.*
>
> *War Department*

I set the coveted letter on the table and hummed one of my favorite hymns, "We Shall Overcome," which always gave me the strength to reach my goals.

On my last day at work, one of the girls made me a big chocolate cake and I received a lot of hugs and kisses along with cards and good luck wishes. After a tearful goodbye to my family, I reassured Mama that I would write often and send home some money. Then, finally, I boarded the train to Fort Huachuca, Arizona.

Chapter Three
Chief Bea
Fort Huachuca, Arizona – Manila, Philippines
1941

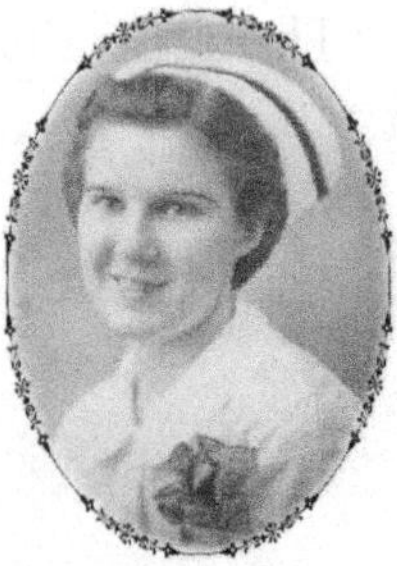

Thank goodness the first part of basic training was finished. We marched to the hospital on base, full of enthusiasm. There we were issued new duty uniforms and several pairs of white stockings.

We attended lectures in the morning and cared for soldiers suffering from various ailments in the afternoon. The month of August 1941 flew by as we took x-rays, did surgery prep, gave immunization shots to new inductees, and filled out charts.

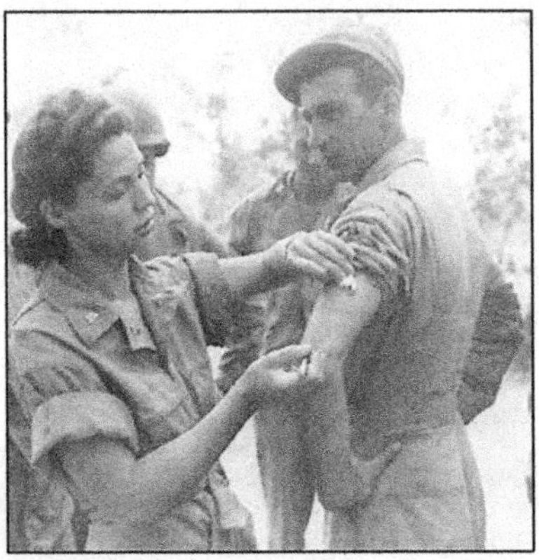

Dr. Ackerman, who was quite a serious man, lectured on malaria. "Malaria is the most prevalent disease you will encounter if you receive an overseas assignment."

Caroline and Molly beamed when they heard the word "overseas."

Dr. Ackerman continued in a deep voice, "Thick jungles, high temperatures, heavy rainfall, swamps, excessive mud, and mountainous terrain create the perfect environment to breed the specific type of mosquito that produces the parasites that invade and reproduce in the red blood cells to cause malaria. Mosquitos bite and infect the soldiers. The first symptoms are fever, headache, and chills, which usually appear 10 to 15 days after the infective bite. The recommended care for malaria is the use of quinine or Quinacrine Atabrine, and bed rest. The use of mosquito netting over beds is another preventive measure. When there is no longer fever or chills, the soldiers may return to duty; however, they should continue to take a low dose of Atabrine every day. If the disease is untreated and reaches the brain, the patient becomes comatose. If it reaches the internal organs, death will occur. I will cover other tropical diseases such as beriberi, scurvy, and scrub typhus, plus the care of patients with gangrene, in the days to come. Venereal disease is the most prolific problem you will encounter, and I will cover it in detail tomorrow and provide pamphlets for you all to hand out to the soldiers in our care. Please take the malaria bulletin to study before you leave today. Class dismissed."

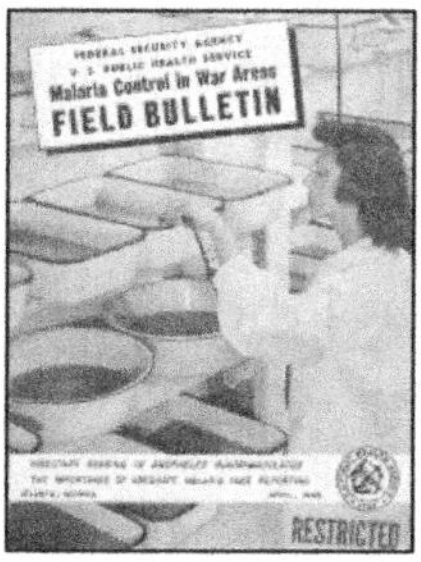

After I completed basic training, I took the train home and waited for further orders. I had put in for a transfer overseas, and every day I looked through the mail in hopes of an exotic location as an assignment.

Mother had missed me and was less overbearing than usual. One day, she asked, "Did you get an assignment letter yet, dear?"

"Not yet, I'll let you know as soon as I do."

I was not used to this much leisure time and reread a few good books in my room.

During my second week home, I received an official U.S. Army envelope in the mail. I slid my finger along the seal as fast as I could to break it. My orders were for a two-year tour of duty in Manila, the capital of the Philippine Islands. A smile spread across my face, then I prepared to tell Mother the news.

Envelope in hand, I went into the sitting room. "I got my orders, Mom. I'm going on a two-year tour in the Philippines."

She put down her newspaper. "Where's that?" she asked in a sharp voice.

"It's an island overseas."

"Why would you want to go there?" Her gray eyes darkened.

"To see the world!" I stood up taller as I thought of the poster of the proud nurse in my *Nursing Times* magazine.

"You should just stay in the States. Why couldn't you go to California or Florida if you need a change?"

"Mom, I'm in the Army now. I have no choice but to obey orders." Annoyed, I left her and went back to my room. I grabbed the "P" volume from my encyclopedia set. My fingers twitched as I found the islands of the Philippines and read eagerly to satiate my dreams of travel.

Mother drove me to the U.S. Army transport, the *SS Holbrooke*. Before boarding the ship, she said, "I hope you find a nice military officer to marry when you're there."

"Of course," I answered, and kissed her pale cheek to avoid conflict. I turned and boarded the majestic, stately ship, and waved a high-spirited goodbye as I stood by the railing.

Our group from Fort Huachuca was sent to a variety of places and we all promised to stay in touch. I had a lovely voyage and roomed with Molly. It took 19 days to reach the Philippines, during which time we gabbed and played cards. Molly went to a dance in the ship's ballroom while I stayed behind and read a good novel.

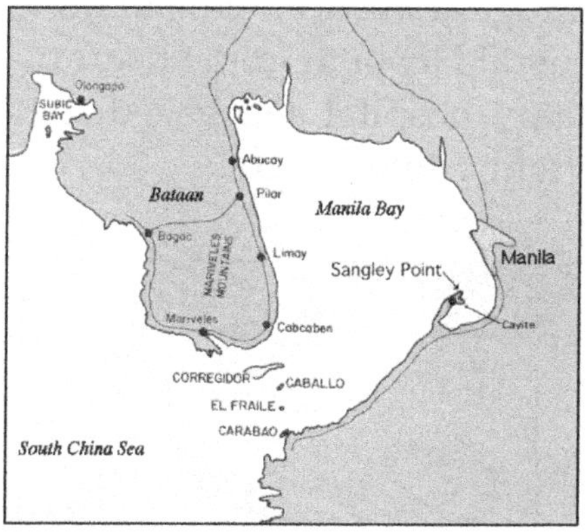

We arrived in Manila Bay in late September 1941, and waited on the deck to disembark. I breathed in the divine salty air mixed with the smell of fragrant flowers. I strolled down the gangplank in my sunset-rose chiffon dress and adjusted my new, large-brimmed straw picture hat, which was adorned with a daisy cluster and a velvet ribbon bow. I observed all the Southern nurses, who fussed with their grand ballgowns, then picked out the Northern nurses, who wore plain cotton flowered outfits with ordinary small bonnets. Molly wore the same dress she'd worn when we went into town back in basic training. She looked darling as usual with her strawberry curls that cascaded out of her bonnet.

At the bottom of the gangplank, a dashing uniformed military band played welcome music with gusto, which heightened the festive mood.

Our commanding officer greeted us. "Welcome, ladies, to the Philippine Islands. I'll have you transported to our Army Navy Club for drinks, then afterward, you'll be given a tour of your new hospital."

A short time later, I sat on a plush lounge chair and sipped a colorful tropical drink. I smiled to myself as my dream of an adventure in a tropical country unfolded before me. Molly flirted with all the handsome uniformed officers.

After our luggage arrived, all the nurses were transported to Sternberg General Hospital in the heart of Manila. I stood outside the military hospital and gazed at the red Spanish-tiled roof and bright-white stucco.

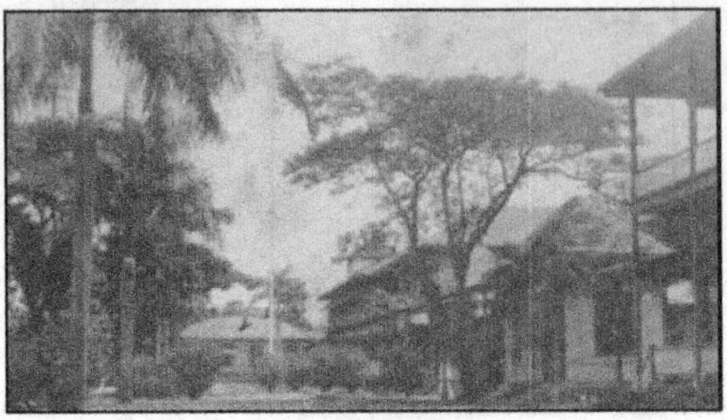

Inside an enclosed courtyard, two nurses sat on wicker chairs and sipped pink-orange drinks. They giggled and chatted away as they paged through the daily newspaper.

Molly and I introduced ourselves, then sat down on the charming furniture and felt the soft breeze from the mahogany ceiling fans that rotated lazily above us in the humid tropical air.

We were escorted to our hotel-like quarters. Molly and I unpacked and finished just as Colonel Margaret Smith came by. She was a sturdy, no-nonsense, elderly career woman I was slated to replace as chief of nursing when she retired in a couple of weeks. She took the new nurses on a tour so we could familiarize ourselves with our surroundings.

"Nurses, due to the tropical heat and humidity, the day shift works only four hours while the night shift works eight."

I smiled. This was a luxury compared to my long shifts at Grady Hospital back home!

"We now have a total of 88 regular and reserve nurses on all the islands in the Philippines. We have had several nurses marry and continue to live on the island with their spouses. I want to remind everyone that once you marry, the Army Nurse Corps will discharge you. Our hospital is the largest of four other hospitals in the Philippines."

Colonel Smith led us to the ward. "We have 450 beds in our ward."

The up-to-date beds had crisp white sheets and I smelled my favorite smell—bleach. A nurse's sign of cleanliness! In the research laboratory, I ran my hand over the many reference books and marveled at the variety of equipment. My mind continued to wander back to Grady Hospital, which now seemed shabby in comparison.

The next day, we received new duty uniforms. Colonel Smith told us we would have surgical as well as obstetric patients both from the military bases and native Filipinos from town. The new nurses attended an orientation class and were informed that many of the soldiers came in with dysentery, tuberculosis, and malaria. We would also treat the many native Filipinos for worms, or ascaris, which they got from eating contaminated food.

The captain took me aside and told me in confidence,

"We've had one case of leprosy— a Filipino soldier who was transferred to a leper colony. Also, most of the emergencies occur on payday when the soldiers in all the nearby bases have brawling accidents because too much alcohol is consumed."

"Thanks for telling me," I said, glad to get any information I could before she retired.

Colonel Margaret Smith had developed well-established routines, which made my work uncomplicated. I was learning everything I needed to know—the tried and tested ins and outs of management and protocols she had put in place—which would make for a smooth transition when she retired in the ensuing days. I was glad that Molly was my assistant since we had worked well together during basic training.

The next week, after a light workload, Molly said, "Chief, let's explore the island today since we have a day off together. I'd love to show you what I saw around the island last week."

"Why, thanks. I'd like that. It will be nice to get to know each other better. There wasn't enough time during basic training to chat, and you were so busy dancing on the ship, I never got to ask you where you are from. Our accents are so similar."

"South Carolina. And you?"

"Georgia. What made you choose nursing as a career?"

"My older sister got me a job as a nurse's aide because my large family needed the extra income. I found the job rewarding and worked while going to nursing school, then got my RN degree."

"Good for you. Your family must be proud."

"I'm pretty sure they are."

"I'm lucky to have you as my assistant. You've been such a hard worker."

"Thanks, Chief, that means a lot to me."

We strolled into town and passed by the municipal golf course. Its green ribbons of grass wound over the hills in front of the nurses' quarters. At one of the many tennis courts, we sat on a bench and cheered as a rousing game of tennis was played by some of the nurses from our hospital. It was an idyllic paradise there in the tropics, and far surpassed the dreamy expectations I'd had at home.

The walk around the island filled my nose with the perfume of tropical flowers. My eyes delighted at the sight of fuchsia-colored bougainvillea that climbed majestically up coconut palm and banana trees. Molly leaned over to smell a multicolored orchid, then picked one and tucked it behind her ear.

The next week, Molly invited me to the Friday night ballroom dance at the Army Navy Club. "Please come with me and I'll spot a tall, good-looking officer for you."

"I'll go with you to sip the drinks, but don't count on me to dance."

I put on my blue taffeta dress and touched up my hair and makeup. Then, arm in arm, Molly and I headed for the club.

"I love your dress," I said as we strolled in the delightful tropical air.

"Thanks, Bea. I saved up for it. I now have two fancy dresses to wear here for special occasions."

We entered the enormous ballroom, which was filled with round tables and chairs, and had a spacious dance floor in the middle. We sat down at a table and I felt the crisp starched tablecloth. I smoothed my taffeta and Molly brushed the wrinkles from her Navy crepe dress. A chandelier above us glittered as we watched people enter.

The women wore lovely ballgowns in sparkling colors of bright blue, emerald green, coral rose, light pink, violet, and peach. The men wore the proud uniforms of their various branches of the service—Army, Air Force, Marines, and Navy.

"I don't like to dance," I said as I hunched my shoulders in an attempt to appear smaller.

"But Chief Bea, look at the full orchestra. It's Glenn Miller's band! They are a dream to dance to!" She flipped her luscious curls about and smoothed her lipstick with her lips.

"I do love that music but I'm so tall, I usually find it hard to find a good dance partner."

"Oooo…look at that dreamboat coming our way..." Molly whispered.

A sharply dressed Navy officer sporting a wide grin asked Molly to dance with him. I watched them as they cut a good rug together. A goofy, crooked-smiled Army private asked me to dance but when I rose from my seat, he turned and walked away. I sank back into my chair and kept my head low while I sipped my tropical drink.

Molly sat down all aglow after her dance and ordered a drink. She bent toward me. "Don't you know how to dance?"

"I do. I had cotillion classes when I was 16."

"Did you have a cotillion ball?"

"Yes. Not that I wanted one, but my parents expected me to find a potential beau for marriage."

"Did you?" Molly's eyes widened.

"No. All the boys were shorter than me and I found it awkward because I towered above them. But it was a fun fairytale party and I got to wear a white, full-skirted gown with matching long white gloves, and had my hair done at the salon. Did you have a cotillion ball?"

Molly snorted. "I wish. My parents didn't have the money. I learned how to dance with my brothers and sisters and practiced every Saturday night."

I nodded. "I was an only child. I would've traded families with you back then." My eyes twinkled as I envisioned a family that danced together.

"How tall are you, Bea?" Molly asked, giving me a curious look.

"A little over six feet." I pulled my shoulders back.

"My oh my, a foot taller than me!"

"Yes, my height is handy as a boss but difficult when it comes to finding a dance partner."

"I see what you mean. I'll keep a lookout for some long, tall officers like I said I would." She looked at me again. "Tell me, do you *have* to wear your glasses?"

"I'm afraid so. My mom always said I needed them because I read too much and wore out my eyesight."

"Your beautiful dress makes you look stunning, but your glasses make you look too studious. Maybe you could put them in your purse…just for tonight."

Another Army officer came by and whisked Molly out onto the dance floor. Her sweet smile and big, twinkling green eyes attracted most of the men to dance with her at the club that night. As for me, I put my eyeglasses in my purse, then sat and watched the dancers and tapped my foot to the music played by the marvelous orchestra.

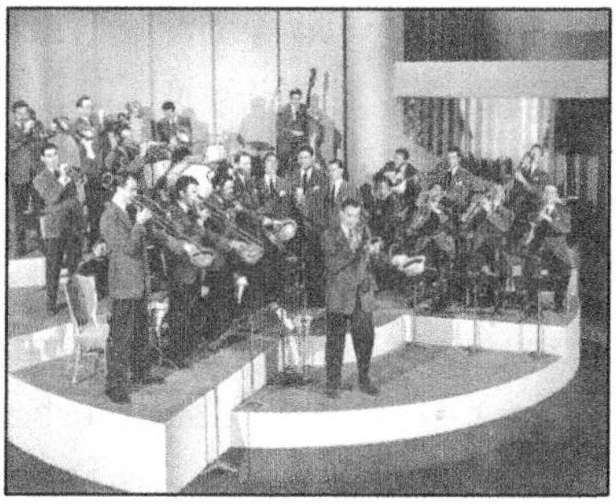

The Glenn Miller Band

After a rousing foxtrot, Molly sat down and scanned the large room.

I touched her arm before she could go talk to an officer across the dance floor. "Molly, I'm fine. I don't mind watching. The music is grand."

She ignored me and disappeared into the crowd, then brought back a tall pilot with silver wings on his uniform that gleamed brightly under the lights.

"Would you like a spin around the dance floor?" he asked me.

"Yes, that would be nice," I answered.

The gallant, sandy-haired pilot held out his hand to escort me onto the floor. I beamed when I noticed that our heights matched up. While we danced the swing to "In the Mood," he added a giddy twirl that made me lightheaded. Then, during a slow dance, he introduced himself.

"I'm Robert Johnson, 1st Lieutenant, Army Air Corps." He breathed in the scent of my perfume. "Tell me about yourself."

"I'm Chief Beatrice Harrington, in charge of nursing at Sternberg Hospital."

"Let's sit the next one out," he suggested. "That way we can get to know each other more." His eyes fixed on mine.

We left the dance floor and found a small table. We sat close so we could hear each other over the sound of the band.

"Tell me, Beatrice, are you worried about the Japanese invading us on the island here?"

His turquoise eyes captivated me.

"Not really," I replied. "The war is far away in Europe, and America is still uninvolved. I don't think the Philippines would take part in a war. Sure, all the nurses have heard rumors of war but most of us feel it's far-fetched. What do you think?" I pulled my chair in closer. "And please, call me Bea."

"And call me Rob. There's plenty of talk where I'm stationed in Fort Stotsenburg. I'm part of the 19th Bombardment Group and I think the Japs could bomb the island and take it from the U.S. at any time, even though we've had the territory since the late 1800s. It wouldn't surprise me any because I think Japan wants all of Asia. They did conquer Manchuria in 1931." His hand made a fist on the table.

"I hope for the sake of our nurses they don't attack the island while I'm stationed here."

Rob softened his tone. "Don't worry your pretty little head."

My face turned a rosy red when Rob called me pretty.

Rob continued, "I heard the Japanese are poor pilots with bad eyesight and balance. Besides, their aircraft are far inferior compared to our powerful planes, which fly faster and higher. Our B-17s, which I fly, can go far beyond the reach of the Japanese. Just between you and me, our outfit has a secret bombsite with pinpoint targets and can destroy the enemy with miraculous accuracy. But others say the islands of the Philippines are secure under the administration of the United States, and war here is just a rumor and shouldn't be taken with much seriousness."

"Thanks for the reassurance. Sternberg is the most up-to-date, modern hospital and I know it can handle any emergencies if we're invaded. And I'd make sure all the nurses did their best if that happened."

"That's very comforting to know, Bea. Our airmen at Ft. Stotsenburg are very confident and have hundreds of 2,000-pound bombs dispersed all around Clark Field. Whenever we come back from a day's leave, we're ready and alert to be in the air within two hours' notice. We have fighter crews on standby, ready in an instant for communications from a network of telephones and teletypes in all remote points of nearby Luzon Island. There are trenches dug all around the base." He patted my hand, which sent an electrical jolt up my side.

"I'm impressed..." I said.

Both of us sat frozen, gazing at each other for a moment.

"Please keep everything I told you confidential," Rob said in a low voice. "I think there's a possibility we might get bombed here in Manila, but we are ready."

"As they say, *loose lips sink ships.* You can tell me anything in confidence." I fluttered my eyelashes.

"Let's dance! 'String of Pearls' is one of my favorites and

you're a fabulous dancer." Rob took my hand and guided me out onto the dance floor right under the chandelier.

After we danced a few numbers, we sat down and I introduced Molly. Rob ordered the fruity cocktail special for everyone.

Molly gushed, "I love those cherries!"

Rob said, "They're called maraschino cherries, and they're nice and sweet."

"They sure are." I pulled in my chair so it touched Rob's seat when Molly got asked to dance. "Where are you from, Rob?"

"I'm from San Francisco. I flew one of the first B-17 Flying Fortresses from there to Clark Field on Luzon Island, 40 miles from here. Where's your sweet Southern accent from, Bea? I could listen to it all night long."

I told him my background and with a dreamlike gaze, cupped my hands under my chin. My insides swam after meeting a real pilot—and a tall, handsome one at that! I asked, "What are your barracks like?"

"I'm quartered with 20 other men and sleep on the porch of a large house that the Army requisitioned."

"Oh, my. That sounds crowded."

"It is but we all enjoy the luxury of native Filipino servants at our disposal to wash our clothes, polish our shoes, and even fetch drinks." Rob's smile displayed his darling dimples.

I took a sip of my drink and looked around to see where Molly was.

"Don't worry about her. She might be a babe, but I only go for tall women." Rob winked at me.

After we finished our drinks, Rob asked, "Would you like another spin around the dance floor? I love dancing to Glenn Miller's Army Air Force band."

"Yes, I do too." I stood.

Rob pulled my chair out and took my hand.

It was a slow dance, which allowed me to breathe in Rob's

aftershave. Our bodies moved in unison as we swayed to the romantic music. With my eyes closed, I became lost in the moment and felt sensuous and feminine for the first time in my life.

All too soon, we finished our dance and joined Molly.

She giggled when she saw us. "I see you two have been having fun."

"Yes, and thanks for introducing us." Rob moved closer and put his arm around me.

We all chatted together as the music rose to a crescendo.

"It's late, we should head back," I spoke over the music.

"I'd love to walk both of you lovely gals to your quarters," Rob offered.

"It's not on your way, is it?" I asked.

Molly said, "That would be wonderful."

"I still have time," Rob grinned. "Besides, I'm curious about where you spend most of your workday."

We strolled back to the hospital in the warm, breezy, starlit night.

Molly announced she was tired and went to bed. Rob and I sat in the spacious Spanish-style courtyard and got to know each other better as the ceiling fans turned slowly in the tropical night air.

"How would you like me to take you on a tour of my favorite places in Manila?" Rob asked. "My next day off is Tuesday. Are you available?"

"No…but I can switch with Molly," I replied. My cheeks reddened in anticipation.

Rob called for a taxi. Even though it was a three-hour ride back to his barracks, he assured me it was inexpensive, just like everything else on the island. We stood outside the hospital, hand in hand, and waited for the cab.

Rob leaned into my neck and whispered, "May I kiss you?"

"I'd love that." With my eyes closed, the sensation of our

kiss floated throughout my body.

The taxi arrived and Rob waved goodbye.

As I lay in bed that night, the kiss lingered and spilled into my dreams.

The next morning, there was a practice drill and evacuation ordered by General MacArthur. We were issued steel helmets, dog tags, and gas masks. All the nurses were blood typed in case of an emergency need for blood. This brought home the reality of a possible war.

Each day crawled by as I anxiously waited for Tuesday and my mind swirled with thoughts of Rob.

Molly helped me with an island patient whose baby was imminent. While we both waited for the birth, she said, "Chief, you have been acting different! Are you in love?" Her green eyes flashed at me.

I put a wet washcloth on the laboring mother's forehead, consoling her as she whimpered. I shook my head in answer to the question but couldn't stop smiling.

Molly whispered with a giggle, "Chief Bea, I think you've come down with love sickness!"

Focused on the task at hand, I said, "Let's see if the baby is close to crowning."

My day off arrived at last, and I waited outside in the lounge for Rob. I wore a casual dress along with my picture hat and diamond watch. I heard a clip-clop noise and looked around to see what it was. And there he was—in a horse-drawn carriage.

Rob climbed off from the back and kissed my cheek. "You look swell in that fine hat, and your perfume smells delicious."

My cheeks flushed. "Thank you," I said, and touched his uniform.

Rob gave me a tiny peck on the lips before he helped me up into the two-wheeled carriage, which was covered on the top and painted with bright colors. I sat on the narrow seat behind a small, muscular Filipino man who held the reins. Rob climbed in and put his arm around me.

I beamed, "I've never been in a horse-drawn carriage. This is a first for me. I can't thank you enough!"

"I wanted to take you in style in a carromata. I've been thinking about you since the day we met."

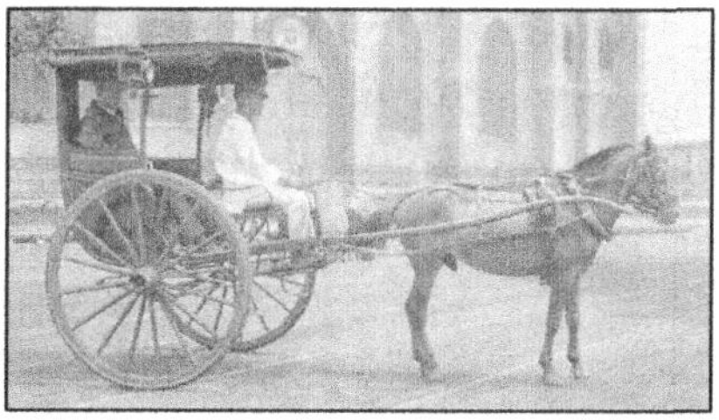

I noticed Rob's shiny gold watch. "What a beautiful watch you have. Was it a gift?"

"My parents gave it to me before I left for the service. It's engraved with my name on the other side. Would you like to see it?"

I smiled and looked at the inscription, *Airman Robert L. Johnson, Love Dad and Mom.*

Rob said, "You have quite a nice watch yourself with all those diamonds."

I beamed and rotated the watch as the diamonds sparkled in the sunlight. "It was my grandmother's. My mother gave it to me right after I joined the Army Nurse Corps."

The driver shook the reins and off we went. A tropical breeze blew my face into a big grin, and I thought that Molly was right about the lovesickness. The closeness of Rob's body sent romantic darts throughout my insides in the same rhythm as the trot of the horse.

"Driver, please take us to the Walled City. Bea, I want you to see the best part of Manila, the Walled City—or in Spanish, it's called *Intramuros,* which means a city within the walls."

"Sounds intriguing," I gushed.

As the carriage entered the old part of the city, I was a bit shocked to see garbage everywhere, which filled the air with a nasty smell. Little brown people scurried in all directions. Most were barefoot and wore shorts and sleeveless undershirts. A few upper-class people dressed in white suits and expensive dresses tried to hail the honking taxis.

"Look, there's the Walled City." Rob pointed to the old sign and an ancient fort. "Don't worry, darling. Inside, the Walled City is a historical wonder, trust me."

I jumped with delight when I heard the word "darling" and gave his hand a little squeeze.

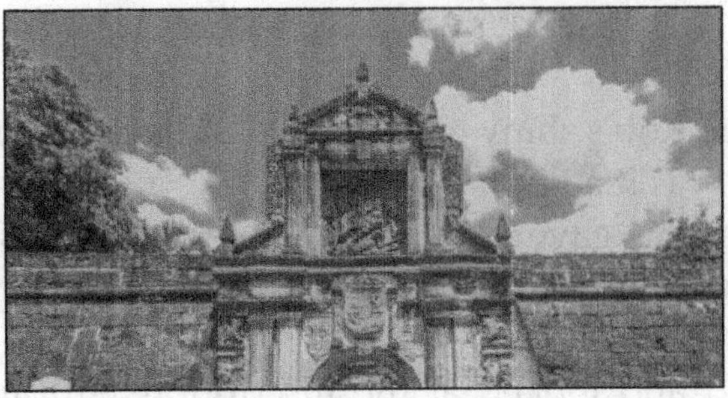

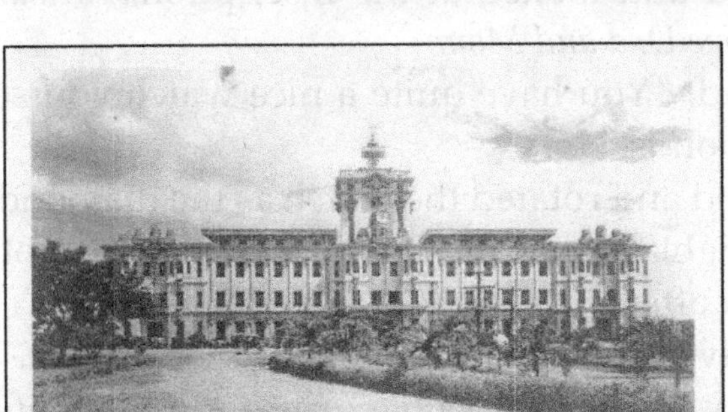

The driver pulled the reins and brought us to a stop. Rob helped me down off the carromata and we walked through an old, dark wooden archway surrounded by brick walls. I looked up at the tall structure in awe.

Rob exclaimed, "These walls are 12 feet high."

It was like I had traveled back into Spanish colonial times. I trailed my hands across the rough walls, which were cool to the touch despite the hot tropical air. "How old is this place? It has an interesting musty smell." I inhaled a deep breath.

"Intramuros was built in 1521 to protect the city from foreign invasions."

"It's hard to fathom that long ago. Georgia didn't even exist until 1733."

"I know what you mean. California wasn't founded until 1850."

As we strolled along, Rob pointed out each building.

"This is San Agustin Church, the oldest of seven churches in the Walled City. The farthest church is Santa Catalina. The streets in here are built in a tight grid and remain contained to prevent attacks from foreign invaders."

As we ambled farther along, Rob said, "This is Fort Santiago. Notice that the walls are fortified with dozens of cannons for protection." He noticed as I squinted my eyes. "Do you wear glasses, Bea?"

I murmured, "Yes," as my cheeks colored.

"I admire a gal in glasses. It shows intelligence—which you definitely have."

I fumbled through my purse and put on my glasses, which provided a much clearer view of the wonderful historical place that surrounded us.

Rob put his arm around me. "I knew you'd look good in them!"

I blushed. "This ornate iron fence has an old, crafted feel to it." I looked through the fence, which faced the boulevard, and watched bicycles, carromatas, taxis, and cars on the street outside, all mixed together and darting about with their drivers shouting and honking. "Manila sure has crazy traffic!"

"Yes, it does for such a small city."

We sat for a bit and basked in the sun before Rob led me to the University of Santo Tomas. We explored the university grounds and my handsome, knowledgeable tour guide explained that it was the largest university in Asia.

"At first it was a seminary college for men, then became a public university for general studies in 1645."

"Tell me," I said, impressed by his knowledge, "how do you know so much about this interesting place?"

"I've been here a few times on my days off and I love history."

"History was one of my favorite subjects in high school. You make an amazing tour guide."

Rob, with his boyish grin, put his arm in mine. We again found a place to sit and watched the many students that milled about, alive with animated conversation on their way to their classes.

It was late in the afternoon when Rob asked, "Are you hungry, sweetheart? I know the best place to eat."

"I'd love to go to dinner." I squeezed his arm in anticipation.

Outside of Intramuros, Rob hailed a carriage. "You'll love the newer part of the city," he said as we climbed in.

My eyes were filled with delight as I grew accustomed to the crowded city. It was bursting with American and Filipino soldiers, and local natives. One young mother nursed her baby on a sidewalk bench while she smoked a long brown cigarette. When the ash got too long, she flicked it onto the ground. It was such an odd sight.

At the Manila train station, a small train jolted to a halt and crowds of military people mixed with locals flooded out onto the platform. There were tiny autos and ancient touring cars everywhere. The drivers honked and plowed their way into the busy streets haphazardly.

The parked taxi drivers called to the passing crowd, "Need taxi, Joe?" "Take bags for you, sir?"

One carromata driver shouted to a young soldier, "You want beautiful girl, Joe? Young, clean girl, two pesos."

This startled me to hear but I kept my thoughts to myself, not wanting to ruin our romantic adventure.

Our carriage bounced across the Pasig River bridge. Modern buildings and hotels came into view along with wide boulevards lined with huge, stately trees and miles of coconut palms. We got off in front of the Manila Hotel and stood in the shade of the acacia trees. A huge American flag waved with pride in the air and the smell of sweet gardenia flowers wafted in the breeze.

Rob pointed out the majestic flag. "In 1898, the U.S. took over the Philippine Islands in the Spanish-American War."

We entered the hotel.

"What a magnificent hotel!" I enthused as I took in the sights around me. "I'm sure the food will be tops!"

The hotel was elegant and spacious, filled with statues everywhere and gold-framed portraits of famous people on each wall. The host escorted us to the dining room, which overlooked the sparkling, diamond-like bay.

While we read over the menu, Rob said, "This hotel is called the Aristocrat of the Orient."

"It sure looks it!"

Rob closed his menu. "May I order for you? The steak dinner is the best."

"Yes, please." I arranged the skirt of my dress, then felt the thick white napkin and touched the ornate silverware.

Rob ordered a pineapple, mango, and orange juice cocktail with rum for each of us.

He held up his drink for a toast. "To many more dinners with you, my love."

The clink of our crystal glasses resonated throughout the luxurious dining room.

Rob whispered, "I know we haven't known each other long, but I think I'm falling in love with you, Bea."

"I feel the same way." Tiny quivers went up and down my arms and my heart thumped in a sudden cadence.

After a perfect dinner, and still basking in the warm glow of the tropical drinks, we took the elevator to the 7th floor to see a panoramic view of the island.

"General Douglas MacArthur, the commander of the U.S. Army in the Far East, has a penthouse here. This large observation deck is used to observe our American Navy stream into the harbor to guard the country."

I looked out at a fort-like structure. "Is that Intramuros… Fort Santiago—where we were today?"

"How right you are. The entire capital of Manila can be seen from here in case of an invasion. There's a ballroom on this floor with a full orchestra. We'll have to come back for a dance sometime. Would you like that?"

"I *love* dancing with you."

Rob's height was the perfect match for me, I mused, as our eyes met and we kissed.

We held each other in an embrace and watched the bright-red sun sink into the distant horizon, its rippling reflection dancing on the water. In the foreground were different types of ships anchored in the bay, their flags waving high in the evening breeze and their multicolored lights blinking signals to the shore. The last of the small fishing boats came in with their day's catch.

"What are those mounds out in the bay?" I pointed.

"The island of Corregidor and the peninsula of Bataan."

"The island looks intriguing. Can a boat be taken there to visit?"

"I'd have to check but I do know we have troops stationed there. I heard there is a secret underground hospital there too."

I raised my eyebrows, intrigued. "Amazing. I wonder what it would be like nursing in an underground hospital..."

Rob put his arm around me and gave my shoulder an affectionate squeeze. "Tell me about your job. Do you only take care of military personnel?"

"No, the natives come in most of the time. Usually with stomach issues, like having worms from eating contaminated food."

"One of my friends at the base told me there is a native tribe here that feeds starving dogs uncooked rice, then after the dogs digest it halfway, they cut the dog open and eat the rice themselves."

I grimaced. "That's horrifying! No wonder we have so many cases of dysentery and salmonella."

"My buddy, Ralph, told me they bury fertilized duck eggs for several months, then dig them up and eat them. The houseboy offered one to me and called it a delicious *balut*."

"Oh goodness, did you eat it?"

"No, I thanked him and said I only like scrambled eggs. We have a lot of steak available for our men, but all the Filipino workers would rather eat fish heads with rice."

Rob and I took the elevator downstairs and stood outside the hotel in the soft warmth of the evening under a coconut palm tree. The sunset colored the sky a mesmerizing purple-pink, and a parrot flew overhead and chattered at us. We waited for a carromata arm and arm in the gardenia-scented moonlit night.

"What type of work do you do on the base when you are not flying planes?" I asked Rob.

"I take care of the map and navigation equipment for the squadrons."

We heard music and decided to wander around the corner from the hotel, and left the wide, new boulevards for narrow walkways. Most of the houses had tiled roofs and were stucco framed but down the alleyways, we saw small, thatched huts that housed the poorer natives.

"Some of the natives here don't look Filipino," I observed as we walked.

"Those are the native Malayans."

The music came from a huge ballroom full of dapper Filipinos who danced and swayed inside. On the sidelines, mothers breastfed their babies next to older children who sat on wooden benches. The very young little girls wore short dresses that exposed their bare bottoms.

We went further down the street and enticing aromas wafted by. Upon further exploration, we saw natives washing dishes in filthy streams, and lost interest in finding a snack.

Rob hailed a nearby carromata. He brushed my hair back with his fingers and gave me a warm, passionate kiss on the ride back to the hospital. "How did you like our date? I hope you enjoyed it as much as I did."

"The dinner was scrumptious and of course, being with you has been a wonderful adventure." I touched one of his sandy curls. "It was quite an educational experience for me to see how the Filipinos live."

"It does take some getting used to. Bea, I don't know when my next day off is because I must go on a short mission. Can I call the hospital to let you know?"

"That would be swell."

All too soon, the hospital came into view.

"Thanks, Rob, for a perfect day."

"My pleasure," he grinned. "I sure like you, Bea. I'll call you soon."

Chapter Four
Chief Dottie
Fort Huachuca, Arizona 1942

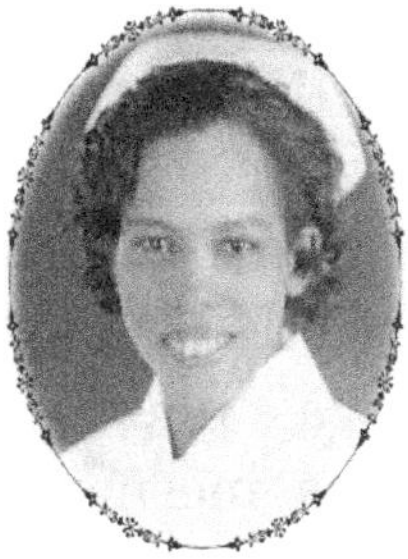

In the hot month of July, 1942, I was on my way to the largest training post for Negro soldiers, located in Southern Arizona, to report for basic training. Every state the train went through made my eyes grow wider and my heart thump faster with anticipation. I sat in the Negro section as the train chugged along, and my mind drifted as I looked at the towns that whizzed by. I was pleased to learn that I would retain my title of chief at the fort.

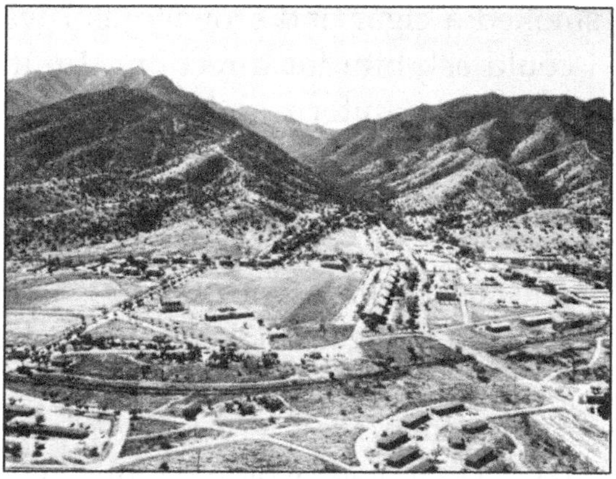

I overheard a passenger say that Huachuca was named after an Indian tribe and meant "place of thunder." I wondered...did that mean there would be a lot of thunderstorms?

After several days of travel, I heard our arrival at Fort Huachuca announced on the loudspeaker. I turned my nerves into positive energy toward a new life. Arizona! At last, I had ventured into a different state.

I looked out my window and scanned the Huachuca Mountains, which encircled the immense U.S. Army base. The vast evening sky was filled with pink, orange, and lavender hues, and I was mesmerized. I wore my white nurse's uniform with my "Chief of Staff" badge pinned on it, and changed into a clean pair of white stockings in the small lavatory. I put on my blue cape with its bright-red lining, grabbed my suitcase, and stepped off the train. I walked with confidence toward a group of massive buildings that lay spread out over quite a few miles. My white shoes became covered in reddish-brown dust and desert sand but I didn't care. My heart skipped a beat as I headed into the same base where my dad had trained as a Buffalo Soldier. I beamed with pride.

Outside the first building I came to stood an older White officer who smoked a cigar and scowled as I walked up to him. Before I could ask him for directions, I puffed out my chest so he could see my uniform and chief-of-nursing ID tag.

He gave my uniform a quick once-over, then barked, "Your barracks are over there." He jerked his fat thumb toward a building.

My voice squeaked, "Thank you, sir."

He blew a big puff of cigar smoke up toward the sky and walked away.

On the door of the long, shabby, wooden shotgun barracks hung a crooked sign that read "Colored Only." I yanked open the door. Inside were 30 gals having a gay old time getting acquainted with each other.

After I walked in and put my suitcase down, the room grew quiet. I introduced myself with a big smile. "I'm Chief Dottie."

A tall, slim nurse spoke up. "Welcome, Chief. I'm Clara. You must be on the bottom part of my bunk." She took my suitcase and placed it there.

"Thank you. I'm very happy to be here, as I'm sure you all are since the Army only permitted a few Negro nurses into the Nurses Corps."

I looked at the women around me, all dressed in an assortment of styles, and my face scrunched into a question. "Does anyone know where we get our nursing uniforms?"

"Nope, we all wondered the same thing. Where're you from, Chief?" Clara asked.

"Outside of Atlanta, Georgia. How 'bout you?"

"New York City."

Everyone came from a variety of mostly Southern states and seemed enthusiastic to be there.

Exhausted from the long train ride, I stretched out and fell asleep early that night in the comfort of a bed. I had a good feeling as I listened to the nurses chatter away into the night.

We were jolted awake the next morning by the sound of a bugle.

The same gruff officer I had encountered the day before hollered through the door, "Ya'll have 20 minutes to wash up and get dressed, then line up outside."

This was a difficult task, what with the limited use of only two showers and two toilets. I was glad I had brought a spare clean nurse's uniform to wear. We were a disorganized group as we scrambled to get in line outside in our mismatched outfits and assorted styles of shoes.

Commanding Officer McDonald pointed out the mess hall. "Y'all have 30 minutes to march to chow, eat, then line up outside again."

As we walked away, the officer shouted, "I said MARCH! And keep your mouths shut. Y'all better remember to never walk when you're on the base. You belong to the United States Army now and that means marching!"

None of us knew how to march and we were a pathetic sight, but with broad smiles pasted on our faces, we did the best we could.

When we entered the mess hall, a group of White nurses stared at us from their table. One of them pointed to the far back of the room, where Negroes were supposed to sit. I led the group to the proper place. I noticed that the White nurses wore one-piece jumpsuits that were too big. The sleeves were rolled up as well as the pant legs.

After a breakfast of putrid powdered eggs, Spam, and weak juice mixed with complaints from everyone, we lined up outside.

Officer McDonald announced, "Report to the auditorium." He did his usual thumb-pointing toward a building to the right. I saw him shake his head in dismay at our awkward marching.

In the old auditorium, Lt. Colonel McDonald briefed us about Army rules and regulations. "Fort Huachuca is the largest training camp for Negro soldiers in the States. We have two separate dorms, fields, auditoriums, as well as hospitals for you Negroes and us Whites. Separate but equal!"

He chuckled with sarcasm and his ugly, pock-marked face turned red. He handed out the curriculum list for basic training, which included drills, map reading, tent pitching, obstacle and infiltration courses, physical fitness exercises, military courtesy, care of equipment and uniforms, property responsibility, military sanitation, how to dig a foxhole, use of camouflage, rifle range, how to advance under a barrage of enemy shell fire, and use of gas masks.

We all read the list and I could tell by the stunned looks on everyone's faces that they wondered why we had to learn how to use rifles or advance under enemy shell fire. We were nurses, for God's sake, not soldiers!

The officer's awful face was hard to look at as he ranted, "You gals have four weeks to learn 144 hours of basic training—that is, if you want to pass and get stationed overseas."

That got everyone's attention as most of us had joined the Corps just to be able to travel.

Bold Clara jumped up and waved her hand.

Officer McDonald snapped, "Whaddya want?"

"When will we get our uniforms?"

The officer huffed in annoyance. "Your uniforms haven't arrived yet. March to field #2 for drills. Times a-wastin'."

After we marched to the field and lined up, a different officer came to instruct us.

Sergeant Nash said, "Begin with your left foot, heel on the ground, then step 12 inches as your right arm swings out, then the right foot, left arm, and swing. Keep your hands cupped and pointed down. The arm swing should be only nine inches. Now, forward, march!"

We all fell into each other with giggles. Half of the group started out on the wrong foot and most of us weren't sure whether we had stepped 30 inches or if our arm swing was the correct length. Our group could not coordinate all the movements, and our legs and arms banged into each other. We mumbled, "Sorry…" or "Excuse me..." as we struggled.

Lorna, a Chicago city girl, whispered to me, "This is hard…"

The sergeant raised his voice. "Keep your mouths shut! Don't y'all know what 'forward, march' means?"

I put a finger to my lips and gave Lorna a *better be quiet and pay attention or else* look.

Sgt. Nash rolled his eyes impatiently. "You *must* learn how to march! It is required on the base that you march everywhere."

The nurses tried to follow his instructions, but their nervousness made it difficult.

"Let's move on to saluting." He clenched and unclenched his fists. "Now, stand up straight—and I mean ramrod straight, ya hear? Bring your right arm up and raise your hand to your brow."

A few of the gals used their left hands and that set him off.

"I said *right hand!* Hold the salute, then slowly lower your hand to your side. Again, salute! Always salute officers and the American flag. And remember that all officers are to be addressed as 'sir.'" The sergeant's face turned crimson red from the heat of the desert and his explosive screams.

After a long day of marching and saluting, the sergeant demanded, "To the rear, march! Report for chow."

Under his watchful eye, our pitiful, tired, grimy group marched to supper.

At chow, there was a flood of protests from the nurses.

"I'm too sore to do this all over again tomorrow," plump-figured Betty announced.

"I can't even salute!" Lorna added. "That mean officer makes me nervous and I forget my left from my right." She was quite a skinny and frail kid.

"I thought we'd be working in a hospital," Hilary whined. "What does learning how to march and salute have to do with nursing, anyway?"

As chief, I knew I had better take the high road and try to keep everyone's confidence up. Just like at Grady, complaints could be contagious and had to be curbed before they escalated.

"I know we're all sore, but we must carry on," I encouraged. "Basic training is only for a few weeks, then we get to do the work we love at the base hospital. Nurses, try to focus on the dream of adventure and travel."

Betty was the first to say, "You're right, Chief Dottie. Thanks for the pep talk. It makes me feel better." She finished up everything on her plate—even the dried-out peas.

"Thanks, Betty." I looked at everyone who had protested. It was nice to have Betty on my side, even though she had the toughest time exercising due to her weight. I forced a smile and waited until the nurses smiled back at me in agreement.

"Nurses, I have a great idea. Tomorrow, put a pebble in your right hand before we must march. This way, you will know your right foot from your left. Then drop the pebble to use the correct hand when saluting."

"Smart idea, Chief!" Polly beamed.

The next day, marching went a bit smoother with the "pebble method" in play. Calisthenics and jumping jacks were difficult in our dresses but at least everyone wore their sturdy nursing shoes instead of heels.

We had to do an hour of awkward and difficult exercises like push-ups and pull-ups on bars. Sgt. Nash would demonstrate an exercise one time, then we'd have to do a set number of them. As the day progressed, we were drenched in sweat and covered with dust from the hot Arizona desert. My white uniform had turned a dirty brown. Some of the girls wore civilian clothes for basic training. Our clothing not only humiliated us but was impractical in the hot climate—especially in white stockings that clung to our legs.

I glanced over at Field #1, where the White girls exercised in comfort and wore one-piece outfits. Their clothes were big, but they didn't have to wear civilian clothes like we did. I hoped we'd get our jumpsuits soon.

The next day, we lined up outside the mess hall and waited for Sgt. Nash. Much to our surprise, a new officer arrived. I was worried he would be as nasty as the last one—but at least he was better looking and had a cute, dimpled cleft chin.

Sgt. Carlson stared at the group with gray-blue eyes that bore a hole through all of us. "Stand straighter!" he ordered.

Most of the gals frowned and their good moods turned

sour. We all stood ramrod straight.

Clara whispered in my ear, "Uh-oh…could be another meany!"

Sgt. Carlson announced, "Proceed to the rifle range!"

At the range, the sergeant handed each nurse a gun and demonstrated the components and how to load and shoot. The gals looked confused, which told me that he had explained things too fast. I also noticed that a few of their arms trembled from the weight of the heavy rifles as they struggled to hold them.

The sergeant announced, "These rifles have terrific range, caliber, accuracy, and power to kill the Japs and Nazis. Has anyone ever shot a rifle?"

I answered, "I've shot cans in the backyard."

"Then you're first. Shoot that round target out there." He pointed.

I was lucky my daddy had taught me and my brothers and sisters how to shoot cans with his World War I rifle. Although I was small, I always enjoyed the satisfaction as well as the noise when I hit the can off the log. I held my breath, squinted one eye through the gun sight, and almost hit a bullseye.

The gals cheered. Lorna held her hands over her ears.

Hilary tried to shoot but her hands quivered and the rifle bobbed up and down, sending a bullet into the dirt. She mumbled with her deep Southern accent, "I can't do this."

Sgt. Carlson hollered, "Damn it!"

Before he could pick on another candidate, I asked the group, "Who here has ever shot a rifle?"

Out of all of us, I was the only one who had. I looked at the sergeant with raised eyebrows in an attempt to make a point.

The sergeant snorted. "Fine, Chief, they're all yours. I'm going to chow. This group is unteachable." He left in a huff.

Once Sgt. Carlson was out of sight, I heard a few of the girls giggle with relief. I called up each nurse, one by one, and with slow, helpful instruction, some of them hit the target.

When Clara hit the bullseye twice in a row, she let out a triumphant, "Yeah!"

Lorna was last. Her skinny body shook as I helped her aim. The bullet hit the rim of the target. Everyone clapped in support but she dropped the gun and walked away, terrified.

"Nurses, it's chowtime," I finally said. "As far as I'm concerned, y'all passed. We aren't combat nurses, and as you know, our job is to bandage soldiers, not help them shoot the enemy."

Never had I imagined that I would teach nurses riflery instead of how to give inoculations or aid the sick. Now I just had to hope that the sergeant would believe my lie that everyone had passed.

A short time later at chow, Hilary asked, "Chief, are all the instructors here White?"

I had noticed that too. "I suppose so. There are certainly plenty of Negro officers here that could teach us, but it's probably the same set-up as I had at Grady Hospital back home. All the physicians were White, and Negro physicians were never allowed to practice there."

A week later, Officer McDonald came by and dropped off several boxes of what they called "fatigues" and an assortment of boots.

After we pulled the so-called uniforms out of the boxes, Clara read one of the labels. "Hot damn! Size 36."

Betty grabbed one. "Yikes, here's a 44!" She was a full-figured gal but the fatigues were still way too big.

"I can't fit in any of these." Thin Lorna tossed aside the fatigues she had grabbed and sulked back to her bed.

Hilary, second to Lorna as a complainer, mumbled, "Us coloreds are always gettin' what's left over."

I wanted to agree with her but knew better than to encourage that bad situation.

We concluded that the uniforms were all men's sizes,

including the big carton of boots.

I went outside and found Sgt. McDonald, saluted him, then asked, "Sir, the boxes you gave us are men's uniforms. Could we have the women's uniforms, please?"

He avoided my eyes and lit his stogie. "Chief Williams, the Army is giving you men's surplus. Take it or leave it. I have a meeting to go to." He stormed off.

The somber atmosphere in the barracks became a party as everyone tried on the men's fatigues. They were olive-drab, one-piece affairs with button-down shirt tops and flies in the pants.

Betty, the largest nurse, had to roll up the sleeves and pant legs only once over. It was easy for her to find a pair of men's boots for her larger feet. She searched for a pair of smaller boots and gave them to Lorna, who took them with a grumble.

I tried on a size 36 but the crotch of the huge uniform hung down to my knees. Handy Hazel got out safety pins so she could hitch in the outfits with Polly's help. Then she took out her Red Cross sewing kit, sat on her bunk, and with a tiny pair of scissors, cut out a back flap in the pants, then sewed on buttons from her kit.

I watched her sew the edges. "Ingenious!" I praised. "A drop seat so we can easily go to the bathroom."

I sorted through the sturdy men's boots and found the smallest pair, size 5, and took Hazel's lead and stuffed the toes with toilet paper so they'd better fit my small feet. Being the shrimp that I was, I kept the size 36 fatigues I had tried on—the smallest I could find. Thank goodness they had attached belts, which helped me find the waist.

One by one, we strolled around the barracks and displayed our creations in an impromptu fashion show. I wore the fatigues with my nurse's hat on, which was hilarious. The star of the show was Hazel, who turned her back, bent over, unbuttoned her drop seat, wiggled her bottom, and displayed her white undies. Rowdy laughter broke out, followed by clapping. Polly copied her and received applause and laughter from everyone.

Clara sang out, "I see London, I see France, I see Hazel's and Polly's underpants!"

Everyone hooted with laughter again until tears ran down our faces. Yes, we did get surplus uniforms but thank goodness my resourceful nurses made the best of the situation.

One day during the second week of basic training, I decided to skip chow when I saw the White nurses doing their calisthenics on a separate field, and slipped over to their barracks. My crazy curiosity got the better of me and I had to see for myself whether our barracks were "separate but equal." First, I noticed that the outside had a fresh coat of paint. After I crept through the door, I saw that the metal bunkbeds and lamps were the same as ours but newer. I had just started to count the plentiful toilets when I thought I heard a noise, so I scrammed out the back door just as someone came in the front. I chastised myself for taking such a silly risk.

As I got closer to the Negro barracks, I spoke out loud, "Mm-mm-mm," sounding just like Mama after she heard bad news. The White women's barracks were just what I had imagined, with us colored nurses getting less, like an unpainted, worn-out building. Images of Grady Hospital came to mind, when I had dared to sneak over to the White nurses' dormitories.

I was the first to get a day-leave pass and looked forward to exploring the town of Huachuca. After I got off the bus and walked down the sidewalk, I saw the usual signs designating

"Whites Only" and "Negroes Only" on the public bathrooms and water fountains. I adjusted my nurse's uniform and made sure my chief-of-nursing pin was level, then straightened the line on my white stockings.

I hummed Fats Waller's ditty, "Ain't Misbehavin'" while I pulled open the large glass door of an enormous department store that did not have a Jim Crow-type sign in the window. It was a hot summer day, and I dabbed a handkerchief across my moist face and sat on a stool at the lunch counter in the middle of the store.

A mean-eyed clerk snapped, "You can't sit here."

I composed myself and ordered. "I'd like a Coca-Cola, please." I repinned my badge to draw attention to my status as a nurse.

"We don't serve your kind of people." His rough fingers drummed on the counter.

"Sir," I persisted, "I'd like to order a cold drink on this hot day before I go back to Fort Huachuca." I forced a smile. "I'm a chief in the Army Nurse Corps there."

"You're breaking the law, lady, and don't belong here. Go round back and order just like all you people are supposed to do. Didn't you see the sign?" He pointed to a small sign on the wall. He then proceeded to wash the counter with a wet rag, swiping right up to my chest.

I picked up the menu.

In a loud voice, the clerk said, "I'm callin' the cops!"

I rose with dignity, flung the menu down, and strolled out of the store, then walked around back and entered through the rear entrance. My stockings stuck to my legs in the heat as I waited a full 10 minutes to be served.

The same soda jerk came through the back and shoved out his palm. I put a dime in it and he returned with an open bottle of soda.

"Put it on the ground when you're done, then get out."

After I downed the soda, I left the bottle. Sweat poured

down my back as I strolled down the sidewalk. I found a "Negroes Only" section in a movie theater, and hoped watching a movie would restore my self-esteem before I got back on the bus to the fort. But I couldn't concentrate on the film and was filled with disappointment that my nurse's uniform did not give me any special rights whatsoever.

I felt degraded as I boarded the bus to go to the base. I walked to the back and noticed how dirty and torn the seats were in the Negro section. Worried that sitting there would ruin my uniform, I moved one row closer to the front and sat in the sparsely populated "Whites Only" area where the seats were in better condition.

The bus driver, who looked sloppy and had a large paunch, stood up, red-faced, and stated, "This is a Whites-only area." He flipped his hand toward the sign.

"But I'm chief of nursing at the Fort Huachuca base," I protested.

"Darkies belong in the back!"

"Sir, I understand the laws of segregation, but the two sections are not equal and I cannot get my uniform dirty." I held my head high and stared straight ahead.

The driver grabbed my arm, pinching it as he jerked me out of my seat and dragged me off the bus.

I shrieked in pain, "Let me go!"

A policeman strolled by and heard my cry. When he investigated, the bus driver explained, "This nigger wouldn't stay in her place."

The cop took hold of my arm. "I'll lock her up."

"Yeah, that'll teach her," the driver said. He lumbered up the bus steps and drove off in a fury.

The policeman gripped my bruised arm and walked me to the police station, where he shoved me into a jail cell. The rancid smell of cigarettes and alcohol overwhelmed me as I sat on a dirty, smelly cot. As time passed, my mind swarmed with mixed feelings of stupidity and disappointment. My nursing uniform did not give me the respect I deserved.

I heard Mama's voice in my head… *"Dottie, you weren't supposed to drink from that fountain, and you know I don't think it's fair, but darlin', I don't want you gettin' beat up. You must obey the law until, one day, Negroes achieve equality."*

I thought that if I served in the U.S. military, it would give me the dignity I deserved, but there I sat, still treated like a second-class citizen, just not in the South this time, but in the West.

I was released early that night for "good behavior." The cop held me tight on my now-swollen arm, led me to the last bus back to the base, then watched to make sure I sat in the correct area.

When I got to the barracks, I ran into Sergeant McDonald.

"Chief Williams, you missed roll call and were AWOL. Report to the general's office in the morning for your penalty."

I could tell when I opened the barracks door that the nurses had heard the officer's reprimand. They all looked frightened.

My bunkmate, Clara, got in my face. "Why were you late?"

I slumped on my bed in despair and told everyone about the sordid events of my day, and showed them the bruises on my arm.

Betty patted my hand. "You poor dear."

Clara spoke with great animation, her hands waving about. "How dare they arrest you and treat you like a second-class citizen while you wore your nurses uniform!"

All the nurses were in an uproar over my jail incident and protested to each other.

Betty diffused the situation. "Chief, please be more careful, especially tomorrow when you report to the general, or the Army will throw you out. We'd sorely miss you."

"Yes, I know that. But I still have a strong conviction in my heart to fight for the equality of races—especially when in the service of helping our country." Before anyone could say another word, I changed out of my uniform and put on my nightgown. "I've got to get some sleep. Good night, ladies."

The next morning, I headed off to the general's office. I knocked on the door and was summoned inside, then stood at attention and saluted the general.

He glanced up from his desk and barked, "Name?"

"Chief Dora Mae Williams, sir."

"It says on your papers that you were chief of nursing at Grady Hospital. Have a seat." He continued to read my file, then stared at me. "Will you follow the laws of segregation while you're in the Army?"

I swallowed hard. "Yes, sir."

"I think you've had enough punishment in jail. Your experience as chief of nursing will be valuable to the Army when you're sent overseas. I don't want to discharge you for being AWOL but remember, obey the laws! Dismissed."

"Yes, sir. Thank you, sir." I saluted and left.

Chapter Five
Bea
Manila, Philippines 1941

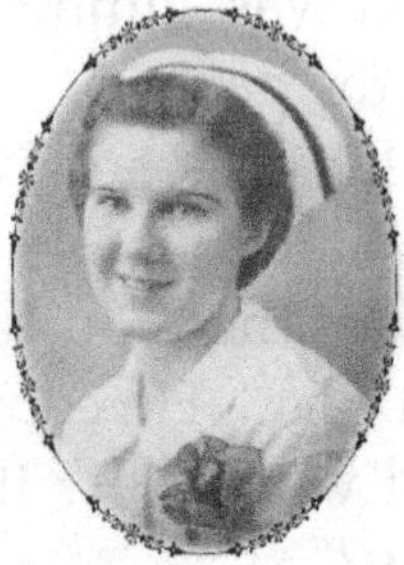

On my next day off, I went into town to look for something to send home to my mother. The shops were filled with native Filipino crafts, and I found an enchanting watercolor of the island at sunset in a handcrafted bamboo frame.

On my way to see a motion picture show, I saw a sign on a small native house advertising private Spanish classes, so I knocked on the door to inquire about it. A petite, creamy-brown-skinned woman answered. She invited me inside and served me fresh-squeezed orange juice while we sat together and spoke in English.

Cecilia's two darling daughters—both with sweet, large brown eyes—stood beside her wooden chair and stared at me with curiosity. After we set up weekly lessons on Monday evenings, I asked, "Cecelia, how do you know English so well?"

"My husband's an American in the Navy," she replied.

"Where's he stationed?"

"Hawaii." She smoothed down her daughters' long, light-brown hair, one by one, then braided it while we talked.

"You must miss him."

"We all miss him but he'll come back soon." She gave each daughter an affectionate hug.

Later that day, after the movie, I bought a cake at a local bakery for Colonel Smith's retirement party the next day.

At the party, there was quite an array of presents from the staff. Everyone congratulated the captain and wished her the best of luck for her future. I was pleased with my new assignment in the hospital and took over her position with ease.

On December 7, 1941, my paradisiacal adventures on the island ended. A phone call interrupted a deep dream about Rob, who was down on one knee with a diamond ring proposing to me. I turned on my small light and looked at my watch. It was three in the morning. *Who in God's name could be calling at such a time?* I stumbled out into the hallway to answer the phone.

"Chief Beatrice Harrington?"

"Speaking," I answered in a small, foggy voice.

"This is Colonel Mannetti. The Japanese have bombed Honolulu."

"Do you mean Hawaii?"

"Chief Harrington, wake up! Prepare your staff in case the Japanese army attacks the Philippines next! This is a direct order from Lieutenant General Wainwright." The phone clicked off.

The phone receiver rattled in the cradle as I fumbled to hang it up. I stumbled back to my room and threw on my nurse's uniform, then scurried into the lounge to hear the news on the Westinghouse radio.

The night shift nurses had tears streaming down their faces as the American mass casualties in Hawaii were announced. Pearl Harbor was 5,000 miles away, but the horrifying radio reports brought it closer to us.

The announcer ended the report, "This was a sneak attack planned by the Imperial Japanese Air Service."

I rose from the edge of my seat and straightened my uniform. "Girls, get ahold of yourselves. Find your helmets and gas masks, always keep them near you. The Japanese are known to use a variety of poison gases." I felt confident that we were well prepared because of our regular drills and practice evacuations.

Five intense hours went by as we sat in the hospital, but nothing unusual occurred. I listened to the radio during my break with a few other nurses.

The radio announcer said in an unsteady voice, "Camp John Hay has been destroyed by Japanese bombers."

An older nurse said, "Oh my god, that's only 200 miles north of here! I hope we won't be next."

Then at 12:43 PM, the radio blasted, "The Japanese pilots of the 11th Air Fleet attacked Fort Stotsenburg and 200 Japanese Mitsubishi Betty and Zero fighters struck Clark Field, our main military airbase in the Philippines."

The announcer's words faded as Rob's face flashed in my mind like a bad dream.

"Our planes were sitting ducks on the runways, fully armed but unmanned as waves of Zeros machine-gunned the entire base. The raid appears to be over now and has left Clark Field littered with shrapnel and thousands of pieces of mangled, burning aircraft. The oil dump is ablaze and the enlisted men's barracks, officers' quarters, aircraft hangars, and machine shops were leveled. Our 12 Flying Fortresses and 30 Curtiss Warhawks were all destroyed. The attack has killed over 100 of our men with over 90 wounded."

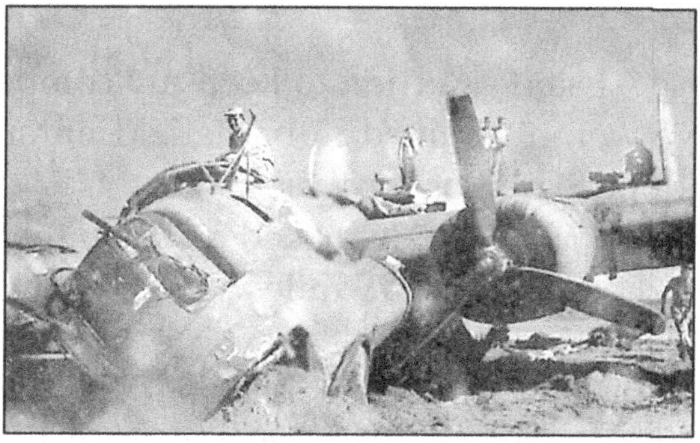

"Oh no!" My voice quivered. "I wonder how my Rob is?" I stood up, snapped out of my thoughts, and barked at the staff, "I see some of you don't have your helmets and gas masks with you. Get them—now! Manila could be next." I walked fast to a group of non-military Filipina nurses who stood close by. "We need you now more than ever. Can I count on your help?"

Carmelita spoke up first. "We'll do our best. Most of us have boyfriends and brothers in the Army here."

All the Filipina nurses nodded, affirming this to be true.

Molly's lips trembled. "Chief Bea, we wanted to know if we could go to the bank and cable all our money home." With downturned eyes, she added, "Just in case..."

Annie chimed in, "Please, Chief, I don't want to lose my savings." She blinked back her tears.

"Absolutely not!" I said firmly. "No one is to leave this hospital. A war has started. I need everyone to stay here." I pressed my lips firmly together.

Three hours after the raid, Department Surgeon Colonel Wibb Cooper rang up from Stotsenburg Hospital near Clark Field and asked if we could take the overflow of casualties they couldn't handle with their small staff of 14 Army nurses and three Filipina nurses at their hospital.

"How many wounded should we expect?" My voice trembled.

"About 80."

"Of course," I said as I tried to keep my composure. But I knew that we weren't trained in battlefield nursing and the Army had not prepared us for war.

After I hung up, I was shocked to hear that wounded patients would be sent from 75 miles away—a three-hour bus trip from our location.

I gathered the staff. "Nurses, make sure all the wards are ready. Medics, get all the cots out of storage and set them up. Everyone be on alert for an onslaught of wounded men from the attack on Fort Stotsenburg and Clark Field," I ordered.

Our first casualty was a small child. The American wife of an officer burst in holding her one-year-old son, who was wrapped in a small blanket. I took off the blanket and the boy howled with pain. His kneecap was shattered with shrapnel and his face was blue, which indicated something was wrong with his heart.

I reached out to take the boy from her protective grip. "We'll take good care of him."

She held back for a minute, then placed him in my outstretched arms. I rushed the child to the operating room and assisted Doctor Santos, who gave him oxygen, but he died on the table within minutes. Stunned, I left to inform the mother. The ambulances began to arrive while I told her the tragic news, which allowed me no time to help her with her grief. I spun on my heels to begin triaging the wounded and left the shocked mother standing in the hallway amid the chaos.

Ambulance after ambulance pulled up and our medics paraded in with the wounded on stretchers. There were so many injuries that Molly and I had to establish an order for which patients were to be treated first. This meant who should live and who should die—something all the medical personnel had only textbook experience with. None of us had ever imagined this would be something we would have to employ.

With every day that followed came more terror to endure as the number of patients increased. There was no end in sight. There were multiple wounds to dress and operations to assist with, and there was little time for breaks. And on top of that, we were supposed to try to comfort the patients.

My trusty assistant, Molly, was my best nurse. She pitched in wherever help was needed and her skills were impeccable. As we assessed patients, I had her point out the worst injuries while two nurses followed behind us and administered morphine for pain.

I put others in charge of wiping dirt off the faces of people who'd had to dive headfirst into ditches during the raids, or had cinders blown into their faces from strafing runs that lacerated their eyes. Grease and dirt were cleaned from gaping wounds and charred burns. We saw legs that dangled on tendons, and partially severed arms. The litters lined up in the hallway, and nurses and medical corpsmen removed blood-soaked clothing and applied clean bandages.

Doctor Willis called me into the operating room from the corridor. "Chief Bea, come here and assist..."

The soldier on the table raised his head and tried to look down at his leg. "It's almost off, ain't it, Doc?"

"Yes, son," the doctor replied.

Doctor Willis glanced at me to see how I was doing. I remained stone quiet and gritted my teeth.

"Will it have to come all the way off?" the patient asked.

"I'm sorry, soldier," Dr. Willis said.

"Please do a good job, Doc." The soldier managed a slight smile.

"Administer the ether, Chief."

I started at Dr. Willis's instructions. "But Doctor, I'm not an anesthesiologist. I'm not trained to do that!"

"We have no choice given the circumstances. I'll walk you through it. We have only two anesthesiologists here."

He gave me brief instructions on how much ether or chloroform to put on the cloth, then how to hold it over the patient's nose and mouth and for how long. I did what I was told and prayed I wouldn't kill the soldier.

Nurse Caroline tended to a soldier on a cot in the hallway.

He told her, "It's horrible out there. On the way here in an open truck, I saw people fleeing into the hills. Some stayed in foxholes that had corrugated roofs and sandbags all around them, or were camouflaged with foliage and tree limbs. Incendiary bombs landed on the nipa huts and their dry thatched roofs exploded, then the whole barrio caught on fire! I'm lucky I'm safe in this hospital with you." He reached out for her hand.

Caroline held his hand for a minute, then cleaned the cinders from his wounds. "We'll take good care of you, soldier. Thank you for fighting for our country." She smiled and moved on to the patient in the next cot in the crowded hallway.

"I saw a dogfight on my way here," he said, "and a Jap was knocked out and plunged straight into the bay." He looked at the frown on Caroline's face. "Don't worry. Our side will win."

Day and night became indistinguishable. Every time a pilot was brought in on a stretcher with wings on his lapel, I'd whisper to him, "Do you know Airman Robert Johnson?" They all shook their heads. One afternoon, after I had bandaged another airman's wounded arm, I asked the question again.

The soldier asked, "What unit was he in?"

Hope sprang in my heart. "The 19th Bombardment Group."

He answered, "Nope, sorry." Then sadly added, "If you see only *one* American plane instead of many in the sky, you know it's ours. Besides, all of our Flying Fortresses were destroyed."

My heart jumped. I knew that could mean Rob's B-17.

A pilot with a head wound next to him added, "All our airplanes were obliterated in just one day by the Japs."

Molly overheard me as I talked to the wounded soldiers and pulled me aside. "Chief, when was the last time you slept?"

"I have no idea." I looked down at my blood-stained white shoes. I felt sick and distraught over all the casualties and was in shock.

"I'll take over," she stated firmly. "Bea, please get some rest. I'll keep asking about Rob for you."

I thanked her and dragged myself back to my sleeping quarters.

On Dec. 12, four days after the bombing of Clark Field, we heard the drone of Japanese warplanes flying overhead to the port area right near our hospital. Then, *kaboom!* The sounds of bombing began as they let loose their weapons.

Commanding Officer Lieutenant General Wainwright stormed into the hospital and demanded to talk to the head of the physicians and nurses. Dr. Willis and I met with him in the only quiet space available—a corner at the end of a hallway. We were informed that our beloved Manila had been set ablaze by over 60 Japanese warplanes. Our ships were sunk, and a flash fire raged in the tall grass all around the perimeter of the hospital.

The general said, "I'm counting on you to take in all the casualties from Manila."

Dr. Willis spoke up, "We're swamped by the overflow from Stotsenburg."

The general's voice rose. "We are at war now! You *must* take every wounded soldier!" His eyes blazed into ours.

"Yes, sir!" Dr. Willis saluted him with a surgical glove on his hand.

The medics were instructed to put cots anywhere and everywhere in the hospital. All the hallways, the dining room, even the lab had cots wedged inside. A bomb fell nearby, which left our ears ringing. I peered out of a hospital window and saw swarms of airplanes with big red circles on their wings flying in over the bay. Our peacetime paradise became a horror movie as the wounded poured in on anything that had wheels: buses, trucks, taxis, hand-pushed wooden carts, even carromatas. Medics carried the soldiers in on blood-encrusted litters. Most of the patients had shrapnel lodged in their wounds. Some poor souls were dead when they arrived.

The surgical nurses scrubbed up and remained in the seven operating rooms under lights that glared in the heat of the day. They dabbed the sweat from the surgeons' brows, anticipated the next instrument that would be needed, counted sponges, monitored vital signs, and reeled off lengths of atraumatic intestinal catgut used for surgical sutures, all the while trying to maintain a sterile field.

A medic on a break poured out his grief. "It's crazy out there. The entire city has no electricity. Criminals are looting. The traffic in the street is a tangled mess of buses, pushcarts, and carabao wagons with no way to obey the traffic laws. And, oh my god, you should see the beautiful parks. They have all been trampled, filled with tents, and dug up with trenches for foxholes." He smoked nonstop like a madman.

I said, "How horrible. But we must keep working!" I went back to my duties, trying to ignore the images of the outside world in my mind's eye and forcing myself to focus on the patients.

The bombing intensified. The heavy chandeliers in the dining room swayed, windows shattered, and glass sprayed onto the patients. Some patients ate under their beds in total fear while the bombs dropped nonstop outside.

That night, the nightmare on the ward intensified when someone yelled, "Bombs overhead! Everyone hit the floor!"

Many of the patients and some of the nurses dove onto the floor and covered their heads. Amid all of this, one wounded soldier growled, "What the hell are you all doing? I need my sleep!"

But sleep was impossible amid the nerve-racking noise of war. We kept working harder and longer, numb with fatigue. Exhausted, several of us crawled into a cement-enclosed cubicle in the basement of the hospital. It had damp, putrid air, but we slept from pure exhaustion and at least felt safe.

The bedlam increased the next day. I helped with amputations, dressings, blood transfusions, and worst of all, dealt with death. We worked day and night. Our soiled, impractical dresses brushed against bloody soldiers on cots in the hallways, but we damn well had no time to wash them.

The enemy kept up the raids as the injured overflowed into our wards and spilled into the corridors, lobbies, and then the verandas. When we ran out of beds and cots, the corpsmen had to lay the wounded on the bare floor. They put them on the lawns and tennis courts nearby, and used old doors and corrugated roofing for makeshift cots after I complained about using the bare floor and ground.

The corpsmen carried out the soldiers who, tragically, had died while waiting for help. Several of the nurses turned their heads away and ground their teeth in agony. I grumbled that we were now wartime nurses whether we wanted to be or not.

When Sternberg Hospital could not fit any more patients, the medics told us that the local schools and hotels had been transformed into hospitals, and new patients could be transported there.

On December 17th, the radio news reported that enemy transports had streamed into Manila with an army of 43,000 Japanese with tanks, field artillery, and flamethrowers. Not knowing whether Rob was dead or alive put me on edge. *Maybe*, I thought, *I'd feel better if I knew he had died*. On the other hand, it did give me a little glimmer of hope when none of the soldiers from his base knew his whereabouts. My sporadic dreams saw him walking into the ward and taking me into his arms, saying, "Everything will be fine now."

By December 23, Manila had been under attack for five consecutive days by the Japanese. On Dec. 26, General Douglas MacArthur, commander of the U.S. forces in the Far East, declared Manila an open city. None of us knew what that meant and didn't have time to find out. By December 23, Manila had been under attack for 16 consecutive days.

Later that day, Major Stevenson came by the hospital and summoned me. "General MacArthur has given orders for all the nurses to leave Manila. It has been declared an open city. Everyone must leave, on the double! Inform your staff to pack one musette bag and report outside, where a convoy of trucks will wait to evacuate you to Bataan. Chief Harrington, after you pack, I'll need to give you a fast lesson in gun handling before you leave. Meet me in front of the hospital at my jeep, then we'll go to the closest part of the jungle to practice."

With a pounding heart, I asked, "Sir, what will happen to our patients and what in God's name is an open city?"

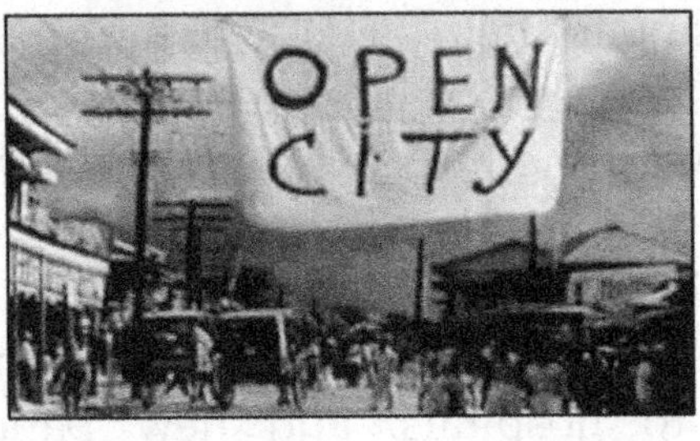

The major answered, "You'll be evacuated to a field hospital. The physicians and medical corpsmen will remain to take care of the patients. Three hundred patients will be transported on an interisland steamer to reach Australia in 30 days. An open city, Chief Harrington, is when military personnel retreat and stop fighting the enemy. This will spare any further destruction of the capital of Manila for the people that remain. The Japanese will take over the city." The major stopped and lit a cigarette. "It's unfortunate but we have neither the men nor the aircraft to defend Manila any longer. Now hurry, pack up, then meet me outside. One more thing—grab as many L-pills or lethal pills that will fit in your pockets. In case the nurses are taken prisoner, they can commit suicide with the poisonous pills instead of being subjected to torture."

In a daze, I mustered up my courage and mumbled, "Yes, sir." The weight of the military laws felt like a pile of bricks on my shoulders.

The officer made a beeline for the front door and left.

I dashed to my room and stuffed my things into a musette bag—a soiled uniform, a pair of white duty shoes, underclothes, and cotton stockings. Of course, I had to leave all my party gowns behind in my expensive suitcases, and felt stupid that I had brought so many.

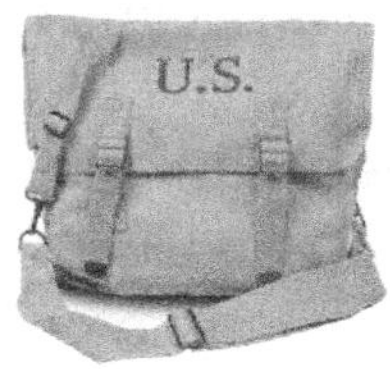

I touched the brim of my fancy picture hat, which I had worn when I first got off the ship and on my date with Rob. I couldn't help myself and stuffed it into my musette bag along with my grandmother's diamond watch and the framed photograph of my mother and father from my nightstand. The glass was cracked from the explosions but I put it in my bag anyway. A feeling of sadness overcame me as I closed the pack and hurried to the hospital supply room. There I found a bottle marked "Lethal Pills" and stuck it into a pocket of my uniform.

I took a deep breath and rushed all over the hospital to tell all the nurses that we had been ordered to evacuate immediately, and to bring a musette bag of their belongings and wait outside for transportation. "Don't forget your helmets and gas masks."

Several nurses asked with tears, "What about our patients?"

I answered, "The physicians and medics will care for them. I'll explain everything outside while we wait to be transported to Bataan. Everyone, speed it up and pack! We must get out of here before the Japanese come!"

With my musette bag on my shoulder, I raced outside to find Major Stevenson, who waited in his jeep. I jumped in and we sped off to a patch of nearby jungle. We got out of the jeep and pushed through a thick area of tangled vines and trees.

The major took out a Colt .45 and pointed it at a large cluster of bananas high on a tree to show me how to shoot. He aimed and fired. Bits of banana exploded into the air. He handed me the gun. I tried to shoot, but it was heavier than it looked. I was exhausted from the stress of leaving as well as the enormous workload, and missed the tree. Dirt spewed all around us.

I looked down at my dirty, blood-speckled white work shoes. "Sorry, sir, I don't know if I can do this." I thought, *I'm a healer, not a killer*. I was not interested in guns. But of course, I had to obey Army orders.

He barked at me, "You have no choice! You must learn how to defend yourself *and* your nurses. Chief Harrington, your nurses are the first American military nurses who will be sent on duty to perform battlefield nursing. We are at war now and you are all severely needed."

I tried again. This time, I shot one of the leaves but no bananas.

"At least you got close. Just remember if you need to shoot the enemy, aim for the gut. That'll kill 'em for sure." He looked at his watch. "There's no time left now. I'll take you to the convoy."

My fingers trembled as he shoved the pistol and a green sock full of gold, silver-tipped bullets into my hands, then ordered, "Keep the Colt loaded and hidden on your person at all times."

Chapter Six
Dottie
Fort Huachuca 1942

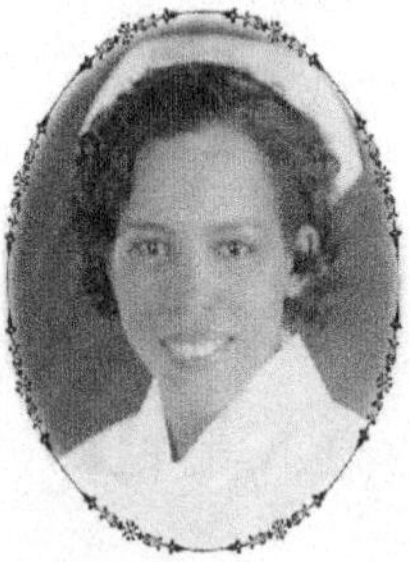

During the last week of basic training in the stifling month of August, our group piled into the back of a large truck. We were driven to an infiltration course and marched to an area 100 yards in length with trenches at both ends that were partially filled with water and mud.

The gravelly voice of the infantry officer thundered orders. "Fall in! Right! Front! At ease!" He handed out helmets and gas masks and told us to put them on.

The nurses watched in awestruck worry as the officer jumped over the ditch and fell prostrate onto the ground, then pushed through the dirt on his belly in an elbow crawl under barbed wire, then over the final ditch.

"Remember to keep your heads, hands, arms, and feet down. And your butts!" the infantry officer shouted. "Tighten your helmets and make sure your gas masks are on correctly."

We looked like a herd of elephants in our snout-like gas masks. I could hear the nervous, muffled laughter from the nurses. On our heads were weighty steel helmets (too big, of course), and we wore pistol belts with metal canteens attached to them to add the burden of extra weight.

The officer announced, "Take your time, but know that the average infantryman's time is 12 minutes. You must do the course in less than 30 to pass. We shoot live ammunition over the course, so when I say keep your body parts down, I mean it!"

I was glad my shock was hidden by the mask after I heard him say that live ammunition would be shot over our heads.

He commanded, "Line up!"

I was first in line and dropped down in an attempt to go through the course. Overhead, the *rat-a-tat-tat* of machine guns sounded, followed by the booms of dynamite explosions from the tower above.

I said the Lord's Prayer, muffled inside my gas mask, and somehow made it to the end. I took off my mask and forced myself to announce cheerfully, "That was fun! You try it, Clara."

As I cheered Clara on, I noticed that the soldiers in the tower shot far away from anyone and it was just a scare tactic.

We all made it through the course except for Lorna, who was last and hung back. I walked over to her and coached her. "Lorna, what would your boyfriend say if you washed out of here?" I squeezed her shoulder and patted her back as she stepped toward the course.

When she got to the end, I heard a sucking noise as she tried to lift her boot out of the mud, but to no avail. Super-strong Betty grabbed her hand and got her out of the muck-filled trench.

"My boot, there goes my boot!" Lorna wailed as she stood there in a muddy sock.

Laughter broke out as Lorna bent over and fished through the gooey mess until she found her boot and pulled it out.

The lieutenant glanced at his watch, gave us a pathetic look, and yelled, "Get into the trucks! You'll need your sleep. Tomorrow's the last test day and it will be the hardest part of basic training."

We waddled to the trucks dripping in mud and slogging with each step in our heavy, oversized, soaked pants and sticky boots. Lorna's face drooped as she held her boot in her lap in the back of the truck.

Oh, the moans and groans on the truck were hard to bear. I forced myself to be cheerful and sang a song to drown out the complaints. A few of the tired gals joined in. Somehow, I think we all completed the course within the allotted 30 minutes because of the sheer fright of getting shot.

In the barracks, we lined up eagerly to take showers. That night, everyone slept soundly, and a cacophony of snores, like bullfrogs in a pond, filled the barracks.

The next morning, we marched to chow. Not much conversation occurred except for quiet Mary, who mumbled, "Are they trying to make women into men?"

Nobody had the energy to answer that one.

It was the last day of basic training. We were brought to the bottom of the Huachuca Mountains and ordered to hike for 10 miles with field packs on. Orders heard, I began the climb but stopped when I noticed that no one followed me.

Lorna, with tears in her eyes, said, "I can't do this. I miss my family and my Tommy. I think I'd rather go home."

Hilary was fueled by Lorna. "My back, arms, and legs are killing me from yesterday. Let's sneak back to the barracks. It's a shorter distance than the hike."

Several of the gals agreed.

Alarmed at what I was hearing, I turned back to intervene. "Girls, we *will* and we *must* do this. It is the final test to prove our stamina to the Army. While we hike up the mountain, keep in your mind a vision—anything positive will do, like your boyfriend applauding at the end, drinking a cocktail under a palm tree overseas, or your family at the finish line proud as fancy peacocks. Now, who can do this?"

There was silence.

"Repeat after me. *We can do it!*" I yelled.

Some of the nurses mumbled, "We can do it…"

Then Clara, my rock, hollered, "We can do it!"

Lorna was tight-lipped.

"I need to hear all of you as loud as possible. Ready? One…two…three… *We can do it!"*

All the nurses shouted, "We can do it!"

I heard Lorna this time and Hilary joined in.

"Much better, nurses! Forward, march! We've made it this far and as you know, this is our last day in basic. In my heart, I know none of you wants to wash out, go home, then never get to see what it would be like in a foreign country."

Lt. Carlson drove his jeep behind us up the steep, magnificent mountain as we walked. In the beginning, we enjoyed the hike. The air was thick with the smell of sycamores, oaks, pines, and junipers. We heard a variety of birds as we wound our way upward. I pointed out what I thought was a butterfly to the gals—its wings hummed and beat so fast, they were a blur.

Prudence exclaimed, "That's not a butterfly. I've studied birds. It's what's called a hummingbird. It's seen in the West."

We all stopped and watched the tiny, five-inch creature with bright-green, glittery feathers and a red throat. Its long, slender bill drew nectar from a tiny, sunny yellow flower with an orange center. We were all mesmerized by this creation from God.

I filled my lungs with mountain air and sang the song of the Army Nurse Corps to keep our energy going and spirits high so we could make it to the end.

We march along with faith undaunted
Beside our gallant fighting men
Wherever they are sick or wounded
We nurse them back to health again
As long as healing hands are wanted
You'll find the nurses of the Corps
On ship or plane, on transport train

At home or on a far-off shore
With loyal heart we do our part,
For the Army and the Army Nurse Corps

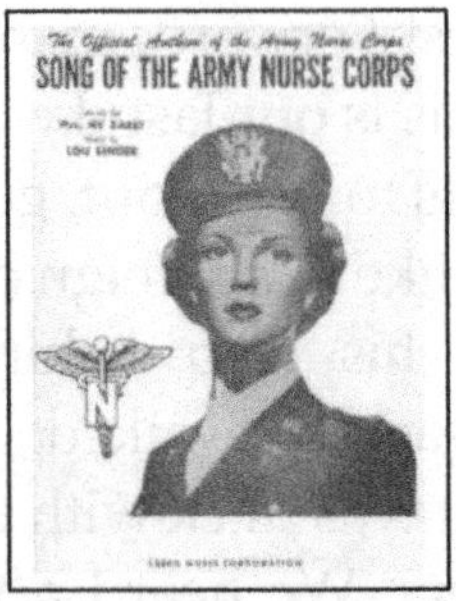

I paused and turned around to face the sullen nurses behind me and sang again. I was overjoyed to hear them join in the refrain, *smile, smile, smile.*

At the home stretch, we were met by a truck and driven back to base. We were dirty beyond description. The heat made the red mud from our coveralls stain the bed of the truck. Some of our faces were unrecognizable. Even our teeth were coated with dirt, and we tried to wash it down with the small amount of water left in our canteens.

There was an unusual silence at the table that night at chow. Nothing could be heard except for the clank of utensils and chewing. After showers, everyone hit their beds. I lay awake amid the snoring, worried that anyone would fail basic training and be sent home in tears.

The next morning, I was startled to hear the wake-up bugle call. I decided to skip breakfast and go to the major's office.

Lorna stopped me. "I didn't pass basic, and I know I didn't try hard enough because I wanted to go home and be with my Tommy. But when I got back last night, I got a letter from him that said he had joined the Army Flying School for Negro Pilots at Tuskegee, Alabama. Now I don't have a reason to go home.

Chief Dottie, I know I've been a thorn in your side, but I do love nursing and it does make me feel like I'm doing something worthwhile for the war effort. Can you put in a good word for me when you see the major?"

"I'll try but I'd better go now. I'll let you know after breakfast."

I was quite concerned on my way over to the major's office. Most of the nurses couldn't shoot a bullseye or march. Then there was the difficult obstacle course and exhausting mountain hike. With a sigh, I knocked on the major's door.

The major said, "Enter. How can I help you, Chief?"

He laughed when I asked for the list of the nurses who had passed or failed. "Everyone passed! The Army's desperate for nurses to care for our wounded soldiers to help end this damn war."

"Thank you, Major. We're anxious to work in the hospital and get an assignment overseas."

The major went back to his paperwork, then looked up and said, "Dismissed!"

I marched to chow and made the announcement. "Congratulations! You all passed. Finish up and head over to the Negro Hospital for the lecture on overseas nursing. Which, by the way, means a whole lot of sitting!"

All my nurses whooped out uproarious cheers that filled me with relief as well as satisfaction and pride.

We had endured the 10-mile hike and were rewarded with a curriculum on jungle diseases and medicine at the segregated Negro Hospital. This would take six weeks and would include patient care. We had classes in the morning and hospital duty in the afternoon.

Dr. Walker, in his intellectual East Coast accent and

bookish, tortoise shell-framed glasses, spoke with authority about gas gangrene. I couldn't concentrate on the medical facts as I wondered whether this handsome man was a White or Negro physician. He wore an officer's cap, which hid his hair—which would have provided a clue as to what race he was. His skin was quite light and threw me off, plus his eye color was difficult to see behind his glasses. He was quite a handsome man in his uniform.

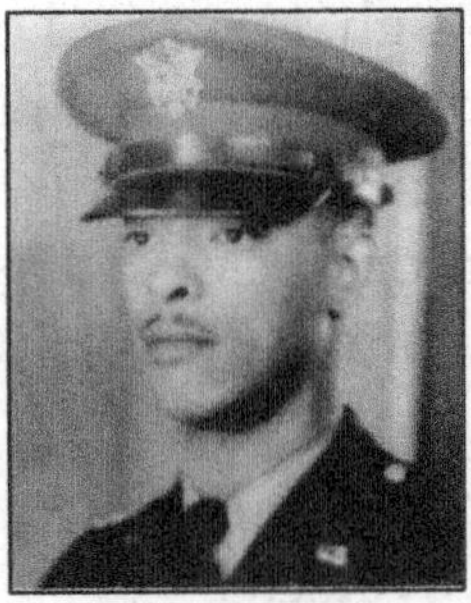

The question rolled around in my head. Then, I turned behind me and noticed the other nurses whispering and giggling to each other. I put a finger on my lips and they stopped talking.

Dr. Walker spoke in a serious voice. "Gangrene is the death of body tissue. Combat soldiers get gas gangrene from the bacteria that live in the soil and infect open wounds. Once within the tissue of an injured arm or leg, the bacteria multiply rapidly. The tiny bubbles created by the bacteria form in the damaged muscle, then press on small blood vessels and stop oxygen-carrying blood from nourishing nearby tissue. Within 72 hours, the bacteria release a toxin that travels along nerve pathways to the spinal column and then to the brain, resulting in the death of the infected person. The only treatment is the amputation of the affected body part. This will prevent the lethal toxin from spreading further in the patient."

After he said "amputation," a few of the nurses gasped.

Clara said a little too loud, "Amputation…how terrible."

Dr. Walker nodded. "Yes, it is. But sometimes a physician has no choice except to complete an amputation when a wounded soldier arrives with a limb that is irretrievably shattered and mangled. It is also protocol to amputate when there is destruction of the arteries. There is a new drug called penicillin that might prevent amputations; however, we might not have access to this miracle drug overseas." The doctor wrote on the chalkboard a list of preventive measures to prevent gangrene.

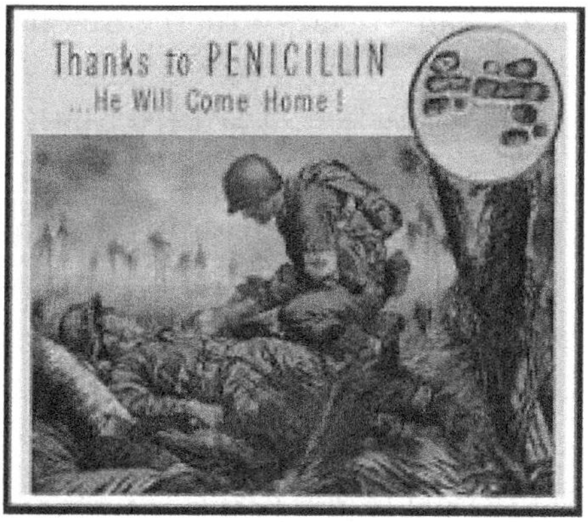

After the lecture, Dr. Walker asked me, "Chief, don't your nurses have new uniforms?"

"No, we were not allocated any. We only have the uniforms from our previous hospitals."

His eyebrows rose. "While you are all at lunch, I will see to it that you get new duty uniforms for work in the hospital."

Sure enough, after chow we stopped off in the barracks and saw that two large boxes and one small one had been dropped off.

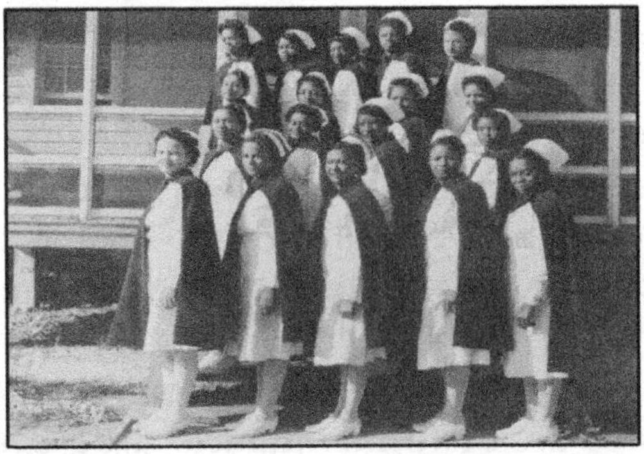

Polly gushed, "What a sweetheart Dr. Walker is!"

I opened one of the large boxes and pulled out a uniform. Of course, the uniforms were used, which caused an onslaught of complaints.

I said, "At least they're clean. Let's try them on and find one that fits."

Hazel got out her leftover safety pins and helped everyone with the sizes. Poor Betty had to squeeze into the largest one, which was still quite tight.

I looked inside several thin boxes, which contained new white stockings separated by tissue paper. The nurses cheered as I handed them out. Everyone loved the new capes.

The following day during class, I sat in the front of the room to keep my nurses quiet for Dr. Walker's lecture. I was pleased to see the enthusiasm on everyone's faces as they lapped up all the new information. The burden of basic training had faded, now replaced by the anticipated reward of practicing medicine overseas. That day, we learned about further jungle diseases, such as beriberi, scurvy, and scrub typhus.

It was obvious to me that Dr. Walker had saved the lecture on venereal disease for last. His feet shifted from one to the other and he sweated profusely, then mopped his face with his handkerchief and coughed nervously.

"Nurses, you may encounter as many as one in eight men with gonorrhea or syphilis. These are the two most prevalent of all the venereal diseases. It can take up to 30 days of treatment for gonorrhea to resolve, and six months for syphilis. During the Great War, the Army lost the services of 18,000 servicemen per day who had VD. Which is why, as medical personnel, we must stress the prevention measures of using condoms or abstention. A booklet is given to every enlisted man. I am passing one out for you all to read. Your job is to remind all the servicemen that VD must be prevented."

Several of the nurses snickered. I looked back and gave them my "stop that" look from my seat in the front row.

Dr. Walker continued, "Tell the soldiers that VD is caught by sexual intercourse with an infected woman. Cooks are forbidden to handle food until all traces of the disease are gone, and military police can lose a stripe if caught having the disease."

He cleared his throat, paused, and took a sip of water.

"Inform the soldiers that if they will not abstain from sexual contact, they must wear a condom and wash with soap and water afterward. This disease is rampant. The Medical Department issues six prophylaxis condoms per month. Troops can purchase more from the PX if there is one." Dr. Walker fumbled as he opened a pack of condoms. "They are cheap and readily available in the States, but overseas make sure you keep them in stock and freely available for all soldiers. Keep in mind that large numbers of men on the march are away from their wives and girlfriends for months or even years at a time, and will encounter prostitutes eager to capitalize on the many potential clients. With our vast number of camps and men on day leaves without condoms, we have ideal breeding grounds for venereal diseases."

He took one out and held up the elongated sheath. "Condoms are put on the penis before intercourse to prevent venereal disease and are made of a polyurethane plastic." His face reddened and he forced himself to say, "All prostitutes and pick-ups should be regarded as infected. The drug penicillin will cure the disease but keep in mind that if you are stationed overseas, it may not be available. The only sure way to prevent venereal disease is to avoid sexual contact."

The doctor passed out a small booklet titled "Sex Hygiene and Venereal Disease" from the War Department. "Every GI is issued an EPT kit, or emergency prophylactic kit. Each kit contains one tube of five grams of ointment, a direction sheet, soap-impregnated cloth, and cleansing tissue." He held up the kit for all to see. "I will pass two around for your observation."

Dr. Walker ended his lecture with a glance at his watch. "Everyone, please take the EPT kit and a packet of condoms from my desk on your way to the hospital. Remember, nurses, education can prevent disease! I'm late for my next class. See you all tomorrow." He dashed out ahead of us and left behind a giggling gaggle of nurses.

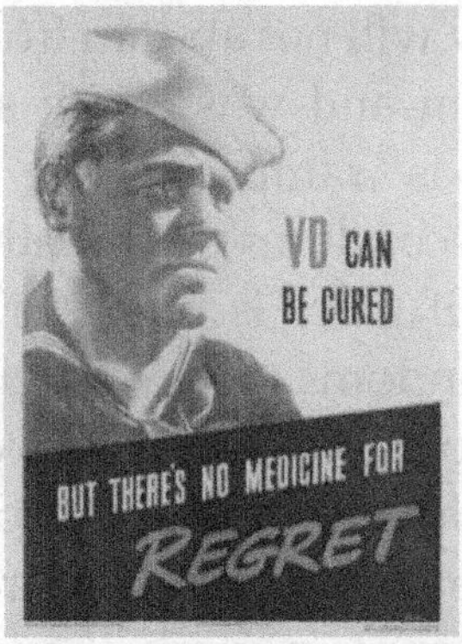

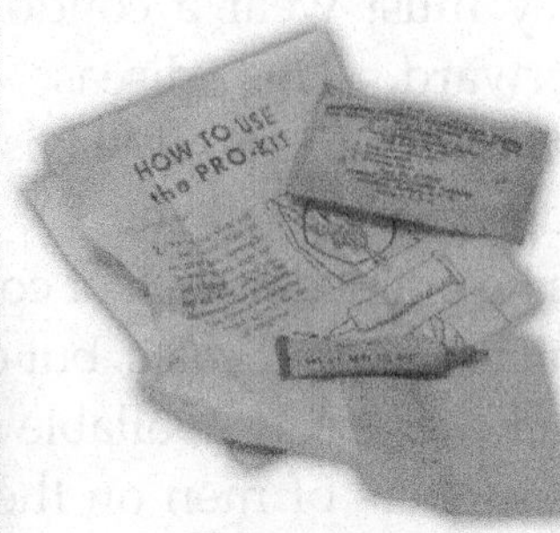
HOW TO USE
the PRO-KIT

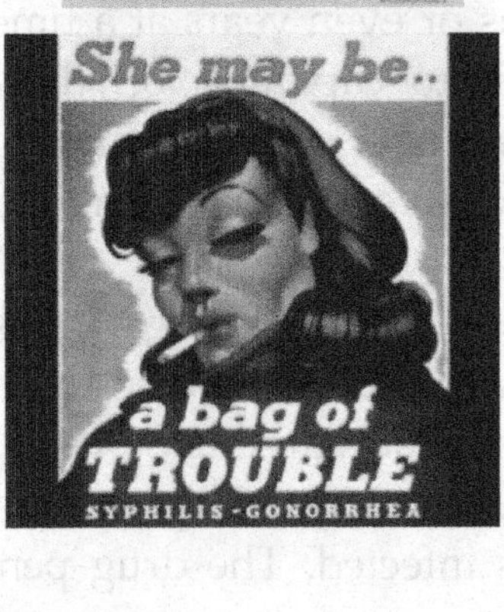
She may be..
a bag of
TROUBLE
SYPHILIS-GONORRHEA

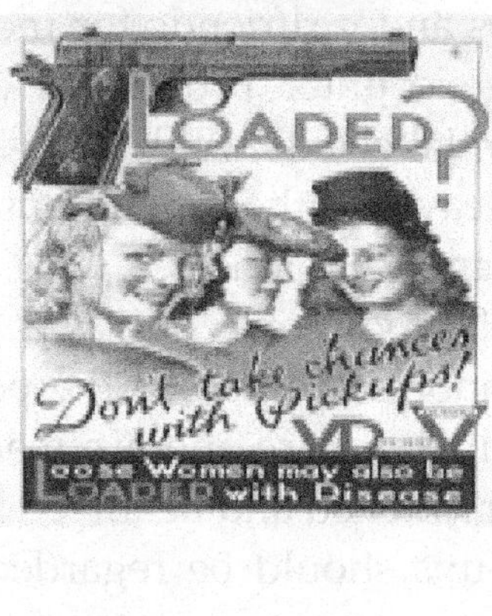
LOADED?
Don't take chances
with Pickups!
VD
Loose Women may also be
LOADED with Disease

Published August 1, 1940
in a brochure:

Manhood comes from healthy sex organs.

It is not necessary to have sexual intercourse in order to keep strong and well.

Disease may ruin the sex organs and deprive a man of his health and happiness.

You have a fine healthy body now. Keep it that way.

Venereal diseases come from sex relations or intimate contact with a diseased person. They are very serious. Gonorrhea and syphilis are two of the worst.

Most prostitutes have venereal disease.

Guard against venereal disease by staying away from "easy" women. Don't gamble your health away.

If you do not have self-control, then do not fail to take safety measures.

If you get diseased, report at once to your commanding officer. Time is most important.

Will power and self-control help to keep a man's body and mind healthy.

A healthy body and a healthy mind lead to happiness.

Chapter Seven
Bea
Escaping Manila to Limay, 1941-1942

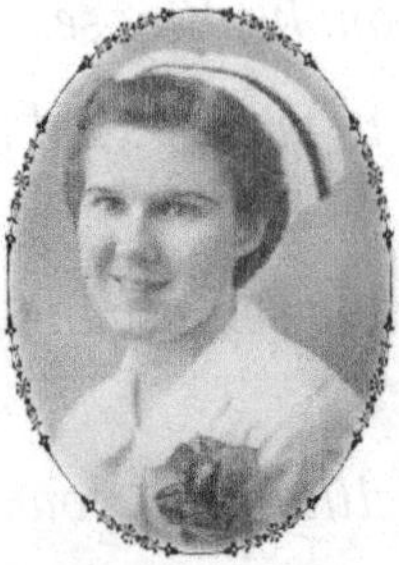

There were 53 Army nurses and 26 Filipina nurses waiting outside to be whisked away from the war-torn city of Manila. We were all issued ID cards, which identified us as non-combatants and were to be presented to the enemy if we were captured. Christmas had come and gone, and none of us had celebrated. Several Filipina nurses called it "Black Christmas."

What a frightening sight we were in our blood-stained uniforms, alabaster stockings, and filthy nursing shoes. Old World War I gas masks were strapped to our waists and we wore man-sized helmets that rocked on top of our heads and hid our faces. While we waited for the trucks to arrive, enemy planes blackened the sky overhead. I felt for the sock of bullets and my loaded Colt .45 in my pockets, but knew I was too terrified to ever use the gun.

Two U.S. Army trucks screeched to a stop at the curb. The first driver shouted out his window, "Get in, now! Pile into the back before the Japs find you!"

I jumped into the bed of the first truck and sat on my musette bag, followed by my assistant, Molly. Half the nurses were in the back of one truck and the rest in the other. We were stuffed in like sticks of dynamite.

The drivers sped off and we raced along the bumpy roads until we came to the heart of the city, where the trucks slowed to a crawl. We saw hordes of refugees desperately trying to flee Manila. Our drivers had to dodge the small yellow taxis that darted in and out of the tangled mess of traffic and people. Brown-faced families fled carrying an assortment of household goods, fighting cocks in cages, and children, all piled high on two-wheeled carts. The constant honking jarred our nerves as the drivers pushed on.

"What about Johnny with the one leg, will he be cared for?" Susie asked as she fidgeted with a strand of her blond hair.

"I'm worried about Ronny, you know, the soldier with no arms. What about him?" Caroline added with a frown.

"What about my brother with only one eye? Will I ever see him again?" Angelica asked in a tearful voice.

"Nurses, I know it's hard to leave our patients—especially relatives—but Sternberg still has doctors and medics to care for them. We're sorely needed elsewhere."

Once outside the city, we traveled alongside rice paddies in the country and followed the Pampanga River, where herds of carabao bathed their huge bodies. The scenery would have been much more enjoyable during peacetime without the worry of where we were headed. We were constantly stopped by patrols and slowed down by roadblocks.

We saw worn-out Filipino soldiers walking down the side of the road carrying old bolt-action rifles. Some of them showed us the V for Victory sign with their fingers and we waved it in return. We passed dozens of bombed-out villages full of the charred remains of unidentifiable objects.

A few of the nurses cried out, "Oh no!" and "The poor people!"

Our truck rattled down the narrow, rocky coastal road toward Bataan, which was surrounded by dense bamboo thickets and coconut groves.

I looked at my panicked nurses, then gave Molly a double-take. I touched her false hairpiece. "Why are you wearing your rat?"

"Shhh," she whispered. "I have suicide pills hidden in it." She refashioned her hair.

I nodded. "Smart idea. I brought some as well."

Molly asked, "Chief Bea, what will our new hospital be like?"

I shook my head. "I'm not sure."

"How long do you think it'll take us to get there?" Annie asked. She wiped the sweat off her brow with her hankie. I saw that she wore a diamond ring on her finger that sparkled in the sunlight.

"I know it's many miles from Manila to Limay in the province of Bataan. It will take several hours because of the mass exodus of people plus the winding roads we have to take to get there."

I was grateful that I didn't hear too many complaints during the onerous journey. Most of the nurses were just tired and hungry. We were all hot and stuffed into the beds of the trucks. Some of the nurses rested their heads on each other and napped.

The jungle on both sides of the winding dirt road grew thicker. There were huge, vine-covered trees with thick canopies and matted underbrush. As we drove deeper into the countryside, the view became more relaxed, with tiny bamboo shacks surrounded by rice paddy fields, and banana, papaya, and mango trees. Brown, round-eyed children came out of the bamboo huts. They waved their little hands and giggled as they ran behind us barefoot and tried to follow the trucks.

Farther down the dirt road, our truck dodged a few water buffalo as they ran amok. We all laughed about the ruckus it made.

I smiled and assured myself, *We'll persevere!* Then I spied a handmade wooden sign on stilts. "There's a sign and it says Limay!" I pointed.

Up ahead, next to the border of the dense jungle, our convoy stopped.

Our driver hollered out his window, "This is it, your home away from home, ladies! You can get out now."

No one moved. All we could see was wilderness. There was no hospital in sight.

I took a deep breath. "Let's go, we've got a job to do," I said, and hoisted myself out of the truck.

Veronica applied lipstick from her pocket before she fetched her musette bag, then followed me off the vehicle. I opened my mouth in disbelief but shut it fast. I was just glad she found a little comfort by putting makeup on. After all, she had been the most popular nurse and had the most dates before the war broke out.

"Where's the hospital?" I said as I walked up to the driver.

He jerked his thumb toward the foliage. "Through there. Find a path and stay on it. Good luck."

I furrowed my brow as I gazed into the thick jungle.

After everyone was off the truck, the two drivers waved and sped away, leaving us in the dust. With a shrug, I led the way as we plunged into the unknown and searched for a building of some kind. The dense jungle was full of strange animal noises. Most of the nurses gasped in fright and looked around with wide eyes.

This place is like another world, I thought as I grabbed a large branch and held it like a weapon to use for protection from wild creatures that might jump out at us. I was still afraid to use my gun.

Our inappropriate, dirty nursing outfits and stockings snagged on the plants and bushes as we struggled through the undergrowth. We pulled off the vegetation and kept moving. I ignored the mumbles and complaints and forged onward. At last, we came to a huge clearing that was full of scattered, crude, rustic shacks.

A large, well-postured man in coveralls came out of one of the shacks. He had gray flecks of hair on his temples, a scraggly short beard, a gray mustache, and a big smile.

"Welcome to Limay, Bataan. I've been expecting you. I'm glad to see the Filipina nurses. Not many of our staff know Spanish or Tagalog to speak to the wounded Filipino soldiers."

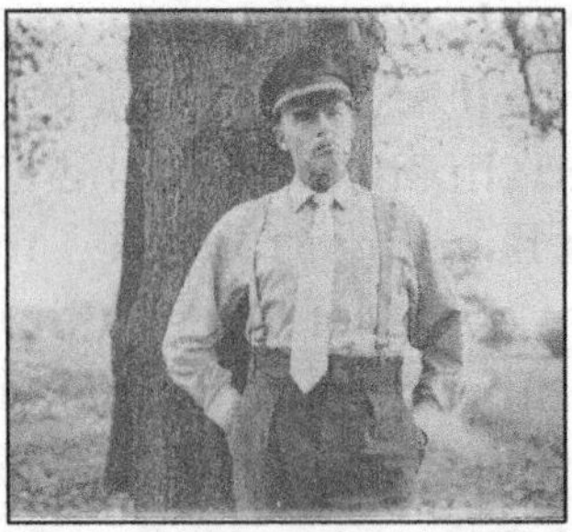

Our Filipina nurses displayed gracious smiles.

He introduced himself. "I'm Dr. Arnold Goldstein. Call me Major Arnie. I'm sure you're all tired, so I'll show you where to set up your quarters."

I stepped toward him. "Chief Beatrice Harrington – or just Chief Bea." I put down my stick weapon and shook his outstretched hand. "Thank you, Major Arnie."

We craned our necks to search for a building that might house us as we followed the doctor along the jungle path, which was profuse with vine-covered bamboo trees. One of the nurses screamed when a large snake wiggled across the path in front of us. Major Arnie ignored it and pushed through as we tried to keep up the pace. My tired group of nurses moved slowly in the thick, humid air but I hurried to catch up to Major Arnie.

"How many nurses did you bring?" he asked.

"There are 79 of us. How many patients do you have

here?"

"The patients have not arrived yet. The war is expected to escalate into Limay from Manila at any time. The Japs will wait for our retreated troops from Manila to move into Bataan before they attack again. I have been informed by the general that we have 14,000 American troops with 72,000 Filipino troops leaving Manila. We're 500 yards from the front lines here and we need to get ready for the possible onslaught of patients from the battlefield."

"How many physicians are at the hospital?"

"Me and Dr. Charlie, who you'll meet later, plus about 100 medics. We expect to receive 40 more physicians."

My thoughts ran wild with this information. *God help us! Only two doctors! I hope more physicians show up.*

Major Arnie stopped in front of an old, long, wooden building. "Here's your nurses' quarters, gals."

He opened the rickety door and we all walked inside the dark, cobweb-infested building. A mouse skittered past our feet and Annie suppressed a scream. She scraped her hand along the wooden wall and gathered years' worth of dirt in her palm, then clapped her hands together, sending up a cloud of dust. Several of the nurses coughed. Most stood in silence and shock at the condition of our new residence.

Susie said, "I hope you don't expect us to sleep on the floor!"

"Where are the beds?" I turned to face the doctor.

Major Arnie answered with a forced smile, "After you scrub this up, you'll find beds and bedding in one of those metal buildings located near the beach. I'll send a medic to bring your cleaning supplies. Come by the mess hall for chow when you're done." He left in a hurry.

I blew out a frustrated breath, then turned to my nurses. "Everyone, change into your coveralls and let's clean up this place," I said, and set my musette bag down in a corner.

Annie whined in her contagious, squeaky voice, "We're

not cleaning maids, we're nurses sent to heal the wounded, for heaven's sake!"

Agnes joined in. "There's rat droppings everywhere, this is disgusting," she said as she looked around.

"I'm tired," Angelica yawned.

Thankfully, Carmelita saved the day. "As nurses, I'm sure we all know how to clean, yes?"

"Thanks, Carmelita. Yes, we do and we will!" I added.

Much to my relief, a cute medic came in and the nurses quieted down. Veronica, our "glamour" nurse who always worried about her appearance, retrieved her lipstick from her pocket.

Medic Davy brought in sponges, buckets, and brooms. He was drop-dead gorgeous with wavy, light-brown hair and big greenish-blue eyes. Not only was he helpful but he was well-mannered. Susie's eyes followed his every move.

While half the nurses cleaned the building, I went with the other half and followed Davy to a large tin warehouse. We pulled out parts of beds that had to be assembled—headboards, footboards, joining bars, and frames. There were hundreds of them packed in newspapers dating from the early 1900s. The nurses lugged mattresses, linens, and bed parts through the jungle to our barracks.

I took out a hankie, pushed up my glasses, and wiped the sweat off my nose. The tropical jungle became hotter and more humid. I caught up to Davy, who carried a pile of sheets and a headboard. "Tell me, Davy, do you know what all these abandoned buildings and supplies are from?"

"Yes, ma'am. This used to be a training camp for Philippine Scouts who were assigned to the U.S. Army in 1901." He dropped the items outside the barracks, tilted his head, gave me a little smile, then went back to bring more items up.

I followed him. "Where are all the other medics? We could use more help here."

"They hide out when there's work to do unless Major Arnie needs them. I'll talk to the doc and get you more help tomorrow."

After we scrubbed down our new "home" and set up our beds, we fell asleep from pure exhaustion. No one mentioned food.

In the morning, we found the mess hall by following the delicious smell of fried chicken. We lined up as the cook and a medic dished out a breakfast of fruit and chicken.

I sat down next to Major Arnie, who introduced me to Dr. Charlie Bartell, a man of small stature who sported a neatly trimmed mustache and smoked a pipe. They had finished their meal and were drinking hot tea.

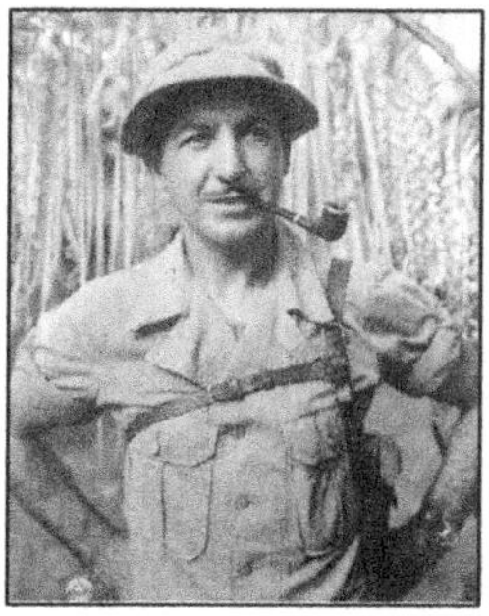

"Your nurses look like they're ready for battlefield nursing now," Major Arnie remarked when he saw our coveralls.

I took a big bite of the juicy chicken. "The fried chicken makes a hearty breakfast. Where do you get the chickens from?"

"Charlie and I go on food-finding tours. I drove my Cadillac here from Stotsenburg Hospital since the war hadn't hit here in Limay yet. Just last week, we drove north of here and in the middle of the jungle was a handmade sign that said 'Chickens for Sale.'"

Dr. Charlie added, "I told Major Arnie to forget it, we don't want worm-infested scrawny chickens. But he couldn't resist and headed down the dirt road."

"Boy, were you wrong!" Major Arnie waved his arms with enthusiasm as he told the story. "At the end of the road were hundreds of chickens in clean wire coops, fat and well cared for. We knocked on the shack and a small Filipino man in a clean white shirt and nice trousers answered. He greeted us in well-spoken English and offered us fried chicken and beans to eat. After that tasty meal, we were sold!"

"The best part was when the farmer said, 'Buy them all, I don't want them killed by bombs or eaten by the Japs,'" Dr. Charlie said.

"We asked the farmer how much he wanted and he said a dollar a bird," Major Arnie chuckled.

Major Arnie's enthusiasm was contagious. I laughed between bites of the scrumptious chicken.

The doctor continued, "We spent the day there and cleaned as many chickens as we could with the help of the farmer. We headed back to Limay with a trunkful of chickens, which we eat for every meal as you'll soon see. Food is supposed to be brought in from Manila, like canned fruits and vegetables, tinned milk, rice, beans, flour, coffee, cocoa, and tea, but of course, it has been unpredictable because of the Japanese invasion." He was quite a fast talker and paused to shove two pieces of chewing gum into his mouth. "Chief, after you've eaten, meet me outside and I'll show you the hospital and wards."

Both doctors got up and left.

I finished my meal and found Major Arnie. As we walked along a path through the jungle, I asked him if he knew Airman Robert Johnson.

He said, "Nope, but if he was stationed at Stotsenburg as a pilot, he's probably dead."

I fought back my tears and glanced away after his blunt remark.

Pinned on the ground in front of the hospital was a large

Red Cross insignia made from bedsheets.

Major Arnie said, "It's to prevent the Japs from bombing the hospital, and since we don't practice blackout procedures, we hope it will help. Besides, it's too darn hard to operate in the dark with flashlights."

"I hope they'll honor our hospital," I worried.

"That's all we got is hope," Major Arnie agreed. "Before I open the door, let me warn you, it's not like the fancy hospital at Sternberg with ceiling fans and all the amenities that you're used to." He paused. "Here it is."

He opened the door and the stale smell of rotten yeast hit my nose. I coughed, then gagged as I spied beer cans scattered all over the dirt floor.

"This used to be a bar." He kicked one of the cans to the side.

"A *bar?*" It was hard to keep my mouth shut from the shock.

We walked through a long shed that had no floors, open sides, and a tin roof. The electricity came from long cords that snaked into each end of the building. Each cord had a bare bulb and there were only a few generators. It was a small operating room of about 14 x 44 feet.

The doctor read my annoyed face. "It's a lousy set-up but we must make the best of it, and we need someplace to patch up our soldiers to win this goddamned war." He stuck another stick of gum in his mouth and snapped it rapidly while he spoke. "In this space we'll have several operating tables with spotlights."

"Where are the operating tables?" My voice rose despite my efforts to curb my distress.

"Everything's in the warehouses near the beach. It's a goldmine in there."

"This building needs to have enclosed walls and a decent floor to maintain a sterile surgical environment." I put my hand on my hip and gave him a stern look.

"How right you are. I'll get some of the medics to fix it up, and you can supervise! But hey, we do have flushable toilets." He beamed.

I wondered about Major Arnie. Would his surgical skills be better than his skills at organizing a medical facility?

"I'll show you the wards." He whisked me away before I could ask more questions.

We went through all the dusty, filthy buildings. Behind the nurses' and medics' barracks was a water tower by an artesian well. Thank goodness there was clean water available for the patients.

When the tour was over, I stood stone still. I could no longer hold my tongue. "Major Goldstein, where are the bedpans? The surgical supplies? The patients' beds?"

The doctor answered, "Like I said, we have a treasure trove of items in the warehouses at the beach. They've been stored there since World War I. It's all part of War Plan Orange, established in 1907 to stock up in case of another war. 'Orange' is a secret word for the Japanese." He looked at his watch. "I've got a meeting with Doc Charlie. Any more questions, Chief?"

"How long have you been here in Limay?"

"Dr. Charlie and I have been here a week."

"I was told by Davy that you have a hundred medics, and we could use their help to set up the wards and hospital."

Major Arnie scratched his beard. "Good idea. I'll round more medics up for you. Let's meet up in front of the mess hall with all the nurses."

On my way back to the nurses' barracks, I was filled with worry about the dirty buildings and lugging equipment through the jungle from the warehouses. We weren't servants, damn it!

In the barracks, I found my assistant, Molly, with the Filipina nurses on their beds, chatting with each other.

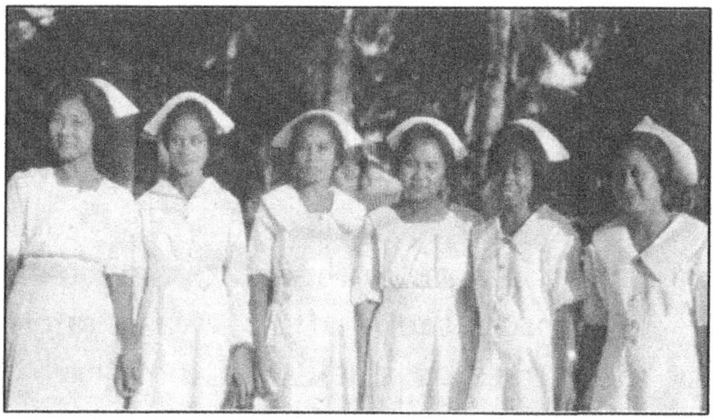

Filipina Nurses

"Where are all the other nurses?" I asked, looking around.

Molly, beet red, answered, "Chief, I tried to keep them here but one group walked into town with the medics to get a Coca-Cola and the other half went down to the beach for a swim with the other group of boys. I tried to get them to stay."

"Molly, please go down to the beach and get them back. We have a lot of work to do before the bombing begins."

I rounded up cleaning supplies with the Filipina nurses. A short time later, the medics strolled in with nurses on their arms. Everyone had a soda to drink.

"Gals, I'm glad you had a fun little getaway but we need to set up the operating pavilion before the Japanese bomb our troops here in Bataan. Major Arnie informed me that we have only a little while before the war starts up here."

I noticed their downturned faces at the realization that their little holiday might end. Annoyed, I sent them all to clean the buildings. Then I waited for the beach bunnies to show up and ordered them to the warehouses with the medics to find the hospital supplies. I gave them my serious speech that the war would reach us any day now before I sent them off.

The warehouses were stuffed with war-reserve medical supplies. We found unmarked cartons that contained bedpans and thermometers, as well as surgical equipment.

With the help of the ambitious, strong corpsmen, we hauled up quite a few supplies to the so-called "hospital" where the clean-up committee was hard at work. Many boxes of operating gowns, linen, gauze, towels, and swabs had to be sterilized.

A few of the nurses put on mascara and lipstick during their breaks to impress the medics. I was grateful that the medics kept the nurses on track, and that their complaints were replaced by flirting and work.

On the way back from the warehouse, I noticed that our two doctors were nowhere to be found and the Cadillac was gone. That evening, I went to chow and sat with them.

Ever the jokester, Major Arnie asked me, "Would you like chicken or filet mignon for dinner?"

I was too exhausted to answer, as well as peeved that they didn't help us set up the hospital facility.

Dr. Charlie laughed at Arnie's joke. "We noticed the great cleaning job the nurses and medics did, and all the supplies and beds have been brought up. Good work!"

"How was *your* day, doctors?" I asked in a sarcastic tone.

Dr. Charlie answered with enthusiasm, "It was a successful day. We found fresh vegetables and fruits and took the road up the mountain near Baguio—a nice drive."

Major Arnie added, "We got great deals because the natives know the war could arrive at any time now. How do you like your fresh fruit salad?"

I gave them a tight grin. "It's fine. When are the physicians expected?"

"The colonel has promised us 40 and they should arrive any day."

I gave them a false smile and suspected they wouldn't help us finish the set-up of the wards and hospital. This seemed to be their vacation time. "How many medical corpsmen did you say are here?" My eyes bored into the doctors' faces.

"About a hundred," Major Arnie answered.

"A hundred? I've seen about 25."

"Not to worry. I'll round up the rest for you, then you can organize the construction of the floors and sides of the hospital." He winked at me.

My patience was wearing thin from exhaustion and the heat of the jungle. "That would be most helpful. We are expecting a war here, aren't we?"

Major Goldstein stood up and cleared his plate, then left without another word. Dr. Charlie followed behind him.

The next morning, as promised, all the medics showed up. The floors and sides of the hospital were completed by the end of the day and a group of nurses and corpsmen helped clean up the entire place.

The next day, a small crew took multi-jet pressure-pumped Bunsen burners and set them up on steel-jacketed pressure cookers to sterilize all the surgical gowns, linens, and gauze. Then, all the nickel-plated instruments—saws, chisels, bone rongeurs, drills, scalpel handles, hemostats of all sizes, retractors, intestinal clamps, and needles—were sterilized.

The operating tables were set up and sawhorses were placed between them on which to set patients on litters, specifically for those who had to be positioned with their feet higher than their heads to allow blood to drain fast from other parts of the body to the heart. Next to the sawhorses were tables with stacks of sterilized blankets and hot-water bottles to keep the casualties who were in shock warm. The sterilized surgical equipment was placed on a large table with a sheet, ready to be brought to any of the operating tables by the nurses.

The hard-working medics pumped pails of water from the well to wash down tables, stands, beds, and cabinets. At last, we were almost ready for the inevitable influx of wounded patients. Vivid shades of my last days at Sternberg flashed through my mind as I supervised the set-up. I knew we could never be prepared enough for what might occur.

On Tuesday, I told everyone that we must cut our long hair because hairpins were in short supply, and we had to keep our hair pinned back. Veronica, a lovely brunette with curls that framed her face, looked like she would cry. She told us she used to be in fashion shows in Virginia and had modeled debutant gowns.

Carmelita sympathized. "I'll cut and style your hair, Veronica. I used to work in a beauty parlor before I became a nurse."

There were plenty of protests about the haircuts, but it was necessary, and with our nursing caps on, I thought we all looked better anyway.

The next day, one of the medics brought in a pile of mail.

"Chief Bea, you have a package," Molly said, and handed it to me.

I wonder if Rob could have sent something… I mused silently.

I took the box from Molly. All the nurses sat on the edges of their beds in anticipation. The postmark was from December 1, and the stamps on the package showed that it had traveled from the United States to Sternberg, then on to Bataan.

I stared at the package until the nurses chanted, "Open it! Open it!"

With care, I opened the box, then pulled off layer after layer of tissue paper and removed an elegant Southern-style hat with a burgundy mushroom brim and deep-blue ribbon binding, adorned with a pale-brown veil in the back.

"It's from my mother." I set the hat on my bed and my tears piled up when I read the Christmas card from her in faraway Georgia.

Veronica snatched the hat off my bed. "Can I try it on, Chief?"

Molly grabbed it from her. "Let Chief Bea try it on first," she scolded.

I took my nurse's cap off, then tugged a jungle leaf out of my hair. As soon as I put on the hat and adjusted the veil, outbursts of delight sounded all around me. I smiled and wondered how silly I must look with this sensational, delicate hat on my head with my short-cropped hair while I wore oversized coveralls. If my high-class Southern mother could see me in this hat in this primitive environment, she'd faint!

Veronica said, "You look so cute. Now can I try it on?"

"Of course, everyone must try it on," I said.

Carmelita, with her jet-black, wavy hair, looked the best as she arranged a few curls to peek out of it. After Carmelita showed it off, I made sure Molly had a turn.

"Molly, you look adorable," Jane gushed.

It warmed my heart to hear the laughter that ensued, and I was thrilled that a fancy hat could bring so much happiness to everyone. The nurses smiled through teary eyes as they chatted about boyfriends in Manila or from their hometowns. This delicate hat symbolized home, going to the theater, and ballroom dances for many of the nurses.

While everyone chatted and fussed over the hat, I heard a soft gasp and glanced over at Annie, who had found a letter addressed to her. She jumped up off her bed and ran away before I could ask what was wrong. Curious and concerned, I followed her.

Outside, I looked around the hospital area but didn't see her. I walked into the jungle, calling for her, but still couldn't find her. I stopped to catch my breath and heard soft, sporadic sniffles, and saw someone on a cot under a sheet next to a papaya tree. I gingerly lifted a corner of the sheet, and sure enough, Annie was underneath it.

"Please tell me, honey, what's the matter?" I said as I knelt beside her.

She rolled away from me and continued to cry into her hands to muffle the sound. Then she burst out at me, "Go away, Chief!"

"Annie, please tell me what's wrong," I said in a gentle voice. I sat on the edge of the cot and rubbed her back.

Annie bolted to her feet and threw the letter onto my lap. When I read it, I understood why she was in deep distress.

Dear Annie,

My husband and I wanted to inform you that your fiancé, our son, was killed in action at the massacre on Clark Field Military Base on December 8. We are grief-stricken and sorry that you will not be wedding our only son. We don't know when you will receive this letter, but please write to us when you can to tell us how you are.

We will always love you as a daughter-in-law and welcome you into our home after this horrific war is over.

Fondly, Mr. and Mrs. Jack Andrews

I folded the letter and shook my head. "No wonder you have been so distressed. You must've panicked when Clark Field was bombed."

Annie's lip trembled. "I tried to find out how my Frank was. Every time casualties appeared at Sternberg, I would look and see if my fiancé was among them." She twisted her diamond ring on her finger.

"I'm sorry, Annie. Stay here and try to get some sleep." I pushed thoughts of Rob out of my mind.

Annie screamed, "I'll never be able to sleep again!" Then she sank onto the cot and cried. With a soft touch, I massaged her thin shoulders.

When her crying subsided, she said, "Oh, Chief Bea, I loved him so much and we were going to get married after the war. Frank wanted to marry me before he enlisted, but I insisted on waiting to have a big wedding since I come from a large family. My mom and dad loved him also. We were high school sweethearts." Then Annie broke down and let loose a floodgate of tears. "I just want to kill myself. Do you have any of those suicide pills?"

"No suicide pills, but I have luminal pills. They will help you get some rest and somewhat help you forget your loss." I went to the barracks and returned with one pill—a small dose because of her petite frame.

While Annie cried and sniffled, I held her hand. "It's the hardest part of life when you lose a loved one."

I thought about my dad and how dazed I was after he died, but felt blessed that his death had brought me to this profession. I pushed my mind away from brooding over Rob. "I promise you, Annie, after you rest for a few days and get back to nursing, it will give you more of a purpose to live."

I sat with her until she fell asleep. I knew in my heart that if I took care of my nurses, they in turn would take good care of the soldiers.

That night I allowed myself to think about Rob. I almost felt that Annie was lucky that she knew what had happened to her fiancé. I tossed and turned, then tried to replace that thought with memories of the glorious time we had as a couple.

At the end of the week, with no Japanese aircraft in sight, the nurses were invited to a dinner and dance on the *USS Canopus*, a 373-foot submarine tender. It was a surface ship assigned to watch over Manila and Bataan on Mariveles Bay, a large cove at the southern tip of the Bataan Peninsula. We were driven by sailors in jeeps, then transported to the ship in four PT boats, which made several trips back and forth until everyone was on board the ship. It was disguised with smudge pots on it that burned as if it had been destroyed and abandoned. The ship was used to manufacture arms for the defense of Bataan and had a machine shop on the lowest deck.

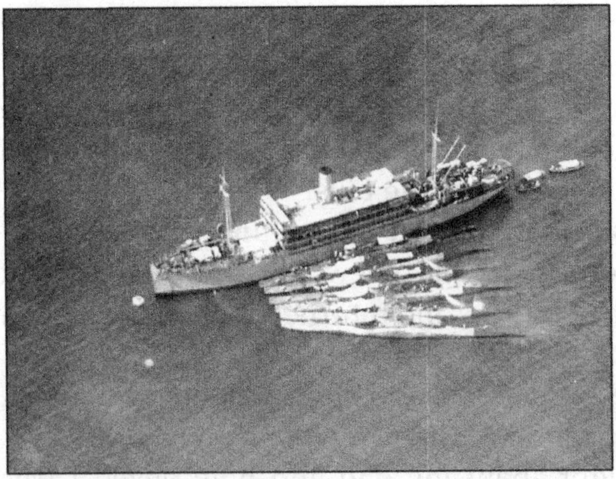

A few of us wore party dresses, and the nurses pooled all the makeup and perfume they had stashed in their musette bags. I wore khaki trousers and a men's shirt, but with glee put on my forgotten picture hat and my grandmother's diamond watch. I convinced Annie to go with us and loaned her the new hat my mother had sent. One of the Filipina nurses wore spike heels and almost fell over from lack of practice on them. Those who had brought dresses had to wear them without stockings and in large boots. What a sight we were in our mismatched costumes! We all looked ridiculous but at least we smelled good! The sailors on board hooted and whistled and were ecstatic to see women. They couldn't have cared less what we wore.

On the ship was a hand-wound portable phonograph and records dating from the 20s. The songs were a hoot! We had an early evening meal of juicy steak, mashed potatoes, and assorted canned vegetables, all served on thick, heavy naval plates with an outer dark blue circle and the letters USN embossed on them. They were placed on real tablecloths with engraved silverware.

A few of the sailors shared their hidden bottles of Johnnie Walker Red. One of them played "Yes Sir, That's My Baby" and "Singing in the Rain" on the phonograph. I sat in a dream and relished watching all the nurses as they transformed into their former selves when they danced. A few of the Filipina nurses performed an exotic rhythmic native dance and received quite the applause.

Dr. Charlie banged out an upbeat rendition of Glenn Miller's "Don't Sit Under the Apple Tree (with Anyone Else but Me)" on an untuned piano. Molly stood close to him and sang everything he played in a beautiful soprano voice.

During the evening, I did notice that a few of the nurses had tears in their eyes, either from missing their boyfriends or from the gaiety of the party. And when it was time to leave, I spied a few long goodbye kisses. It worried me some, but I shook it off. Actually, I was a bit envious.

The sailors gave us each a lollypop for the short journey back. It seemed like years since any of us had tasted candy. On the boat ride back to shore, we were treated to a blaze of colors from the tropical sunset. It had been a glorious night, and we all fell into a deep sleep that night in the barracks. Even Annie.

Chapter Eight
Dottie
Fort Huachuca – Camp Florence, Arizona
1942-1943

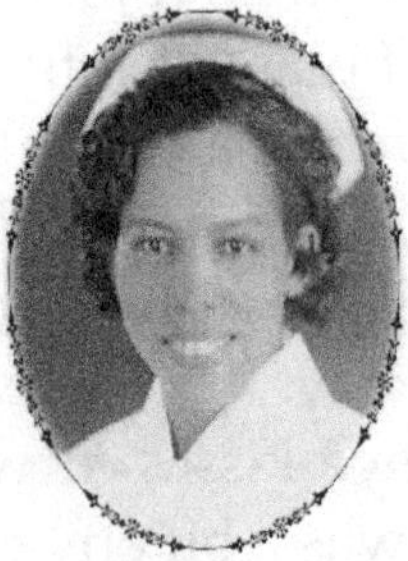

It was a pleasure for all of us to attend the morning lectures by the handsome Dr. Walker, then in the afternoon, take care of the soldiers on the ward. The patients we cared for were those who required long-term hospitalization that was not practical in the hospitals overseas. These soldiers were severely injured and it was our job to heal them so they could return to battle.

Some of the men were discharged and sent home due to amputations, or were blind or deaf from the battlefield and could not continue to serve. It took compassion on our part to listen to and help these soldiers. We were amazed by their patriotism, and most of the men insisted on returning to their platoons even though that was impossible. I checked on my nurses frequently to make sure they were expressing the needed empathy in these situations, and they did their jobs well.

There were soldiers at the base who had syphilis and gonorrhea, and we had to hone our bedside manner to deal with and prevent these personal diseases. My shy nurses, like

Emily from the Midwest, were not as adept, and I often had to call on other nurses who could better handle these sensitive matters. Clara from New York City was quite experienced and had cared for patients with VD at her hospital there. I was grateful for Dr. Walker's helpful lecture on this touchy subject.

It was rewarding to see my nurses laugh and flirt with the ill soldiers, but I did have to rein them in. On one occasion, I caught Clara strolling by a soldier, and she let him feel her white silk stockings as she passed by. But I knew that the men were lying at eye level with the nurses' legs and had nothing to do except watch attractive women stroll by day and night. It was a difficult situation that I had to talk to my nurses about more than once. It was a top priority for me to make sure no one got pregnant, then discharged without the opportunity to travel overseas. But despite the challenges, I was filled with pride as I watched my gals apply their nursing skills after the tough time they'd had in basic training doing useless calisthenics, marching, and riflery.

Lorna became less homesick and more focused on the rewards of her job. I overheard her when she spoke to a patient with one arm, who told her all about the tropics of the beautiful Philippine Islands. I knew my nurses wanted to know where we were going, but I was not permitted to tell them until the day before we were to leave.

The nurses handed out a base newsletter for the soldiers to read. The men kept themselves occupied and wrote articles for the newsletter and drew sketches for posters. There were many requests for paper, which I tried to accommodate as best I could with our limited supplies.

Fort Huachuca Army Base Newsletter

At the fort's hospital, the staff is mainly treating rampant venereal disease. All soldiers receive the War Department's Army booklet "Sex

Hygiene and Venereal Disease." Every patient is required to read this. You will also be given a packet of Trojans and a Pro-kit.

The Base newsletter will pay $10 for every article written by a soldier on how to prevent VD. Winning sketches will also be paid for, and silk screened by the art department of special services, then made into posters.

Keep in mind the following themes: how to avoid the disease; a defense worker loses man hours, including time and money; the dangers of gonorrhea and syphilis.

We couldn't enjoy ourselves in town because of the Jim Crow laws but did have the Negro Mountain View Officers' Club located right on the base. The first night we went to the club, there was a dance. Excited, we dressed up as best we could with what we had.

Prudence, the prettiest nurse, said, "I miss my one fancy dress. It's a shame none of us brought an outfit to wear to the club."

Lorna added, "I hope my boyfriend doesn't find out if I just have one dance."

Clara chastised her, "That's a stupid thing to worry about. How could he possibly find out? Stop sittin' around and poutin' about a boy, Lorna. Dancing will be good for you. Here, borrow my midnight-rose lipstick."

Lorna smiled. "I think I will. Thanks, Clara."

"I can't wait to feel a soldier's jacket pressed against my chest while we're slow dancing," Jane swooned.

Betty chimed in, "I love how our boys always wink and tip their hats when we walk by them on the way to the hospital."

"One of the soldiers saluted at me in basic training when

we wore those huge overalls," Polly chuckled.

What a night! All of us gals were chosen to dance over and over because the gorgeous soldiers outnumbered the nurses. Later, as we walked back to the barracks under the starry night sky, everyone felt popular and acted like they were in love with one soldier or another.

"I wanted to keep dancing with the tall one. I think his name was Sammy, but it was hard for me to find him again," Hazel said.

Hilary gushed, "I liked the boy who put the 33s on the phonograph, but he was so busy he never did ask me to dance."

"Did you hear that Lena Horne will come to the base to sing to the troops next weekend?" I asked all my nurses.

"Oh gosh, I hope she sings 'Stormy Weather'! That's my favorite," Emily said.

"When she sings the verse *'keeps rainin' all the time'*..." Betty sang it out, "...it makes my romantic heart flutter."

The nurses were overcome by the quality of Betty's voice and asked her to sing the entire song, which she did, and added gestures and swayed gracefully even though she was a bit on the heavy side.

"Betty, what a terrific voice you have! Sing us another one!" I said to keep the jolly mood alive.

Clara rang out, "I'll sing with you. 'Boys Take the A Train' by the Delta Rhythm Boys—it's about Harlem, my town."

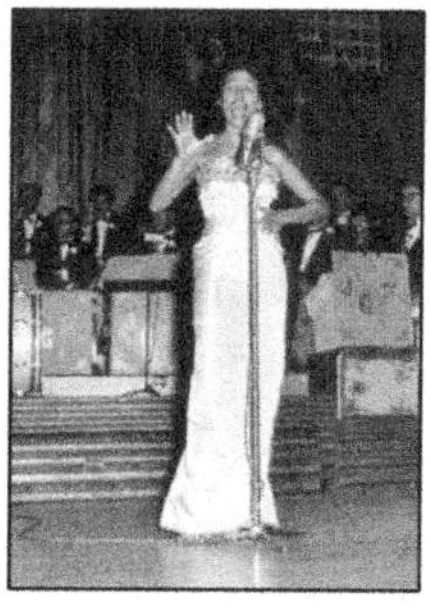

The following Saturday, Lena Horne came to perform. This time it was in the White officers' club because it had more room. We borrowed lipsticks and perfume from those who had some, then marched over to the shared auditorium. The White personnel sat in the front, and we sat in the back with our Negro soldiers.

The highlight of the evening was when Lena floated down the aisle to our Negro section and sang "Stormy Weather" just for us.

On the walk back to our barracks that night, Clara announced what all the nurses felt, "I think I've died and gone to heaven!"

It was our last week of work at the hospital, and everyone was anxious to receive the assignment to travel overseas.

Sgt. McDonald handed me an envelope and let out a raucous laugh. "Good luck!"

I opened the letter in private. It read that our assignment was Camp Florence…Arizona! Not an overseas assignment as expected. I decided not to tell my nurses until I talked to Dr. Walker.

The next day at the hospital, I spotted him as he made his rounds. "Hi, Dr. Walker. Have you ever heard of Camp Florence?"

The doctor replied, "Yes, I have. Why do you ask?"

"My group is transferring there."

"That's unfortunate, Chief. It's a POW assignment."

"What's that mean?" I tucked some of my wiry curls into my cap.

"POW stands for prisoners of war. Camp Florence is one of many camps where captured Germans are sent to work for free until the war is over."

"Me oh my! Germans are brought all the way from Europe to the United States?"

He nodded. "That's right. From what I heard, the US recently agreed to take 50,000 captured German and Italian prisoners from Britain because they had a housing shortage after the Blitz. We have POW camps in almost every state.

White nurses have POW assignments as well. Each time the quota gets raised to accept Negro nurses, they are sent to the POW camps and the White nurses are swapped out, then sent to Europe."

"Nursing the enemy is hard for me to believe."

"It has to do with the Geneva Convention of 1929, which states that after an enemy is captured, they are required to work for the Allies until the war is over. The prisoners are used for cheap, unskilled labor like building military installations for the Allies. And even farmwork."

"Dr. Walker, what duties do you think our nurses will have at Camp Florence?"

"You'll be needed there to care for the prisoners because, in exchange for free labor, the captives must be given any necessary medical treatment."

I frowned. "I'm sure my gals won't like that."

Dr. Walker chuckled. "You're in the Army now, and like it or not, I'm sure you know that when ordered, you go where you're needed."

I frowned. "It will be hard to explain all this to my nurses without a big upset. Everyone had counted on an overseas assignment."

Dr. Walker sympathized. "Just tell them Camp Florence is a temporary assignment until an overseas position becomes available, which is probably true. I'm waiting for a new position myself. Also, the Army Nurse Corps still has strict quotas as to how many Negroes are allowed to join. I know for a fact that the Army has not permitted Negro nurses for overseas assignments yet because there are not many all-Negro hospitals there."

"Thanks, Doctor, for all your help," I said, somewhat dejected and thinking about how I would break this news to my nurses.

Dr. Walker said, "Good luck, Chief."

Later in the barracks, I took a deep breath and waved the

envelope. "Look gals, I got our new assignment."

They gathered around me like bees on the lookout for their hive.

I opened it and read, "Camp Florence, Florence, Arizona."

A groan spread throughout the group.

"I guess we're not going overseas *yet*." I emphasized the word *yet* and tried to move the conversation in a positive direction.

Hilary initiated the first complaint. "I don't want to stay in this humid state any longer."

Lorna agreed and added, "It's too damn hot here."

With a deep breath, I blurted out the last vital piece of information. "Girls, Camp Florence is a prisoner-of-war camp, and we will be caring for German prisoners."

Further outrage ensued.

I took another deep breath and explained the Geneva Convention, then said, "Girls, we have no choice. We're in the Army now and that means we are required to obey orders." I was thankful for the talk I'd had with Dr. Walker earlier that day.

Polly said in her upbeat voice, "Camp Florence might be in a better part of Arizona. It might be fun there."

The next week we packed our meager bags and said our farewells to our patients. It was a two-hour train ride to Camp Florence. All we saw out the window was desert, desert, and more desert set against the distant mountains. The landscape was dry and desolate with no green foliage in sight. Polly was wrong. Camp Florence was indeed *not* in a better part of Arizona, and seemed to be in an even more remote area of the desert.

When we arrived, we saw three rows of barbed-wire fences that surrounded the entire camp. White military guards with vicious-looking dogs safe-guarded the compound. The nurses' emotions ranged from fright to anger.

A short time later, we entered the hospital, where we

found a cheerful-sounding bunch of White nurses who were happy to be leaving for the Philippines. We were their replacements. Before she left, the chief of staff showed us to our own individual rooms. Each had lamps and tables, and had been previously set up for the White nurses. This was far better than the rustic, crowded barracks at Fort Huachuca!

I asked her how many prisoners were housed there. She said over a thousand. My eyes bulged.

She added, "Don't worry, very few need hospital care. They are a fit group of men." With that, she left to pack.

That morning in the hospital, Major Mahoney, chief of surgery, introduced himself and in a low voice told me, "I want you to know that we have had trouble with the White nurses fraternizing with prisoners who tried to develop flirtatious relationships. I warn you that under no circumstances should your Negro nurses do the same."

I hid my surprise at hearing this information. "It's part of my job to prevent that from happening. And besides, it is illegal for the two races to have a relationship. But of course, any nurse doing so would be automatically discharged from the Army Nurse Corps."

He gave me a small smile, changed the subject, then took me on a tour of the hospital.

"Major Mahoney, my nurses are worried that this is a dangerous assignment, nursing enemy German soldiers. I heard that Nazis consider all non-white people subhuman, and we are the only people of color on this entire base."

"I assure you, Chief, that they are not a threat and work long hours picking cotton on the nearby farms. All German prisoners must sign an honor statement denouncing fascism. Rest assured that if there is any uncooperative prisoner, they would be transferred to Camp Rupert in Idaho. I will make sure a guard or physician is always on the floor with the nurses." Dr. Mahoney shook my hand and left.

We were required to be on duty from 7:00 a.m. to 7:00

p.m.—a 12-hour shift a few days a week with breaks, even when there was no work to do. There were several White physicians and for the most part, they were congenial. Negro physicians were excluded from the POW camps.

The German prisoners wore loose-fitting, button-down cotton jackets and matching pants with "Prisoner of War" printed across the back of the garment in large letters. They were brought in by Army guards if they required medical care. Many of the patients suffered from anxiety attacks, chronic intestinal problems, and malaria from combat overseas. We provided routine physical exams to check for scabies, venereal disease, and hernias. The majority of the Germans were in good health.

One young, baby-faced German who had a cold spoke to me in broken English after I took his temperature. He told me he liked it there and was well fed, and could buy items such as soap and cigarettes with "money" he earned in the form of coupons. The POWs worked as waiters, cooks, and janitors in the hospital, but most worked on the nearby farms.

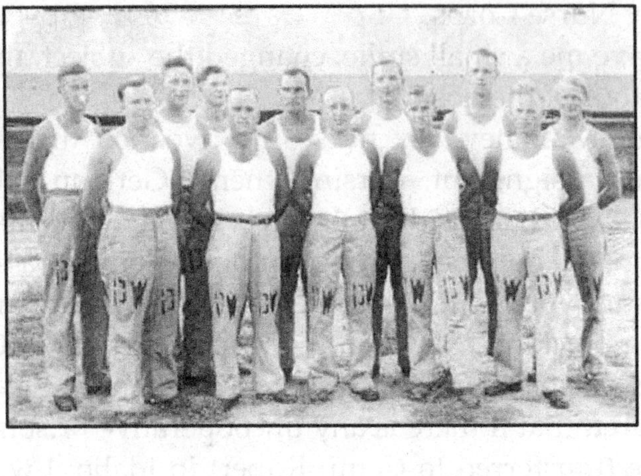

The White physicians had only a few operations to perform, like appendectomies, and played card games most of the time.

On my break one day, I asked Dr. Mahoney, "What's the cotton used for that the prisoners pick?"

"Cotton is a vital resource for us to make uniforms and tires for military vehicles and airplanes," he replied.

"We've noticed that the prisoners' hands are sometimes torn up. Is that from picking cotton?"

"Yes, it's hand-picked and extracted from thorny bushes. In a way, we're very lucky to have the prisoners because of our severe labor shortage. This is important work since our own men are in combat overseas and many women work in factories. These Germans are a tough bunch who bend over in the blazing hot sun and pick thousands of bales all day long."

"I noticed they work in the kitchen too, and the meals here are terrific."

"Everyone here at this base is well fed. Wait until you see Christmas dinner! Have you been to town yet? There's one good restaurant."

"No, but I'd like to go with my assistant on our day off."

"I'd be happy to show you both around."

I smiled. "I'd like that."

On our day off, Dr. Mahoney took Clara and me into town for lunch.

In the jeep on the way, I asked, "What's the tattoo that the men have on their left arms just below the armpit?"

"It identifies the SS Nazi German soldiers' blood type, with the letters either A, B, AB or O." He noticed my frown after I heard "SS Nazi" and said, "Remember, I told you they do have to sign a form that denounces Nazism."

I pressed my lips together and thought about our safety risk there. After all, the Germans were White and we were NOT!

The small-statured Dr. Mahoney parked his jeep near the mom-and-pop café in the one-street town of Florence. Clara towered over him as she stood beside him on the sidewalk.

A moment later, Clara whispered to me, "Chief, there's a

sign."

I noticed the "Whites only" sign that perhaps Dr. Mahoney didn't see.

The doctor pulled open the heavy glass door to the café and spoke over the ringing metal bell, "Try the fried chicken. And you'll love their milkshakes."

We walked behind the doctor and were glad we had worn our new nursing uniforms with our caps and capes.

An older couple with sour faces and pinched lips stared at us.

"We don't serve coloreds. Didn't you see the sign?" said the man.

Dr. Mahoney said firmly, "These are my nurses, who would take care of you at the hospital if you became sick."

The old man said, "We can serve you, Doctor, but those colored women will have to go around to the back door to get food to eat elsewhere."

Dr. Mahoney nodded. "Let's go, ladies. This establishment looks dirty anyway."

We followed him out and the three of us stood on the sidewalk in silence. All over town were German POWs who laughed and conversed with the gas station attendants and residents. They all smoked together and seemed to be having a swell time. Two of the prisoners walked by us, went into the café, then sat down and were served by the owner.

At this point, Clara couldn't contain her New York City temper. "This is outrageous! Prisoners with labels on their backs are served a meal and we were refused!"

Dr. Mahoney turned red in the face. He walked back into the café and returned with three bottles of Coca-Cola. "Here's a soda. We should go back to the base now."

As we walked back to the jeep, I noticed another small sign in the hardware store window, "Whites Only." It made my blood boil and I gritted my teeth to prevent my anger.

When we got back to the hospital, I thanked the doctor,

who mumbled, "I'm sorry it didn't work out."

Clara opened her mouth and started to say something, but I nudged her to be quiet.

I don't think we'll ever get used to segregation, but we're required to develop a thick skin… I thought.

When the doctor was out of earshot, Clara flew into a rage. "Those enemy prisoners are treated better than us, and we're nurses in the Army! How long do we have to stay at this hospital, Chief? At least at Fort Huachuca we could care for our own kind and have fun in the officers' club."

"I'm not sure how long we'll be assigned here but let's make the best of it. Dr. Mahoney did try his best," I replied.

That night, my nurses asked how our trip to town had gone. Clara blew up again and upset everyone. I tried to put a positive spin on our trip but I was too tired. I also hid the fact that I agreed with Clara.

Polly optimistically said, "At least the White doctors respect us. I come from a small town in Massachusetts with mostly White folks and a few Negro families. There's no segregation there."

"I thought all the states were segregated," Hilary, who was from Mississippi, piped up.

"I didn't even know what segregation was until I wanted to become a nurse and couldn't get into most of the nursing schools. I had to attend the private all-Negro Lincoln School for Nurses in the Bronx," Alma from Maine added.

Most of my nurses felt betrayed by this second-rate assignment to care for captured enemy soldiers instead of our own wounded men. And I didn't blame them.

Months crawled by with nothing to do for entertainment, and going into town was not an option. There were only a few emergency surgeries. Our full potential was not utilized. I was surprised that many of the German prisoners were not fascist bigots as I had expected, and were friendlier than the White guards. Plus, they showed gratitude for our care.

One afternoon, I made an announcement to the gals. "Nurses, I've decided to write a letter to Mabel Staupers, who is the executive director of the National Association of Colored Graduate Nurses, to tell her about our situation, and that we were promised an overseas position and were unaware that we'd have to treat German prisoners of war."

Some of the nurses were grateful for this gesture, but conversation ensued about the fact that there was not enough to do.

The next day, Emily from the Midwest mentioned that she had seen horses in the camp and wondered whether we could ride them. I told her I didn't know how to ride. But we had a day off together and I agreed to at least go with her and look at them. I followed her to the stables.

Emily approached the soldier in charge of the horses. "Hi Harry, how are you today? This is my boss, Chief Dottie. Do you think we could ride two of the horses?"

Harry seemed to know Emily and brushed his blond bangs aside with his hand. "Sure, I'll saddle them up for you gals."

I looked at the long, tall animals. It was my first time being that close to a horse. "I'll just watch…" I said with apprehension.

Harry helped Emily into the saddle and she lit up with glee as she rode down one of the trails.

He waved to her, then turned to me. "Here's an apple, Chief. Give it to the brown one. Her name is Chestnut."

The muscular horse towered over me as I stood next to her. I felt quite small. I held the apple up and the horse gobbled it, then whinnied softly. I was surprised by how much fun it was to feed the horse once I got over my initial fear.

Harry asked, "Have you ever ridden before?"

"No, I'm from Atlanta. I've only seen a horse once."

"I'll help you up on Chestnut. She's a gentle mare. Just sit on her and enjoy the scenery. I'll hold the reins."

Harry was right and I felt grand as I sat in the saddle. I watched a black-and-white butterfly flitter about as he led Chestnut around the stable area.

Emily galloped back to the stables and asked me to go with her on another trail, but I politely declined. We thanked Harry and left.

The next week, Emily got Clara to ride with her. Clara was a fast learner and as they rode down the trail together, I stayed behind and fed the horses. The horses turned out to be a good social outlet for our nurses and I was grateful to Emily, who helped alleviate some of the boredom since we couldn't go into town.

At work in the hospital the next day, I checked a German patient's bandages after his hernia operation, when, out of the corner of my eye, I saw Emily and the German cook go into one of the three operating rooms that was not used often. I gasped, then clamped my mouth closed. *I will have to have a talk with her about this when I get off duty. We sure have too much free time here,* I thought.

That evening after dinner, I took Emily aside and told her what I had seen. She denied it at first, but then admitted it.

"Emily, not only could you be court-martialed with a dishonorable discharge for mixing with someone who is not your race, but you could get pregnant! What were you doing in there?"

She fiddled with her hands and glanced down at the floor.

I said as I tapped my skirt, "Did you use a condom?"

She said nothing for a moment, then pleaded, "But…he loves me."

I sighed. "Emily, he probably doesn't. Do you want to get

kicked out of the Corps?" My face burned.

She answered, "I don't think so."

"Go to your room and stay there, and think about everything I just told you."

I looked in on Emily the first day, but she wouldn't talk to me. The nurses asked me what was wrong with her. I used the opportunity to talk to everyone about flirting with the prisoners and reluctantly added to use condoms and where they were kept. I ended the conversation with, "Pregnancy in the Army Nurse Corps would mean an immediate dishonorable discharge."

Two guards caught the cook when he tried to sneak into Emily's room the next night. They pulled him out of the room and beat him up. Some of the nurses woke up and looked out into the hallway. They watched the guards hold him down and shave off his hair to mark his shame.

The following month, Emily knocked on my door and between sobs, told me she was pregnant but the cook did not want to marry her. Not that that would have been possible, anyway.

"You know, Emily, it's against the law to marry a man who is not your race…don't you?"

She let loose a flood of tears, then returned to her room without a word.

The next day after much contemplation, I went to see Emily. "Emily, have you written to your mother about this?"

Emily sobbed with shame. "I did. My mother's a very religious person. In a letter she said that he most likely did not love me and was probably using me to get a permanent visa in this country. She also wrote that the sooner I admitted this, the sooner I could come home, and she would help me take care of the baby. My daddy's furious."

I consulted with Dr. Mahoney, and a few days later, the nurses watched sadly as he drove the poor girl to the train station.

I announced to them, "Let this be a lesson to all of you. I've noticed a lot of flirting going on with the prisoners and I want it stopped. We're here to work, and we certainly don't need another pregnancy."

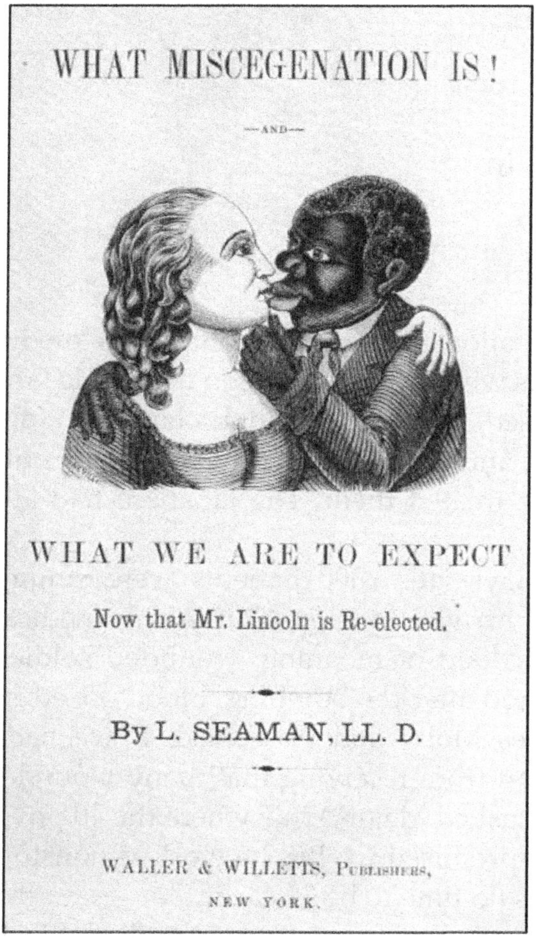

WHAT MISCEGENATION IS!

—AND—

WHAT WE ARE TO EXPECT

Now that Mr. Lincoln is Re-elected.

By L. SEAMAN, LL. D.

WALLER & WILLETTS, Publishers,

NEW YORK.

Chapter Nine
Bea
Limay 1942

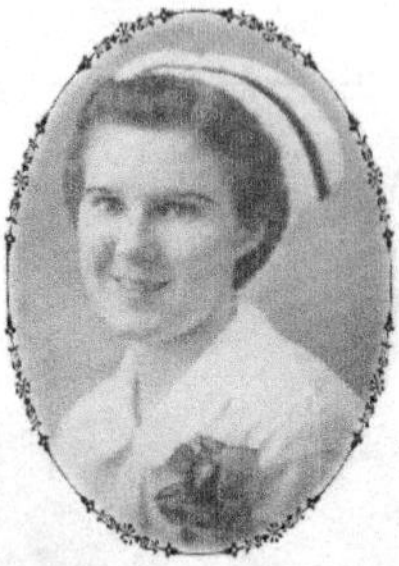

Our "vacation" ended abruptly when medics drove in patients who were in battles in the jungle far from where we were based. Soldiers in foxholes had been found hungry, dehydrated, and bleeding out. The men cried out for food or water as we treated them. The Japanese had attacked once again.

A few days later, 300 patients were smuggled out of Manila and arrived by ship. Our Army medical corpsmen carried in a flood of moaning, wounded soldiers who had been neglected after the bombing. Blood oozed from most of the casualties Molly and I assessed. If we hadn't been so overwhelmed from receiving that many wounded at once, I would have asked Major Arnie where the 40 physicians were that he had promised us. But he worked nonstop in surgery and this was no time to be sarcastic.

"Here we go again, just like in Manila," I sighed. "Molly and Jane, please help me triage all these patients."

Our two physicians wore baker's hats since there were no surgical hats in the warehouse to be found. It would have been hilarious had we not been surrounded by so many wounded soldiers.

Molly worked with Jane and on a clipboard, listed the soldiers by order of severity of their injuries. I went to the operating room and assisted Major Arnie, who held a surgical saw and stood over a patient. For eight and a half hours I assisted him with continuous surgical cases and gained a new respect for the man. He was a powerhouse and never once did he act tired or make a mistake. Dr. Charlie held up just as well.

I took a quick break when Annie came to relieve me. I went to chow and ate a few pieces of chicken, then elevated and rubbed my legs, which were swollen from standing for so long. I had just leaned back against the wall and was starting to nod off, thinking I should find bigger boots and more socks, when in walked the promised 40 physicians in well-pressed uniforms.

I got up and introduced myself. "We sure are glad to see all of you. Yesterday we received 300 patients all at once from Manila."

Dr. Harry Wilson said, "That's why we were sent here. Where's Major Goldstein?"

"I'll take you to the hospital," I said with a song in my voice, happy that relief had finally arrived. "Where are you all coming from?"

Dr. Wilson said, "We've been at the Baguio Hospital north of here."

The physicians took over for Major Arnie and Dr. Charlie, who left for some much-needed nourishment and sleep.

Recordkeeping was essential in nursing care, but we couldn't keep on top of it with such a huge influx of patients arriving at the same time. I asked Molly to find a medical corpsman to enter the basic information for each patient, and the available nurses had to fill in the rest.

On January 15, Commanding Officer Colonel James Duckworth, who was housed there, came into the surgery hut. He stood over 6'2" tall and with a stern jaw and piercing eyes, announced to Major Goldstein in a booming voice,

"General MacArthur has sent thousands of American and Filipino troops, plus hundreds of planes, to Bataan. The soldiers have been told to never retreat and fight every attack. I expect your hospital to be ready for any casualties."

Major Arnie didn't look up. "Yes, sir," he answered. He did not salute because he was in the middle of surgery.

After the colonel left, Major Arnie finished up with his patient, then went to visit the ward. "Get prepared for more patients to arrive," he told us. "Our honeymoon's over. Everyone roll up your sleeves and continue working."

I thought we already had more than enough patients but kept it to myself.

Two days later, we heard American bombers flying overhead, followed by Japanese aircraft that dropped leaflets all over the hospital area outside.

On a break, I picked one up. It read, *Roosevelt is your enemy!*

The medics went to the front lines with litters to bring back more casualties. Ten more patients arrived that day. Eight were wounded and two needed surgeries. One of the patients informed me that the Japanese were bludgeoning the American and Filipino troops that tried to escape from Manila into Bataan.

We couldn't hear or see the battlefield because we were over 13 miles away. But we knew the fighting was fierce when hundreds of wounded soldiers streamed into the hospital by ambulance, truck, bus, car, and on horses and by mule trains. Within a few hours, our "new" hospital received an additional 200 casualties. Flights of bombers appeared overhead. Most of the nurses stood for long hours and assisted any surgeon who needed help.

On a brief break, Molly said, "I thought Sternberg was horrendous battlefield nursing. That was a baby compared to this."

Weary-eyed, I mumbled, "That's for sure."

The dirt floors in the wards were soon covered with

wounded on litters. Many of the soldiers had massive wounds that seeped all over everything as the patients waited to be put on the table for surgery. The surgery tables were occupied 24 hours a day. On one day alone, the operating teams performed 182 major surgeries—the most recorded so far.

As we worked through the chaos and the piercing sounds of the planes overhead, out of the corner of my eye, I looked at the operating table next to me. Nurse Annie kept dashing outside for a minute, then would come back in. Each time she did this, Dr. Willis gave me a stern stare. When I was able to leave the surgery hut for a second to find her, I heard retching sounds and saw her throwing up behind a nearby bush.

"What's wrong, Annie?" I asked with concern.

"It's the airplane noise," she said, wiping her mouth with her sleeve. "It upsets my stomach. Even when I was in Manila, I threw up when I was sick with worry about my Frank."

"Go take a break and find one of the nurses on the ward to replace you," I instructed.

Annie squared her shoulders. "No, Chief, I'm needed here."

She washed up and returned to assist Dr. Willis. I admired her for trying to be such a dedicated nurse.

In the days that followed, we lost all sense of time. The operating tables became an assembly line and we took breaks only when sheer exhaustion forced us to. Two of our doctors set up a receiving station outside, where ambulances loaded with sick and wounded patients stopped first. They took care of minor casualties, like jagged flesh wounds, amputations of fingers and toes, or facial lacerations. With this many casualties, we had to be inventive because we ran out of supplies. We even had to use small tin cans for drinking cups.

As more enemy planes flew overhead, I thought about the bedsheets on the roof of the hospital and in the middle of the compound with the Red Cross symbol on them, and prayed that the Japanese would not bomb us.

The roar of low-flying planes rattled our tin-roofed hospital. All the assisting medical personnel at the operating tables ducked under them and held their gloved hands above their heads to avoid contamination.

When the noise of the planes stopped, Major Arnie boomed out, "Everyone keep it together! We have lives to save and for God's sake, stop crawling under the tables or we'll never get any work done!"

I was amazed to watch him perform surgery. With the noise of bombs dropping above us, not one muscle would tighten on his forehead. But under his mask, I heard him nervously popping his chewing gum.

I overheard a soldier with a partially severed arm say to Susie, "Fix my buddy first. He needs help more than me. Besides, I'm getting ready to go back to the battlelines."

After I heard that, I told the nurses that they were not to release any patients until they were well, with no exceptions.

At one point, I saw Susie standing frozen in front of two patients trying to decide how to triage them.

I ordered, "Just wrap up the one with the severed arm, and for God's sake, don't let him leave! Then wash up the other man to ascertain how severe his wounds are."

Young Sonny was next in line to have his leg amputated. I gave him a shot of morphine to subdue the pain.

He spoke in a sugary-sweet Texan drawl. "I have a swell girl back home and we've been planning on getting hitched when I get back there. Will she still want me with one leg?" He chewed his nails and waited for my answer.

I rubbed his shoulders until he stopped fiddling with his fingernails. "Sonny, I'm sure she'll marry you and will be proud of you for serving our country and sacrificing your leg. Of course, you'll get married."

Medic Bobby placed him on the operating table and I administered the ether. He asked, "Chief Bea, do you really think she'll marry him?"

I shrugged. "I don't know, but I do know the poor boy needs all the encouragement he can get."

Our job as battlefield nurses was an endless one of changing dressings. Some bandages were stuck onto raw flesh from blood and pus, which acted like glue. I gave several nurses the job of giving morphine shots to ease the pain of the patients while they waited for surgery. The chaos of trauma nursing made our minds numb and we worked in an almost automated state, like robots. Like any good nurse, we did whatever we could to get a patient stabilized. The remarkable spirit of our soldiers kept us working with very few breaks.

Between procedures, Major Goldstein hollered at me, "Chief, we need clean operating gowns!" He put another piece of gum into his mouth.

He exhausted me but I reminded myself of his valuable skills as a surgeon and how he kept track of all the physicians while he operated. I hurried into the utility room and saw haphazard mountains of dirty operating gowns and sheets stained with blood and feces.

"Ronnie, get in here—fast!" I called to one of the medics, frustrated to see the mess. "I need you and another medic to sterilize all of this. We're running out of sheets and gowns. You must stay on top of this!"

With a sheepish face, he mumbled, "Yes, ma'am."

I knew I had lost my composure and needed either food or sleep. Or both. Later, after a much-needed rest, I went back to apologize to Ronnie for yelling at him.

He flashed me the sweetest smile. "Don't worry, Chief Bea, I understand. The doctors scream at us all the time."

Major Goldstein stopped after he finished with a patient and attempted to organize the chaos in the hospital. His deep, powerful voice blasted over the noise of the operating room. "You take this brain case, Dr. Smith. Dr. Willis, remove the bullet near this one's spine." He turned to me and ordered,

"Chief, we have only two nurses trained to anesthetize. I need you to train more of the nurses to do this. The wounded are piling up!"

"Yes, Doctor," I said. I rushed outside and found Molly returning from a break. "Molly, who do you think is capable of administering chloroform or ether?"

"Our nurses aren't trained for anesthesia," Molly said. Her voice cracked with stress.

"I know that. But we both know which nurses could learn how to do it. I learned from Sternberg before we were moved." I squinted and looked up through the trees at the sound of planes flying overhead. "We have no choice, just look at our burgeoning population of patients!" I said with a tinge of panic in my voice.

"Yes, Chief, you're right. Caroline and Agnes can learn fast." She listed a few others and spoke in a soothing voice to calm me down. She then rounded up Agnes and Caroline and I hoped for the best.

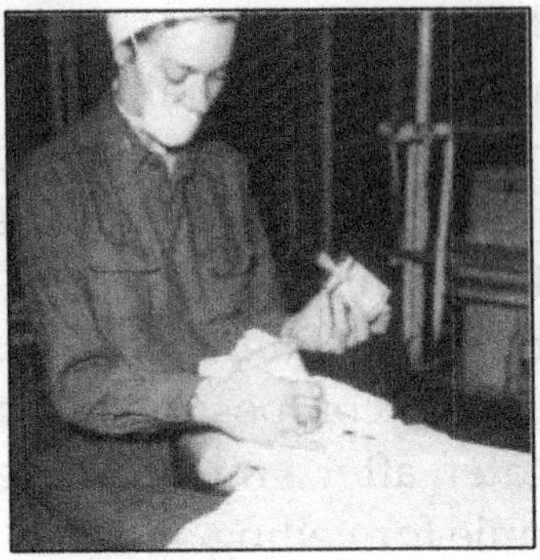

As the days and nights melted together, we all slept and ate at a minimum. Because of the inadequate number of physicians—even with the addition of 40 new doctors—and the mounting number of casualties, our nursing abilities were forced to expand. We diagnosed tropical diseases, gave intravenous injections, and administered medication all without the consultation of a physician. We had more medical corpsmen than nurses, and the medics took over many of the nurses' jobs when necessary, like administering blood transfusions.

When I watched Major Arnie, I was astonished by his incredible talent not only as a surgeon but as a commanding director of the surgeons. The major could be gruff and mean but seemed to balance those qualities with an unusual sense of humor. Plus, he was the king of multitasking and was admired by everyone.

Amid a flurry of activity, Major Arnie focused his eyes on a soldier and yelled, "Who unwrapped this massive bandage on a dead patient, for Christ's sake? Davy, take him out of here. Bury him!"

Davy hurried to get an unoccupied stretcher and took the poor man out to bury him in the base cemetery.

Medic Tom brought Major Arnie the next patient, who was a Filipino soldier with a gaping hole in his face from a machine-gun burst.

Major Arnie shook his head and rolled his eyes. "We don't do jaw wounds. Send him to the dentist over there, damn it to hell!" He moved over to Dr. Andrews' table. "That patient's pulse is too fast. You'll kill him if you operate now. Give him some blood and let him rest, then he'll snap out of it." In a blur, he moved to another table and began sewing up a leg wound. He glanced over at Dr. Smith's patient and barked, "Quit stalling, Doc! Are you going to take off his arm or leave it on?"

With his leg stitched, the patient was removed and replaced by a man with an abdominal wound and intestinal perforation. Major Arnie looked at the patient and shouted out in his thundering voice, "Nurses, for Christ's sake! Inspect everyone first before you bring them to me. If they have worms, get rid of as many as you can before you put them on the table. This wounded man has roundworms as large as earthworms!"

I walked over to the operating table to look at the patient. Indeed, a huge number of worms crawled out of his intestinal perforation and spilled onto the table. "Oh, my!" I yelped, then clamped my mouth shut.

Dr. Charlie said for all to hear, "Look at those goddamn worms crawling out of his gut. Makes me wish I was fishin' in the Tallahatchie at home!"

Major Arnie exploded with laughter and gave Dr. Charlie a thumbs up. His laugh was contagious and a few of the nurses giggled as well. If we hadn't been inundated with patients, it would have been an uproarious joke.

Nurse Agnes, who had a stomach as strong as steel, attended to the patient with the worms and cleaned him up while Major Arnie moved to another table to sew up the next soldier.

Dr. McCarthy—a young, green physician—stood staring at the dead patient on his table.

Major Arnie looked over at him. "Why didn't you stop his bleeding? I saw you fumbling."

Dr. McCarthy tightened his lips and mumbled, "I couldn't find the bleeding vessel."

Major Arnie swore. "You couldn't find the goddamn bleeding vessel? I knew it! You killed him. Get the hell out of here and get something to eat and some sleep before you kill someone else."

Nurse Agnes motioned to him that his abdominal patient was ready. Major Arnie moved back to his table and yelled, "Davy, we got another one for you! Get this dead body out of here, we need the table."

Dr. McCarthy slunk out of the room. A short time later, Dr. Charlie relieved Major Arnie for a break.

Flights of Japanese bombers flew closer over the hospital. Our own anti-aircraft guns opened fire on them, and shell fragments fell all around our area. Our first attack was a bomb that landed outside the nurses' quarters. Glass windows blew out, shrapnel hit the walls, and dust spun around like little tornadoes. I heard the sharp whistle of a second bomb. This one threw me and several patients to the floor. We heard explosion after explosion and saw flames all around us. Thank God the wards were missed, but other buildings that had cars and trucks in front of them were on fire. I worried...would the hospital and wards be next?

On my break outside with Molly, we saw several of our P-40s as they zoomed back and forth high above the treetops. They opened their machine guns against the Japanese planes, and it was a hot and heavy fight with our boys shooting several enemy planes down.

Molly smiled. "Chief Bea, maybe there's hope that our side is winning and the war will be over soon."

I shook my head. "Perhaps... We'd better go back inside. It's dangerous out here."

As we dashed back into the safe cover of the hospital, we heard a full force of airplanes flying overhead, followed by the booming sound of the big guns. The battle zone was getting closer.

The nurses had their own battle to deal with—malaria. We lived in a thickly vegetated jungle surrounded by malarial swamps. Several of our nurses came down with the disease and many of the soldiers came in suffering from it. If not treated, a patient could easily die. The fevers, chills, headaches, nausea, and vomiting kept the sick nurses from performing their jobs and the soldiers from fighting. Both the soldiers and nurses were difficult to keep in bed. I put Carmelita in charge of dispensing Atabrine every day as prophylaxis for every medical corpsman, nurse, and physician.

One morning, Veronica came to me with a complaint. "Chief, look at me…I'm turning bright yellow!"

I glanced at her face and rolled up her sleeves to check her arms. It was true. "What do you think caused it?" I asked, perplexed.

A tear fell down her cheek. "I think it's the Atabrine. Ever since we had to start taking one every day, I became yellower and yellower. Chief, I can't look like this! I used to be a beauty queen!"

"I'm sorry, Veronica. It seems to be a side effect of the drug."

"Well, I refuse to take it any longer," she pouted.

"You only have to take it until the war's over, which will be soon," I lied.

After Veronica left, I flagged down a few of the nurses and found a variety of yellow-pigmented skin. The nurses who were the whitest showed more color from the drug. Carmelita, whose skin was a darker shade, had the least. I took Carmelita aside and told her to make sure that each nurse took the Atabrine, and to inform me of anyone who refused. I felt thankful we had no mirrors.

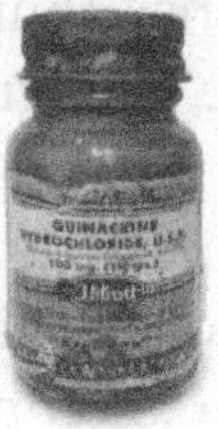

We had two fatal cases of a cerebral type of malaria in patients who were brought to the hospital in a convulsed, unconscious state. Quinine had to be given intravenously but nothing seemed to help.

Major Arnie and Dr. Charlie screened off an area in the woods where they could perform autopsies to learn more about the disease. One day, Ernesto, a curious Filipino patient, wandered out there to see what the new structure was. He saw a patient on a table under a sheet, and lifted a corner to see a body with an exposed abdominal cavity. He ran out of there howling, with a frightened look on his face. After that incident, I had Davy post a sign in the area that read *Danger! Keep Out!*

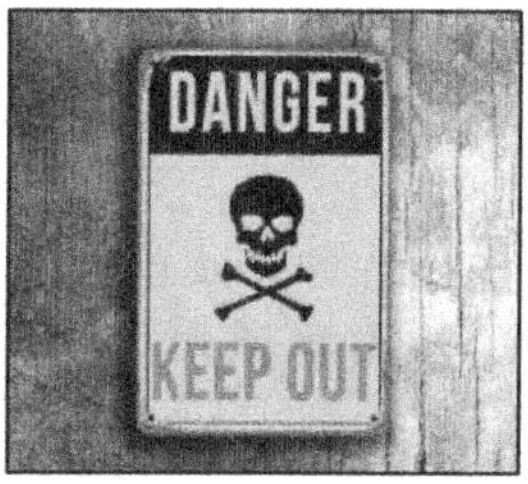

Our environment was full of chaos as the medical personnel tried to stay organized. In the operating room, hours burned into days, and eyes blurred and stung from the constant stress under the harsh operating-room spotlights. The overflow of wounded soldiers had to be left on litters outside in the jungle. Most didn't cry out or yell—they just quietly gritted their teeth in pain while they waited.

The respirations of soldiers with chest wounds ranged from gasping to strangled. The moans and screams were heartbreaking for the nurses. Thank goodness for the shots of morphine.

I assisted Dr. Frank in the operating room frequently. He was a seasoned surgeon with gray sideburns that poked out from under his baker's hat.

Dr. Frank examined a patient with a blown-up leg, then ordered, "We can't save this leg. Chief Bea, put him under so I can amputate it."

Medic Bobby interrupted, "But Doc, he's just 17! He'll be a cripple all his life!"

I sympathized. "Let's put the leg in traction. Maybe it'll heal."

"Look, both of you, his bone is crushed to hell. Get the saw," the doctor demanded, not especially thrilled about our medical suggestions.

After that sad, stressful case was over, the next patient was lifted onto the table.

Dr. Frank examined his head wound. "His skull is as thick as a gorilla's. I wish we had electric drills. Jesus, my hands are tired." He took the hand drill and did the best he could.

One of our favorite patients, Billy, was just 18 years old. Both of his arms had been amputated. Nonetheless, he was such a cheerful fellow that even the ambulatory patients loved to visit him.

One afternoon, I stopped by to see him. "How are you today, Billy?"

He answered like he always did. "I'm fine, thank you. And how are you?"

One patient gave him a radio. Nurse Annie checked in on him every day because we couldn't tell by his cheerful disposition alone whether he felt better or not. Billy was skilled at diverting attention away from himself. No one could pity him; he wouldn't stand for it. When Pastor Miller read to him every day, his face lit up with joy.

Billy brought much joy to everyone's lives—both nurses and patients alike— and we were grateful to have him in our care.

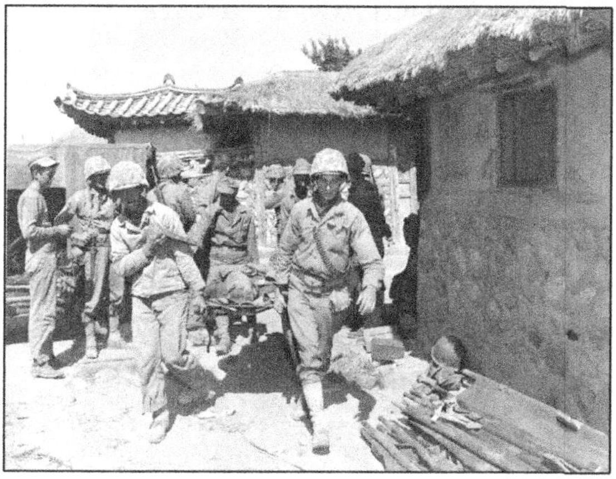

Medical corpsmen

Poem by Alfred Weinstein, M.D.

A surgeon on Limay and Little Baguio

The zzz-zzz-zzz of a saw as it cut through bone…the plop of an amputated leg dropping into a bucket, the grinding of a rounded burr eating its way through a skull, the tap, tap, tap of a mallet on a chisel gouging out shell fragments…the hiss of the sterilizer blowing off steam, the soft patter of the nurses' feet scurrying back and forth, the snip of scissors cutting through muscle, the swish of a mop on the floor cleaning up blood…the gasp of soldiers with chest wounds…the snap of rubber gloves on out-stretched hands, the rustle of operating gowns being changed. Rivulets of sweat washed away the nurses' rouge and powder, leaving only lipstick to match the ruby-red blood.

Chapter Ten
Dottie
Camp Florence, Arizona – Liberia
1943

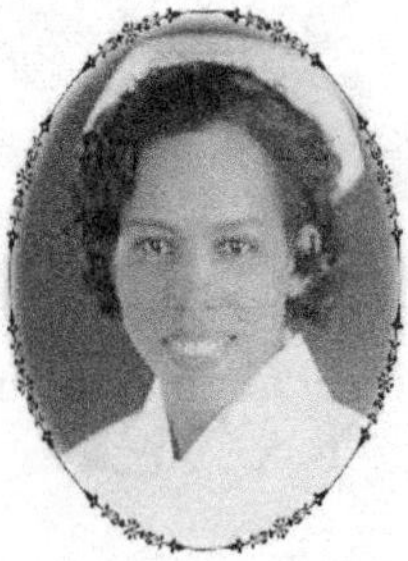

We were at Camp Florence until January 1943, at which time Dr. Maloney gave me a letter from the War Department.

> *By command of Surgeon General James C. Magee, US Army Medical Corps*
> *The quota for Negro nurses has been raised by the War Department. The nurses stationed at Camp Florence will be the first Negro unit to be deployed overseas to Liberia, West Africa to the 25th Station Hospital. Report to Hoboken, New Jersey to take a troop transport ship.*
>
> *War Department*

What an honor it was to be the first Negro unit deployed overseas! I wondered whether perhaps my letter to the National Association of Colored Graduate Nurses had enabled us to receive this promotion.

That night, when I told the nurses we were to be deployed to Liberia, they cheered. I did have to remind them that we were sworn to secrecy and to not tell anyone. This brought on more squeals of delight. We felt truly valued at last. I was as proud as a mother hen with chicks that we had stuck it out at basic training and Camp Florence, and were finally being rewarded by going overseas. There was quite the celebration during the train ride to Hoboken—and there was the bonus of a cruise on the Atlantic Ocean! We were told it would take 30 days to cross the Atlantic to West Africa.

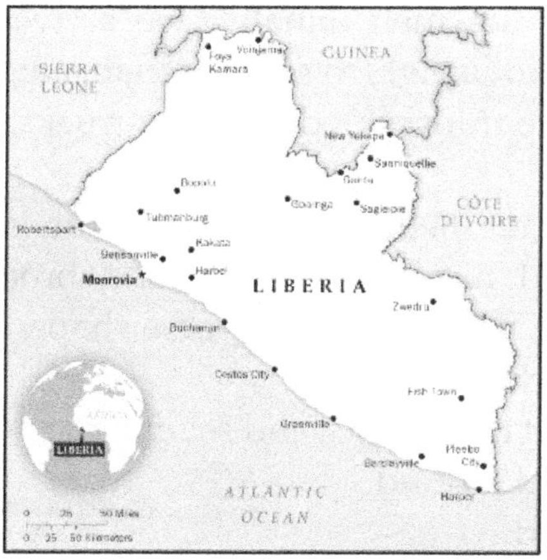

In New Jersey, we boarded an enormous ship that was part of a convoy to West Africa. None of us had ever been on a ship before, and we were honored to be there. The ship's massive size filled the nurses with exhilaration as we congregated on the deck and breathed in the intoxicating smell of salt water while awaiting our departure. Our American flag flew high on the mast and swayed in the breeze. The best part for most of us was that we were the only women on board among hundreds of sailors and soldiers of our color, all dressed in their dapper uniforms.

After a week on the sea, we stopped dead in the water.

Clara asked one of the sailors, "Why have we stopped?"

The sailor whispered to her, "It looks like enemy submarines were detected in the area."

Sure enough, over the loudspeaker a message was relayed: "Everyone is ordered to remain below deck. All crew report to battle stations."

I rounded up my 30 frightened nurses and we all went back to our bunks.

Our ship sat off the coast of Casablanca for a week to wait for the protection of an armed escort so we could move on to Liberia. But none of us minded and most delighted in nonstop flirting with all the men. Finally, we arrived safely at the Freeport of Monrovia, which was the main commercial port in Liberia, and were transported by army trucks to our barracks at Roberts Field.

A short Negro medical corpsman with a cute, crooked smile introduced himself as Larry and brought us to our shabby barracks, which were in worse shape than what we'd had at Fort Huachuca.

Larry showed us our cots, and several rats scurried past our feet as we walked around.

Jane screamed.

Lorna crossed her arms over her skinny frame and yelled, "Yikes!"

Larry scrambled to grab a nearby broom and pushed the rodents out the door. "If you gals see any more, just beat them with a broom and sweep them outside."

I grimaced.

My gaze was drawn toward the rafters after I heard a scratching noise. Everyone looked up to see two big, short-necked creatures with small heads and long tails crawling from one rafter to another on four legs.

My eyes widened. "What are those…and are they dangerous?" I pointed above me.

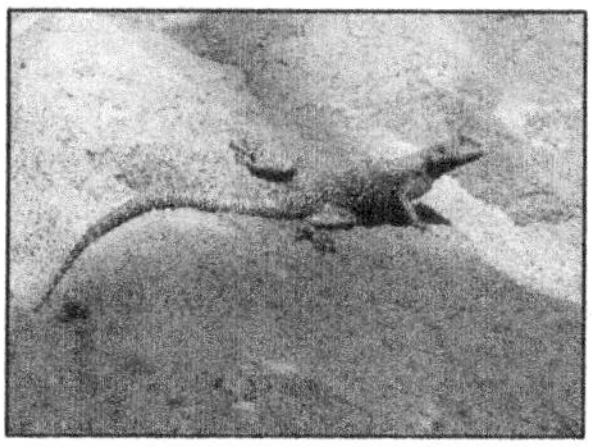

"They're harmless," Larry grinned. "They're called agama or lizards. That red one is called a red-head rock agama. They're from the reptile family."

"We have lizards in Mississippi but not foot-long ones like those. Ours are plain green or brown," Hilary exclaimed.

"Welcome to the tropics," Larry smirked. "We have a lot of colorful creatures here."

"That bright-blue-and-red one is adorable." Prudence batted her eyelashes at Larry.

"Excuse me, medic. Where's the bathroom?" I interrupted to break up the flirtation.

He led us all to the latrine, which was quite a distance from the barracks.

"Make sure you always go in pairs at night when it's dark. You never know what creatures you might encounter. Here, I'll leave a flashlight for you." Before we could look inside the latrine, he said in a hurry, "I've got to get back to the base," and left.

I opened the rough wooden door to the small building. The smell overpowered us and frail Lorna ran and threw up behind a tree. Inside the latrine was a wooden bench with five holes cut into it. This place was ungodly primitive. Beyond the airfield, I saw a dense tropical forest where more creatures most likely lurked.

The next day, another medic dropped by standard nursing uniforms along with helmets and gas masks. We also wore armbands with the Red Cross symbol on them, which indicated that we did not carry weapons.

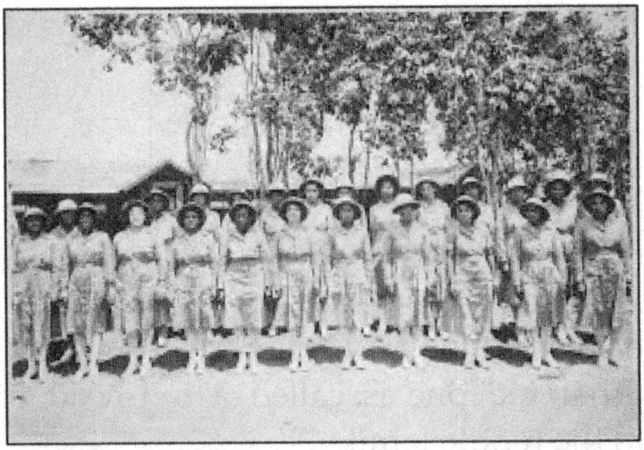

The work at the 25th Station Hospital consisted of taking care of the U.S. Negro soldiers from a nearby base who were there to protect strategic airfields and valuable American Firestone rubber plantations. We were to provide medical care for American and Royal Air Force troops and a substantial number of native Liberians. The hospital consisted of eight barracks—one surgical, one psychiatric, and other medical buildings. There were only White physicians, just like at Grady.

Our nurses took care of both Negro and White patients with ease and proved that integration was possible. After all, patients, regardless of color, were people who needed our medical attention. There were over 20 Negro medical corpsmen who cared for the patient population plus a few who stood around with nothing to do.

As weeks went by, we found living there to be a crude existence. One day after work, we returned to our barracks and heard a strange sound when Clara opened the door. Clara and I peered inside and saw that a monkey had joined the agamas. It swung from rafter to rafter and made a loud hooting noise. The nurses refused to go inside, so I sent Clara to find one of the medics to get it out.

Medic Larry came to help. "I wonder how it got inside?" He looked around and saw that one of the windows was open, then took a broom, climbed onto one of the beds, and swatted the noisy monkey out the open door. "Better keep the windows shut, ladies," he said before he left.

Many of the patients were quite ill from malaria, and we treated them with Atabrine tablets. I caught up with one of the four White doctors on the staff, Dr. Martin, and asked him why malaria was so rampant in this country.

Dr. Martin answered, "It's the damn mosquitoes. They bite and attack everyone, then spread parasites within the body."

"I'm worried about my nurses getting it," I frowned.

Dr. Martin said, "Keep the mosquito netting over the beds at night and wear clothes that keep you covered, and long-brimmed hats."

"But we have to wear nursing uniforms that expose our legs, even with white stockings on."

He nodded. "That could be a problem. Make sure your nurses take Atabrine every day. It's an excellent prophylaxis."

"We've been taking Atabrine, but the nurses don't like the side effects of the pill, like the headaches, nausea, and diarrhea."

"Well, we all must deal with that. See Corpsman Willie, and he'll show you where you can get more pills." He left and continued with his rounds.

Medic Willie was an E-7 level medical corpsman who oversaw all the medics. He did an excellent job and had a corny sense of humor. After he showed me where additional Atabrine was located, he spontaneously asked, "Why did the monkey fall out of the tree?"

I played along with him. "I can't imagine. Why?"

"Because it was dead."

I smiled and gave him a false little laugh.

The food was horrible and we missed Camp Florence's flavorful, abundant meals. The cooks at our new place only made food that came out of cans. On top of that, the month of May began the monsoon season. This was quite a shock after enduring the dry Arizona desert. We were given small men's raincoats, which were still huge on most of us. Handy Hazel showed us that we could cut them to size, then hand hem them up. The mosquito netting was helpful and kept the insects off us for the most part.

I overheard Jane asking Corpsmen Willie when the rain would end. When he answered November, she said, "Oh no, that's terrible! We have leaks in our barracks!"

Willie avoided the problem. "I've gotta check on Allen to see if he still has a fever," he mumbled.

That night, all the nurses joined in and complained about the rain that dripped from the leaky roof and onto our beds. I was beside myself with worry about our living situation and didn't know what to do except sing "You are my Sunshine." Betty and I made a duet out of the song, and soon the others joined in. We got through the night and endured the misery of the climate.

The next day, I obtained extra raincoats to put over our beds to keep them dry during the day, and at night they were useful to shield us from the drips from the roof.

As the first month crept by, I realized we were overstaffed for the hospital's minimal workload. The medics did a terrific job caring for the patients but adding nurses to the equation made for too many caregivers. Our nurses had too much free time—which would have been nice had there been anything to do. There were no officers' clubs or recreational activities of any kind. So, we were left to play various card games for entertainment.

Sometimes we were called to work at the clinic in a nearby native village, which was home to over 15 indigenous tribes of people. The official language of Liberia was English, which made it easy to talk to and care for most of the natives. We enjoyed their brightly colored, patterned fabrics. The women wore long wrap skirts called *lappas* and loose tops called *bubas*. Their head wraps were also multicolored. The men wore long pants and long, loose, colorful shirts with white head wraps. The tribes' clothing made for a beautiful visual experience for all of us to enjoy.

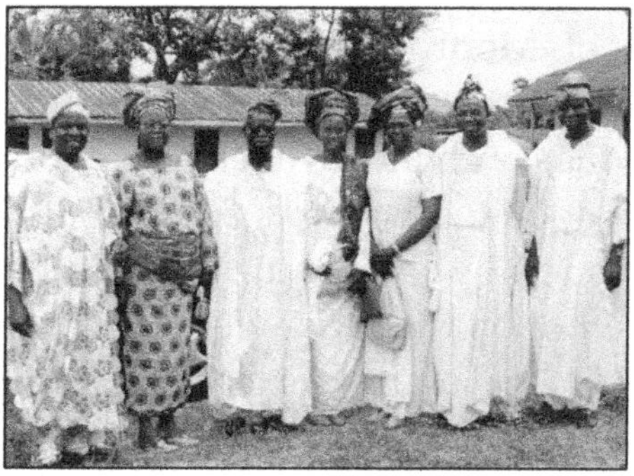

When the weather was good, a few of us hitched a ride with a soldier in a jeep to the port city of Monrovia on the Atlantic Coast. To get there, we traveled 30 miles through the Firestone Rubber plantation.

Sergeant Kingman, who had a deep, intellectual voice, told us about the 65-foot-tall rubber trees as we passed by row after row. "Tappers milk the trees for their sap by collecting what comes out in small metal buckets. See that milky white liquid dripping into the container on that tree?" He pointed. "It's called latex. That's what natural rubber is made from."

We looked up toward the sky at the tree's leaves, which grew only at the very top.

"The trunk of the tree is a soft wood, which makes it easy to tap."

"Tell me, Sergeant, what is the rubber used for?" I inquired.

"Mostly tires for all the U.S. Army vehicles and aircraft, plus, of course, rubber bands and pencil erasers."

We observed the many natives putting taps in the trees as the jeep whizzed by.

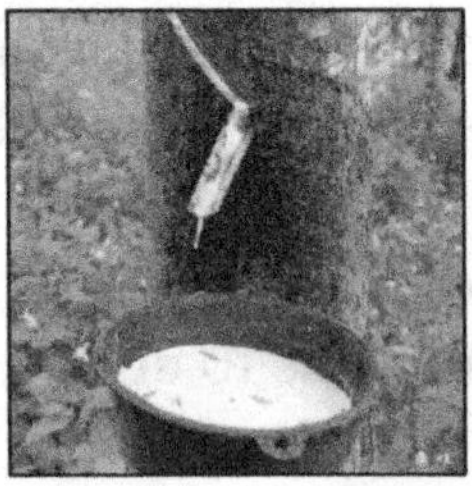

At the port of Monrovia, the open-air markets were a colorful, visual feast for our eyes, with exotic carvings and painted ritual masks plus artifacts in ebony, mahogany, camwood, sapwood, soapstone, and natural hardstone. The city was surrounded by the beautiful, dark-green rainforest. We walked barefoot on the sand, waded into the crystal-clear sea, and watched the abundant sea creatures. Beyond the shore, the ocean was speckled with native wooden fishing boats.

The nurses found the city a much-needed escape, but because it was the wettest capital of the world, we were not able to venture there often. Sergeant Kingman told us the city could get over 18 feet of rain a year, which turned the dirt roads into mud. And the floods after the fierce rainstorms made the city impassable.

The next week, we were invited to lunch by the U.S. Ambassador to Liberia, Lester Walton, who was appointed by President Roosevelt. The nurses listened attentively to stories about the ambassador's accomplishments, which included negotiating the terms of Roberts Field airbase and helping Liberia build a market for its rubber exports. We all sat around a grand table inside an elaborately decorated dining room that had artifacts displayed on the wall, and were served tea by a native staff.

The ambassador was a clean-shaven man in a handsome tailored suit who spoke in an animated voice. "Would you ladies like to know the interesting history of Liberia?"

I spoke up, "I'm sure we would." I took a sip of the flavorful exotic tea.

"Liberia became a free and independent African republic in 1847, the first of its kind. Between the years of 1853 and 1903, hundreds of Negroes left America to come here to start a better life. It was a haven for freed slaves from the United States and the British West Indies."

Nurse Hilary interrupted, "Why did our people move this far if they were free?"

The ambassador answered, his enchanted brown eyes sparkling. "Most of the emigrants departed for Liberia during the uncertainty of the post-Civil War years, especially from the South. Although slavery was abolished, the Negroes were still poor and discriminated against, and moved to escape the tortures of the Ku Klux Klan, plus many of the other hardships they had to endure. They were promised greater opportunities for prosperity here."

Prudence piped in, "My mother had relatives who left the United States at that time. She said they did not get equal treatment as expected after the Civil War. I'm from Alabama and I heard they moved entire large families here."

The ambassador continued, "Yes, that's true. The American Colonization Society, which was publicly funded by White Americans, was the primary sponsor of the Liberian emigration movement. They used it as an opportunity to spread Christianity throughout Africa. Its capital, Monrovia, was named in honor of President James Monroe, who had procured U.S. government money for the project."

Ambassador Walton asked if we would like to go outside and see how *dumboy*, the national dish of Liberia, was made. There was an enthusiastic response from the nurses, and we all followed the ambassador outside to an area behind his residence.

We watched the native cook pound a white substance with a mortar and pestle. The ambassador pointed to a pile of potato-like vegetables. "Those cassavas are a root vegetable that has a nutty flavor. The cassavas are washed, then peeled like a potato, then grated and pounded by a pestle in a mortar for over 15 minutes until they turn into a pliable dough."

He continued, "Many different stews and soups can vary the dumboy recipe, like using goat, beef, chicken, or fish."

We watched the strenuous process and listened to the thump of the pestle until the substance turned into a bright-white mound of dough. The cook kneaded the dough into balls and put them into a large serving bowl.

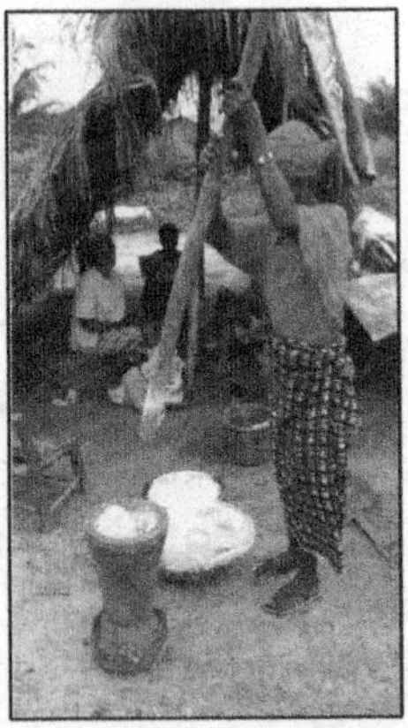

We all headed back into the house and the cook brought in the serving bowl. At each place setting was a soup bowl in which the servant placed a ball of dumboy, then poured Liberian pepper soup with codfish, lobster, and shrimp over top of it. Mr. Walton told us to cut up the dumboy with our soup spoons, then spoon up pieces of it along with the soup.

I enjoyed the flavorful, hearty, steamy fish stew mixed with the dumboy. Betty gobbled up hers in a flash and politely asked for another bowlful.

Chapter Eleven
Bea
Limay – Baguio 1942

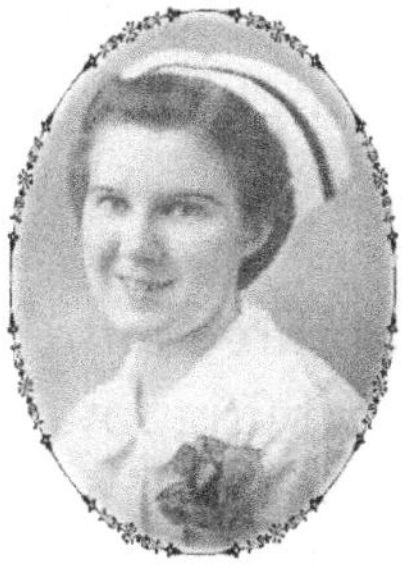

I jerked upright in my bed when I heard the warning bell ring. It was two in the morning and a medic announced over the loudspeakers, "Gas attack! Gas attack! Everyone out!"

We all scrambled to put our gas masks on, then ran outside and stood together in the dark, looking around the compound. The Japanese had huge supplies of gas bombs. Would they use them on us?

While we stood there in the moonlight, we heard liquid splattering on the ground. A closer look revealed that it was coming from the physicians' barracks. There was Major Goldstein, naked in the light of the full moon with his gas mask on, urinating out the open window. Everyone roared with muffled laughter. After a few moments, it was announced that this had been a practice drill and we were allowed to go back inside.

We had been in Limay for a month, but it felt more like a year. Food was limited since it could only be delivered when the bombing had ceased, and oftentimes we worked while hungry. The heavy fighting continued. Some of the patients ate their meals under their beds when they heard bombs dropping all around us. Our two chaplains, Pastor Miller and Father Garcia, quit giving sermons on Sundays due to the incessant bombing but continued to administer last rites.

We lost patients with dysentery, malaria, and battle casualties at an alarming rate. We treated over a thousand patients, with a quarter of them forced to wait for medical care on stretchers in the jungle. We all kept our World War I gas masks on our belts in case the Japanese used gas to try to knock us all out.

Early one morning at three a.m., we were awakened by one of our P-40 airplanes flying low overhead. It circled and crashed nearby. Two medics ran out to find it and search for survivors but returned with long, dejected faces.

"Burnt to a crisp," one of the medics said with tear-filled eyes.

The Japanese did not honor our big Red Cross hospital insignia as we had expected. Later that day, a 50-caliber bullet went through an empty bed on the ward. As it hit extremely high decibel levels, it made a few of the nurses cover their ears with their hands. One patient went outside to go to the latrine and narrowly missed getting killed by shrapnel. He came back weeping with body shakes. Shell fragments rained down everywhere. When a fragment pierced the foot of one of our already wounded soldiers, my face beaded with sweat and I squeezed my clammy hands together, fearing the worst as I thought, *Will the nurses be next?*

I glanced at a few of my nurses. They stood motionless, with blank faces, obviously in shock. Several medics rushed into the ward with more wounded patients who helplessly moaned in agonizing pain. I forced myself to snap into action as Davy pointed out each case.

In a trembling voice, he said, "The mess hall got completely showered with shells. This cook caught an unexploded shell in his chest, and that Filipino kitchen worker got hit in the skull and—"

I interrupted him with orders. "Davy, most of these men need to be taken to the operating room. Get them out of here. Leave us only the minor wounds and have your medics take the rest to the surgeons, for God's sake." I turned to my nurses. "Girls, come over here and start cleaning the wounds. Molly, help me ascertain which patients need to go to the operating room."

One afternoon, the dogfighting outside became quite loud and we could hardly hear each other in the operating room.

Major Arnie commanded, "Strap all the patients down, then everyone out! Find a foxhole and stay in it until the fighting stops!"

The nurses had to obey orders but dragged their feet and looked back at their patients with somber faces, then left to find foxholes in the cover of the jungle.

I did the same and soon found myself lying in a grave-like hole in the ground, covered in dirt and jungle debris. The sharp, high-pitched whizzing noise of a bomb zoomed over my head. Oh my god, it sounded so close! I scrambled to arrange jungle foliage and branches around my foxhole for camouflage from the enemy while I waited for the bombing to end. I needed to get back inside to help the wounded.

At the end of January 1942, our hospital commander came into the surgery room. "Major Goldstein, the Japanese are approaching. You have two days to evacuate this hospital and move to Baguio. It's safer there. I'll send transportation. Pack up the patients and leave."

After the commander left, Major Arnie barked out orders for everyone. I was amazed by how he seemed to take everything in stride. But I protested as my gaze bounced from bed to bed. We had over a thousand patients to pack up.

"We've only been here for six weeks and now we must leave a good working hospital?"

Major Arnie stared at me. "Let me put it to you this way, Chief." He counted on his fingers. "One, how can we do our jobs from foxholes? Two, the Nips are on their way here and *will* take us to their prison camps and leave all the patients to die." His fiery eyes bore into mine.

"Where is the Baguio Hospital?" I asked in a whisper, hoping to calm the volatile situation.

"It's several hours from here to Baguio on the island of Luzon—two acres in a mountainous area that will afford better protection from the enemy. Now, for God's sake, start packing up the patients!"

God Almighty, here we go again. This will be the second move since Sternberg. It's a good thing we'll move with our patients this time, I thought as the enormity of the task began to sink in.

The front lines were now closer. We could hear tanks rumbling by, troops on the march, and persistent rifle shots and exploding bombs. Amid the cacophony of war, the medics and nurses helped the surgeons apply protective plaster casts and ambulatory splints to replace traction for the patients who needed it. This made them transportable. The serious casualties were given morphine shots so they could endure the rough ride to the hospital. Stripped-out buses transported the patients, and we loaded them as fast as we could, trying not to traumatize them further.

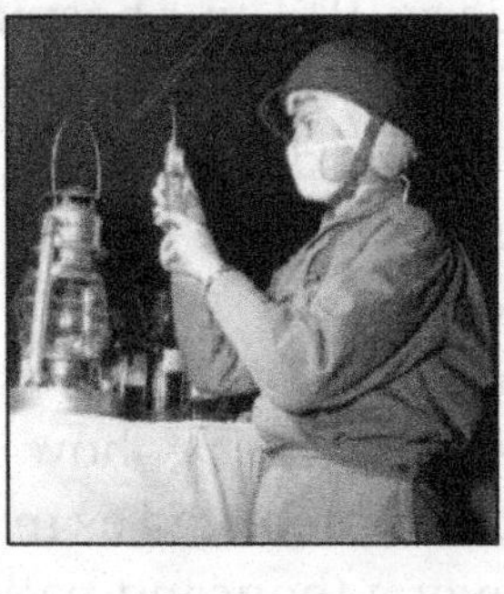

When drivers came back for more patients, the nurses barraged them with questions.

"Can you tell me how the little Filipino soldier, Juan, did? He was the one with a large abdominal wound," Angelica inquired of one driver.

"What about our blind soldier, Carlos, did he do all right?" Caroline pleaded, peering over Angelica's shoulder hopefully.

The driver gripped his steering wheel in silence.

I frowned. "Could you please just tell us if anyone dies during transport? We won't bother you anymore if you can do that."

"I'll try," he said and sped off up the rough road with another full load of patients.

I was proud of my nurses and how they handled the stress. We were all frightened and worried about ourselves and our patients. Between loads of patients, the gals boxed up all the medicine, surgical instruments, and bandages, and stacked them outside to be loaded onto trucks. That night, after the last of the patients had been transported, we saw flashes of gunfire in the distance and heard the grind of tanks close by. We collected our meager belongings and headed to our trucks, and wondered how close the fighting would be in Luzon.

As we passed by the hospital cemetery, the nurses waved goodbye to the 64 white crosses as we bounced into the jungle high in the mountains. The overhanging branches of mango, papaya, banana, and hardwood trees scraped the roof of our truck as the driver sped along the dirt road. We drove past pine forests and inhaled the fresh, heady smell. We sped past bamboo shacks and heard the sound of rushing water from a mountain stream that flowed between two inactive volcanos. It would have been a beautiful ride if there hadn't been a war going on around us.

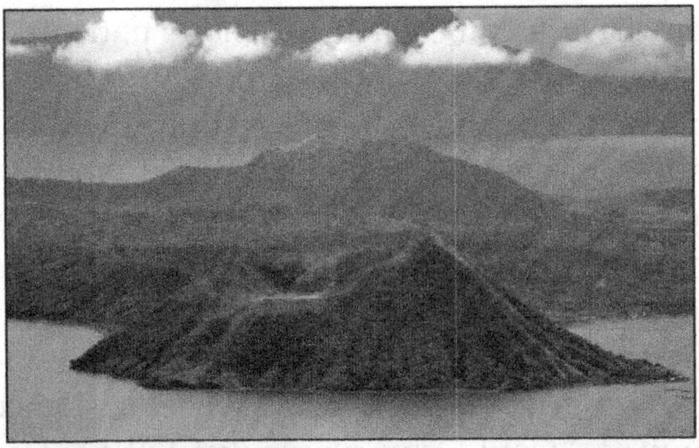

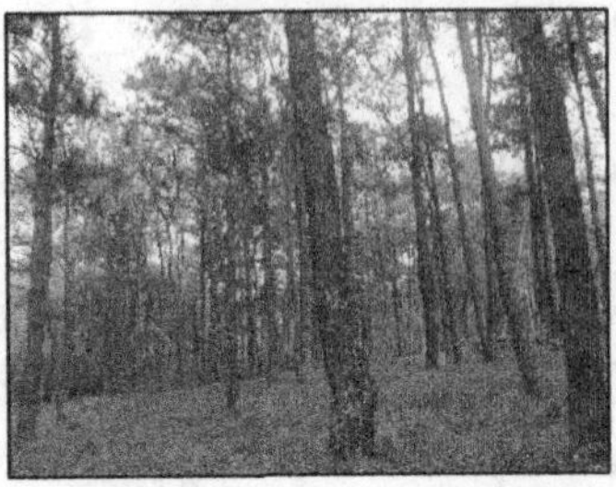

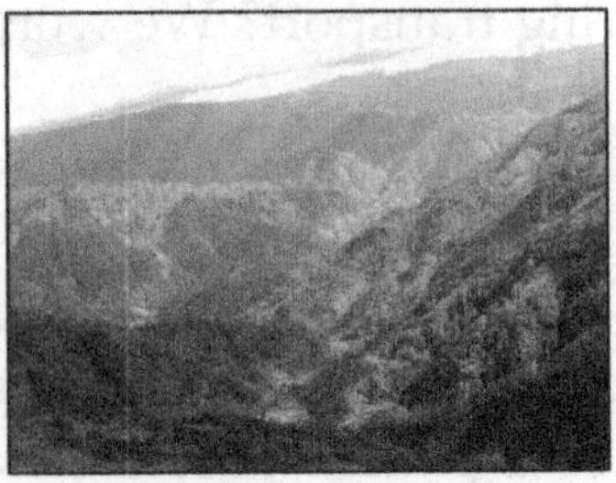

The trip felt like an eternity. The nurses fretted over the state of our patients and what the hospital would be like.

When we finally arrived, our favorite medic, Davy, greeted us. "Welcome to Baguio in the province of Luzon. I'll show you to your barracks."

The barracks had the same rough exterior as our barracks in Limay. Before Davy opened the door, he saw my wrinkled brow and grinned. I pressed my lips together and held my breath, wondering what sort of mess we would be walking into this time. But, as the door opened, a smile of relief replaced my frown.

"There's electricity and plumbing…and a bamboo floor!" I enthused.

Molly flopped down onto one of the many made-up beds and the other nurses put their bags down and stretched out.

I said to the nurses, "After you unpack, half of you need to go to the hospital ward."

They nodded in silent agreement as I left with Davy for a tour of the two-acre compound.

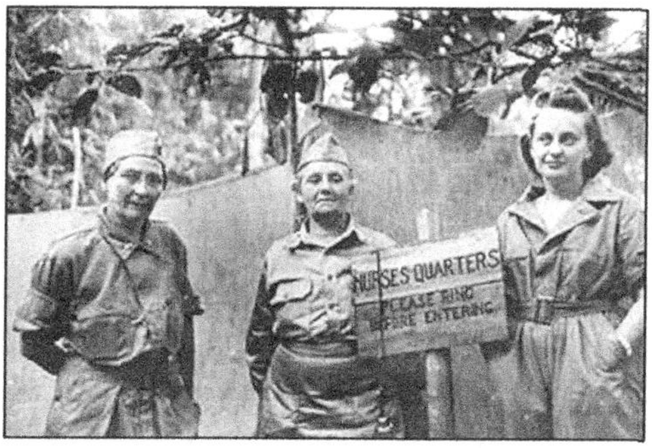

"Nurses Quarters. Please ring before entering."

"Chief, you'll be pleased to know that all the buildings are finished and clean!" Davy's grin was contagious, and I flashed him a big smile back.

"Who finished them?" I asked, astonished.

"While we were in Limay, the Army officers and medics planned for the possibility of retreating here and constructed a workable compound."

"Did this used to be a scout training camp, like in Limay?"

"No. Before the war, it was used to serve the Philippine Army motor pool and was a motor-repair shop for troops on maneuvers. The garages, repair shops, and barracks have all been converted into buildings needed for a hospital."

I followed Davy to the surgery building and admired the working water faucets and decent electricity. I greeted the surgeons and medics, who helped settle in our patients.

"I'm sure my nurses will be delighted to work in a finished hospital," I said happily as I took it all in. The thought of another site to scrub and haul supplies to was not something I wanted to put them through ever again. "I'd better get back to my patients. Thanks for the tour, Davy."

Back in the ward, I could see that the nurses were doing a

fine job settling the patients into their new beds. We left for chow and the medics took over. I poked my head into an old garage shed that was now a kitchen. The mess attendants were retired Filipino Scouts. The stove they used was a crude sort of affair that was placed over a hole, where wood burned for heat. The cooks served us rice and various canned goods on tin plates, which we carried to outdoor picnic tables under large acacia trees.

"Remember the fried chicken?" Annie said as she shoved rice into her mouth and drank tea from a tin cup.

"I loved that chicken. But can you remember what you used to eat at home for Christmas dinner?" Jane asked.

The conversation spurred everyone to reminisce about their culinary pleasures back home. Ice cream, candy, and oven-roasted turkey were the hot topics. It was a comfort to be hidden far away from the noise of the battlefield in Baguio. We could enjoy the jungle sounds of the tropical birds and hooting monkeys instead of the terrifying whistles and piercing explosions from the bombs. I hadn't heard one airplane fly over, which put a broad smile on my face.

Dr. Charlie came by and sat down with Molly and me.

"Hi, Doc," I greeted. "It's beautiful here surrounded by these luscious green mountains, and it's so peaceful with no bombs or airplanes flying over us."

Dr. Charlie nodded. "The best part is that the mountain breeze prevents the malaria mosquitoes."

I commented, "That's a bonus!"

Molly leaned closer to Dr. Charlie. "It is really beautiful here…" she said.

On our way back to work, we saw Major Arnie, who asked, "How do you gals like our new place?"

Molly spoke right up. "I feel safe here in the mountains and am grateful for the move."

"We got out of there just in time. Lieutenant General Wainwright informed me that the Nips obliterated our entire site in Limay. We'll have a break in the war now before the next wave of the battle and can get organized before the Japs wake up from their naps!" He chuckled.

"Obliterated? Thank the Good Lord we all got out of there,"' I said, amazed, and thinking what a close call that was.

The nurses were in high spirits during our first week on the ward. Nurse Carmelita had the idea to have recovering patients who could not sit up or get out of bed fold gauze. This kept the soldiers occupied until we could release them to return to the front line.

Maria came up to me while I checked to make sure all the records were in order, and said, "Chief Bea, I have an idea. There is a lot of gauze to fold. Can I organize a contest to see who can fold the most?"

"That's a terrific idea. Thanks, Maria."

Maria's contest got all the gauze folded, then she collected used cardboard to make playing cards and puzzles. This clever idea helped the soldiers pass the time and got them through their convalescent period with less worry about hurrying back and helping their troops in battle.

Our two chaplains followed Maria's example and saved old magazines to give to their patients to keep them occupied. A few of the almost-recovered Filipino soldiers were quite clever and carved pipes, cigarette holders, decorative flowers, and vases, all from bamboo. Manuel gave me a charming, intricately carved flower, which I treasured and put on my bedside table.

The positive attitudes of our convalescing boys made our nursing job a delight. Pastor Miller and Father Garcia read to the patients with eye injuries, distributed cigarettes, and conducted uplifting sermons on Sundays. In the outside chapel were boards laid across wooden sawhorses, which could seat about 75 people. Clever Manuel fashioned carved communion cups out of bamboo and made wooden vases to put his handcrafted flowers in.

We had many pet monkeys outside the ward. A group of nurses on break would put canned peas in their palms and the monkeys would pick them off one at a time and pop them into their mouths.

Molly laughed until there were tears in her eyes. "That one's cute with its adorable eyes and long tail. Let's name him Curious George!"

"Who's that?" asked Imelda.

Molly told our Filipina nurses about *Curious George*, a children's book about a monkey's funny antics.

"This one's aggressive and sneaky. I'll name him Tojo, after Japan's prime minister!" Susie laughed with glee.

Angelica joined in. "That one's Homma, after the Japanese general. He's ugly enough!"

Animals wandered around in the darkness, like wild pigs and lots of small geckos with their suction-cup feet. A large carabao frightened us one night, even though it was a harmless, gentle water buffalo. A short time later, Annie screamed when she was smacked in the face by a bright-green snake that swung down from an acacia tree. I examined her face and she was fine, just shaken. As time went by, we learned to live with the creatures and there was less shrieking heard among the nurses.

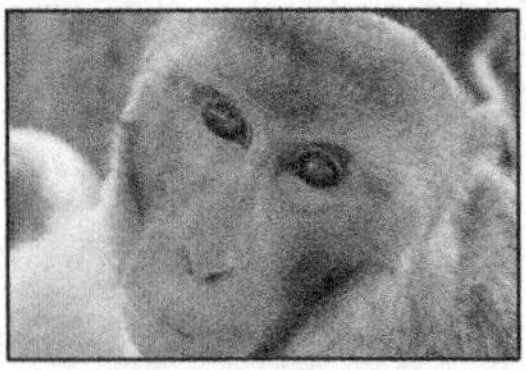
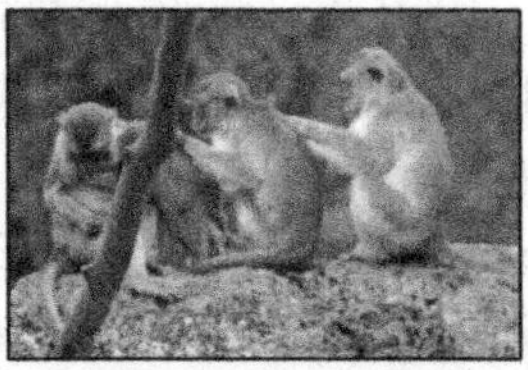

One morning, Medic Davy complained to me, "The ants here are out of hand and are crawling all over the patients."

"I've noticed…but what can we do about it?" I asked.

"I have an idea. What if we put the empty tin cans from the kitchen on the legs of the beds and fill them with water? It might stop the ants from joining the patients in bed for companionship!" Davy chuckled at his own joke.

I laughed. "Great idea. Let's try it."

Several medics helped with the ant-prevention plan, and to everyone's surprise, it was a great success. Davy also got some of the medics to paint Red Cross flags on every rooftop in the entire compound with the slight hope of preventing the Japanese from attacking us. I knew it didn't help at the Limay hospital but if it made the medics and nurses feel more secure, it was important to do.

In March 1942, a young pregnant Filipina woman was picked up on the road while fleeing Limay. A truck driver brought her to the ward and grumbled, "This is no time to have a baby, in the middle of a war, for God's sake. You'd better keep her!" He rushed back to his truck.

The baby-faced mother was ready to pop. Her breasts swelled through her thin pink slip. As I helped her into a bed, she said in broken English, "My baby soon want to leave me."

I found Angelica to help with the labor and birth. She was the most knowledgeable in these matters, and had assisted her mother in delivering her siblings. We palpated the mother's abdomen and knew the birth was imminent as her contractions became stronger, so it was decided to move her to a quiet place on the ward. Angelica told me it was time to get Major Arnie.

The doctor came to her bedside. "The baby is crowning. Angelica, tell her to push."

After a quick, uneventful birth, the umbilical cord was cut and the baby was wrapped in a clean sheet. The proud-as-a-peacock doctor held the babe up as the newborn cried her first breaths of life. When the nurses heard the wail of the infant, they swarmed around the new mother to see the precious miracle.

Major Arnie put the bundle in the mother's arms and said, "You have a lovely girl!"

After the young mother nursed her baby, she gave her to Angelica to be the first to hold the tiny infant. Angelica held the babe in the crook of her arm, rocked her, then kissed her forehead and breathed in the baby's smell. "I love to smell the heavenly scent of a newborn." She put a finger in the baby's tiny hand and the infant gripped it. "She's a strong one!" Angelica gushed.

Major Arnie lingered. "I'd rather deliver a new life than perform an amputation any day." He kissed the infant's cheek, then slowly left.

The nurses took turns holding the baby. The cooing of the new mother was heard throughout the ward. The Filipina nurses got out their sewing kits and made tiny outfits from whatever old clothes they could gather.

The grateful mother refused to name the baby. Angelica translated that it would be up to the nurses to decide. They were delighted and discussed it for an entire day. After a vote, it was decided to name the baby Eleanor, after our president's wife, and for a middle name, Baguio.

Major Arnie let us keep the sweet mother and baby until a native village was found for them to live in. It was a godsend for the nurses to have an infant to play with and fuss over—a much-needed respite from war—and it warmed my heart to see them so happy, for however brief a time.

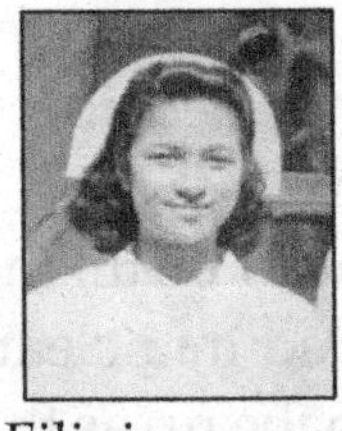

Filipina nurse

Chapter Twelve
Dottie
Liberia – Camp Livingston, Louisiana
1943-1944

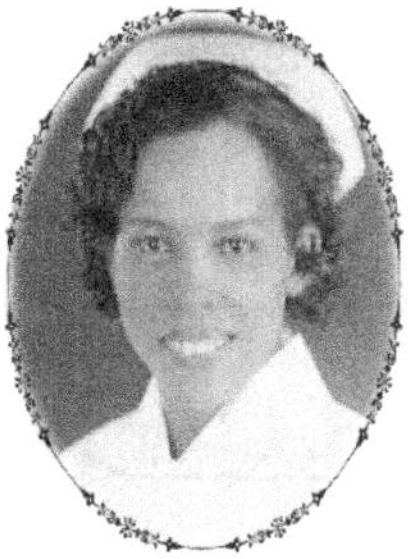

Jane was the first of our nurses to get the dreaded malaria. When I saw her shivering with chills, I took her temperature.

"Jane, it's 105. Do you have any mosquito bites?"

"Of course, we all do." She rose from the bed and almost fell over.

"Stay where you are, you're a patient now," I admonished, and helped her back into bed.

By the end of December, half of our staff fell victim to the parasitic infection despite the use of Atabrine, and they suffered from fevers and chills. Every time one of the nurses came down with the disease, Clara would say, "Those mosquitoes are voracious!"

At night, I heard the constant sound of bites being scratched.

When Dr. Martin came to the hospital with an envelope, I knew what it meant. Sure enough, the letter stated that we were being recalled back to the States due to our staff having malaria. The well nurses were to report to Camp Livingston,

Louisiana. Those who were sick were sent home to recuperate. I worried about my nurses. I knew that if malaria was not treated with bed rest, pulmonary edema—a dangerous accumulation of fluid inside the lungs—could develop, which interfered with breathing and could cause kidney failure.

We had been overseas for just 10 months! I felt like a failure but faced the fact that not only did many of the nurses get sick, but the hospital was also overstaffed and we weren't really needed. The medics did a terrific job taking care of the few patients we had, and would continue to do so without us. Besides, West Africa was not a major scene of fighting in the war.

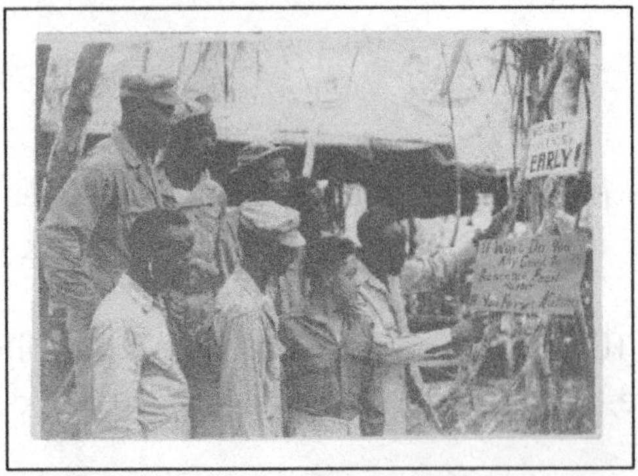

"It Won't Do You Any Good To Remember
Pearl Harbor If You Forget Atabrine"

I asked Dr. Martin in private if he knew about Camp Livingston in Louisiana. He told me, "It's one of those POW camps with Japanese prisoners."

Shocked, I turned away to hide my surprised expression and mumbled, "Thanks."

Back at the barracks, I made the decision not to tell my nurses right away that Camp Livingston was a POW camp. They would not like returning to the States, even though I heard constant complaints about the boredom where we were. I wished we could have been sent to England or France to better help with the war effort.

On the voyage back home, I finally informed the nurses who were assigned to Camp Livingston that it was a POW camp.

Hilary was the first to complain. "I'm *not* going to take care of our enemies again!"

Clara added, "I agree. We put in our time doing that job already. Besides, Louisiana is in the Deep South...and we all know what that means."

I said, "You've heard me say this before. You volunteered to join the Army Nurse Corps, and that means you go wherever they assign you, regardless of your personal feelings."

Lorna exclaimed, "I'm not going! I'll only go where our Negro soldiers need us."

I raised my eyebrows. "OK, then you'll be court-martialed for disobeying orders." I went below deck to my quarters to get some needed rest.

Prudence, one of the sick nurses who would be sent home, continued the conversation the next day. "We should've been sent to England where we could have really helped the war effort. There's no malaria in England and I know for a fact that American White nurses are stationed there."

Clara added, "It was fun going on a ship to a distant country, but we weren't needed. I think we were only sent to Liberia to make a showing that the government was willing to send Negro nurses overseas."

We arrived at Camp Livingston in January 1944. It was another isolated camp and was located on the edge of the Kisatchie National Forest in Louisiana, 12 miles north of Alexandria on a vast expanse of rolling wasteland and bogs.

Most of our 16 nurses were a grumpy bunch with mixed feelings about leaving Liberia. In retrospect, I thought we were being placated by being sent overseas to a country that didn't need our services. Were we a failure in Liberia, and being punished by this assignment to a POW camp once again?

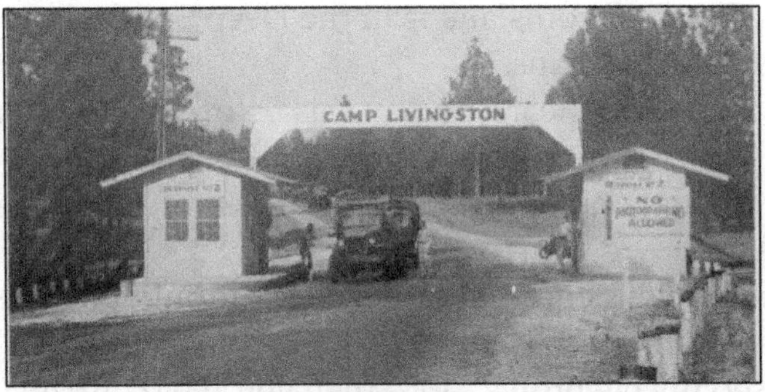

After the nurses settled into the comfortable, leak-free barracks, I left to visit the large hospital to meet the Negro chief of nursing, Ethel Jackson. I introduced myself and shook her hand.

Chief Ethel welcomed me warmly. "Nice to meet you, Chief Dottie. We can use the extra help at our hospital."

I glanced around at the expansive number of patients. "There are a lot of Negro soldiers here…" I observed. "Where are the POWs?"

Chief Jackson answered, "The Japanese American people have been transferred to nearby Camp Claiborne. Your nurses will take care of Negro soldiers only. We have many Negro servicemen stationed at Camp Livingston for infantry training. It is a large base with a population of over 17,000 soldiers."

I was happy to hear that we would not be caring for any POWs. The nurses would be overjoyed to hear that because it might have been a precarious situation dealing with that population.

"What type of cases do you have in the hospital, Chief?"

"We deal with many accidental infantry injuries. Our camp here has a training exercise that involves two imaginary countries that fight each other. The site is known as the Louisiana Maneuvers. Our base is one of the largest training facilities for Negroes."

"What a practical way to train our men to fight overseas. But I can understand why there would be many accidents with this type of training exercise," I remarked.

Chief Ethel's voice became serious. "Chief Dottie, I do need you to know that there has been serious violence here against Negroes and we are not permitted to go into town for recreation anymore."

"What kind of violence?" my eyebrows knitted with worry.

"Louisiana is in the Deep South, as you know, and we do have a large contingency of White soldiers stationed here—in separate facilities, of course. Last year, a group of unarmed Negro soldiers from our camp went to the Ritz Theater and various bars. When they came out, an altercation occurred."

"What happened?" I asked as my eyes widened.

"I heard a variety of stories. One of our soldiers told me that a Negro soldier was accused of approaching a White woman in front of the Ritz Theater. Either a White police officer or a White townsperson accosted him. A riot broke out and over 60 White armed military police were called in to break up the brawl. The police threw gas bombs, and wounded and supposedly killed many Negro soldiers."

"Oh my god, how horrific!"

"It was. I checked 29 of our soldiers into the hospital that day for critical medical treatment. The town newspaper reported that the riot lasted for over three hours and involved 3,000 unarmed Negro soldiers and 60 military police. No deaths were reported. But I heard from the many wounded soldiers who were brought to the hospital that many Negro soldiers were killed. Another rumor, which I think is true, is that the dead soldiers were gathered up by the military police and buried in unmarked graves with no documentation. I think it was an obvious cover-up." She shook her head. "Our soldiers must fight the enemy for our country overseas and at the same time fight the Jim Crow laws while on leave."

"That's for sure. It seems our people try to break down the color lines and the Whites attempt to preserve them."

Chief Ethel sighed. "Well, I wanted to inform you about the incident to make sure your nurses do not go into town on leave."

"I'll make sure they don't. Tell me, Chief, is there a Negro officers' club on base here?"

"No, I'm afraid not."

"That's a shame. We couldn't go into town when we were stationed in Fort Huachuca, but we had a terrific officers' club there. We heard Lena Horne sing."

"You were lucky to have a club. Not many of the segregated camps do."

"It was nice to meet you and I'm looking forward to working with you tomorrow," I said, grateful for Chief Ethel's time.

I went back to the barracks and gave my nurses the lay of the land. Everyone was disappointed that there were no social outlets, but they were all pleased that we would not have to care for any POWs because it was an all-Negro Hospital.

We were stationed at Camp Livingston for quite a few months when Chief Ethel handed me an assignment envelope. I opened it in private and discovered that we would be deployed to Tagap, Burma, in one week. I put the letter back in the envelope, then held my tiny gold cross necklace and said a private prayer that this assignment would be more rewarding than Liberia.

Chapter Thirteen
Bea
Baguio, Philippines 1942

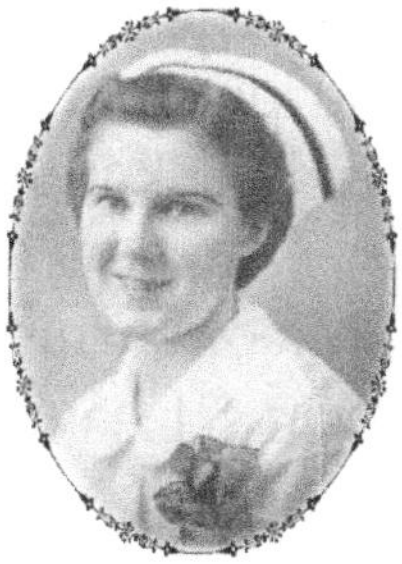

The war had not started back up yet. Major Arnie joked that the Japanese were taking a rest to celebrate their victory. He invited me to join him for a trip into the mountains in his Cadillac. The black exterior was a bit beat up due to Bataan's rough roads, but the interior was a marvelous red leather. My hair, unrestricted by my nurse's cap, flew free as we rode with the convertible top down. The doc was a terrific adventurer, which he had proved already from his food-finding tours. He told me during the ride that he was in search of an ancient tribe.

We became better acquainted with each other on this impromptu trip, and I asked him why he chewed gum all the time.

He laughed. "I had to give up smoking because of a chronic cough, which was disruptive when I performed surgery. Chewing gum was the trick to quit. I buy stacks of gum anywhere I can find it."

I was impressed. "That's a remarkable way to quit."

Major Arnie asked me if I had a beau. I told him about Rob and how he was probably missing in action. He touched my hand gently and told me he was sorry to hear that.

We rounded a sharp turn, and the doctor spun the steering wheel and yelled, "Damn it all to hell, these roads are insane!" He noticed my perturbed face and said, "I didn't say I gave up swearing!"

I chuckled as we continued up the mountain roads, which were not very wide for his large automobile. He swore again when he almost hit a wild pig that ran out into the road in front of us, then scampered back into the forest to avoid the collision.

A short time later, Major Arnie spied a well-defined footpath and parked the car. "I have a feeling this is it!" he enthused.

We got out and followed the path through the forest. Soon the trees thinned out and there, in a clearing, we saw a few doll-like bamboo shacks.

The doctor couldn't contain his excitement and whispered to me, "I think we found it. It's a tiny pygmy settlement. I heard they are a tribe called Negritos or Batas, and that Bataan was named after them."

As we crept to the edge of the clearing, we saw three teeny-tiny gray-haired men who squatted on their heels and wore black-and-red-striped loincloths. They each attached small pieces of limestone to branches to make darts. One stood up and I held my mouth in surprise. He must have been less than four feet tall! We edged closer and spied several tiny women wearing black-and-red woven skirts. They suckled their babies with their miniature, pear-shaped breasts. The dark-skinned children were naked and played with a sparsely furred dog in a coconut grove and bamboo thicket full of huge, vine-covered trees with wide canopies and matted underbrush.

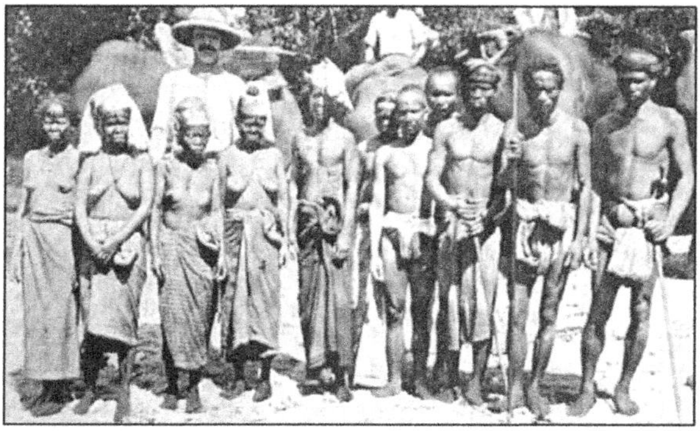

Major Arnie whispered to me, "By golly, aren't we the lucky ones to see this rare tribe!"

He tossed a pack of cigarettes at one of the Negritos. The startled elder emitted a strange wail, then scampered away into a deeper part of the forest. I almost said something but Major Arnie put a finger to his lips. We waited a few minutes, then he tossed another pack. This time, the elders picked up the cigarettes. Doc encouraged me to follow behind him, and together, we walked slowly toward them.

When the children came up to us, Major Arnie handed each one a stick of chewing gum. Soon everyone was chewing gum or smoking cigarettes while they chit-chatted in their native language.

I stood next to Major Arnie. I was much taller than him, and the petite natives stared up at us in awe, scanning our heights like they had seen a ghost. I squatted down, and with a forced smile, tried to make them feel more comfortable with me. One of the elders offered us each a small banana, which I accepted and ate, and found it to be sweeter than the larger ones we were accustomed to.

Another elder spoke one word of English, which was "hello," then showed us his spear and used sign language and noise to explain wild pigs and hunting.

Major Arnie, always ready to bargain, went back to his car and got more cigarettes, gum, and combs, which he traded for coconuts, bananas, and papayas.

I walked hunched over to make myself appear shorter and approached a circle of breastfeeding mothers. I sat down and kept a smile on my face. When they smiled back, I smoothed a baby's head with a finger. They were as small as the premature babies I had seen in incubators back home at Grady.

Major Arnie came over and I got up. It was time to go. We waved farewell to the adorable, petite natives, and they waved back while chewing and smoking their new presents. Doc and I hopped back into the Cadillac and weaved our way back to the hospital, full of delight after our brief getaway.

The break in the war continued. Our patient load held a steady pace, then went down. So, several medics and physicians arranged a swimming party at a cove on the bay that faced Corregidor Island. Half of the nurses went one day and the other half the next. The cooks packed carabao sandwiches for us and made up a delicious tropical fruit drink to take in canteens.

We piled into the hospital trucks and drove to a high bluff. I watched as the group whooped and galloped down the gently sloped beach and dove into the calm blue tropical waters in their underwear. As I sank into the warm sand, I reminisced about viewing the island from the hotel in Manila with Rob. I brushed a tear away from the faded memory.

With the battle at a standstill, romances bloomed. The nurses and medical men flirted, giggled, and teased each other as if we were in the States where there was no war. Dr. Charlie and Molly splashed each other in the water, which made my heart sing but left me with a twinge of jealousy. I missed Rob once again. But I shook my blue mood away. I sat back against a papaya tree and delighted in the sound of cheerful camaraderie. It was a needed calm away from the sound of combat.

When we got back to base, many of the nurses told me

they were in love with medics, and even a few physicians had uttered the forbidden phrase *I love you.* Back in the States, the average man would never say that until quite a lot of time had passed. But we lived in close quarters and the pressure of wartime sped up the romance. Love gained an intensity never experienced during peacetime, born from the desperation of not knowing whether we would die, or worse, be captured by the Japanese. The nurses were giddy and the men were testosterone-driven.

As chief, I listened to my nurses but reminded them how valuable they were to the U.S. Army, and that pregnancy resulted in immediate discharge. After Susie confided in me that Doc Harry told her he loved her, I gave all the nurses a lecture on pregnancy and reminded them that it was illegal for a married woman to be in the U.S. Army. As an afterthought, I also told them where the condoms were located.

Molly had become smitten with Dr. Charlie. I saw them as they sneaked deep into the jungle for trysts. Major Arnie even loaned the lovestruck couple his Cadillac for further private getaways. One night, Molly came into the barracks, starstruck, and told me the doctor had asked her to marry him. I pleaded with her not to consent, but she wouldn't listen to me.

All the nurses were aflutter with the arrangements. The wedding would take place in the chapel. They rounded up whatever hoarded cosmetics were available and curlers with two bobby pins were found. I gave the bride the pretty new hat my mother had sent, and added, "I hope the Army doesn't find out about this or you'll be discharged. And what would I do without you?"

Molly hugged me and kissed my cheek. "Oh, Chief, you worry too much!"

The bride's dress was the biggest concern until one of the officers said he had a parachute he'd found in the jungle.

Malaya was the finest seamstress. She took the parachute from Officer Mac and got the rest of the Filipina seamstresses to work on it.

We all scrubbed up our old nursing uniforms and stained shoes for the wedding. Both chaplains presided over the ceremony, given the fact that Dr. Charlie was Protestant and Molly was Catholic. Dr. Charlie wore his Army medical uniform, which transformed him into Prince Charming. Molly's parachute wedding gown was a beautiful, knockout creation. She looked like a fairytale queen with her strawberry-blond curls adorned by my hat. Many tears of joy streamed down the nurses' faces. And mine as well.

Nurse Annie did not attend the wedding. After the service, I found her crying and gave her a sleeping pill. I thought that maybe later I would see if she would attend church services with me, which might give her more faith to get through the grief of her fiancé dying.

A few days later, I was in the middle of spoon-feeding a soldier carabao stew when I heard a baby crying. I looked up and there was Sgt. Robinson with a three-month-old Filipina baby in his arms.

The broad-shouldered sergeant smiled and brought her to me. "I found this baby in the jungle, wailing." He rocked the babe in his arms, soothing her while I watered down some stew and poured a little down her tiny throat while he held her.

Nurse Annie appeared after hearing the baby's cries. "Can I take a turn feeding the little darling?" she cooed.

"Of course," I said, happy to see her up and about. "I'll get some oatmeal."

When I returned, Annie had taken some spare fatigues

and wrapped the baby in them like a sling. She swayed back and forth, and the baby fell asleep. I put her in charge of keeping her alive and was overjoyed to see the satisfaction it gave her. It was a wonderful distraction for her.

The next day, I checked in on Annie as she fed the baby oatmeal.

"Sweet thing," she said. "I'll care for you. I'm going to call you Angel."

"Make sure you feed her every two hours around the clock," I said.

"My pleasure!" Annie said in a high-pitched voice.

The next week, the poor babe died in Annie's arms. Her tears rolled onto the baby's face as she held the child to her chest. It took a while to coax Annie to give me the child, but she finally did. I handed Angel to the medic at my side, then put my arm around Annie as he quietly took the baby away. Sadly, the loss of the baby caused Annie to revert to the state she had been in after losing her fiancé. Not knowing what else I could do for her, I gave her the last of the luminal pills I had.

That week, one of the medic truck drivers brought us news. "The Japs are on the march again. Get ready for a rush of patients!"

Our soldiers were fighting deep in the heart of the thick jungle, on cliffs, and on beachheads. The medics brought them in haggard, hungry, dehydrated, and bleeding out. They also arrived by mule pack over the mountains. The first words out of most of the wounded, beaten-down soldiers were, "Water," then "Food!"

I questioned an undersized Filipino soldier who had a mortar shell fragment stuck in a compound fracture in his thigh. "How many days has it been since you've had water?"

"I think three days," he managed to say.

"Susie, clean up his thigh, then take him to one of the doctors and tell them this soldier is dehydrated. I'm sure he'll give him an IV."

I got to thinking that with such a constant influx of patients, our nurses should be trained to do this procedure. That way, it would free up the physicians to do their necessary operations. *I'll mention this to Major Arnie,* I thought. *He has taught the nurses how to administer anesthesia successfully. Surely they can learn how to start IVs as well.*

The medics brought in a few captured Japanese POWs that were injured, and a compound outside was made for them surrounded by barbed wire. After a week of fighting, we ended up with a total of 42 Japanese casualties at our hospital. Then, one morning Davy reported that four were missing. Major Arnie and I went to the compound to have a look and sure enough, a hole had been dug under the barbed wire with bare hands. Davy suggested putting secure boards into the ground. Major Arnie told two medics to guard the captives.

As the weeks went by, it was reported that our infantry and tank units were holding and beating back more than 2,000 enemy troops. News spread that perhaps we were winning.

With a slight smile, one of our new patients told me, "Look what I retrieved, nurse." He pulled out a Japanese saber from under his bed. "I was almost stabbed to death with this sword but wrangled it from him and killed him with it."

Agnes said to him, "Hurray for our side!"

Later, I noticed a few patients gathered around a bamboo table and went to see what all the commotion was. Agnes stood next to the table with a grin on her face. I frowned when I saw rubber-rimmed Japanese spectacles, beautiful sabers, tiny Buddha figures, a Japanese flag, watches, and Japanese helmets, among other assorted Japanese paraphernalia.

"What's this all about?" I asked.

"Chief, the soldiers take objects from the Japanese after they wound or kill them to prove their conquest. They are proud that I have collected them and made a trophy table."

"Hmm." My forehead wrinkled. "I don't know what to think about this..."

"Just watch our soldiers while they look at the trophies," Caroline said.

I stood back and watched our patients, who touched each item and boasted about the souvenirs.

Private Jack, who was recovering from a wound, bragged, "I got this diary. Look, it's written in Japanese." He opened it and showed it to the others with a sparkle in his eyes.

Ronald, with a bandage where his arm used to be, added, "I brought in this Japanese food kit and it's got real Jap food in it—tea balls, dried fish, and rice."

After I heard the laughter and fun the trophy table produced, I told Agnes, "It seems to have a healing effect on the men. This is a clever idea. Let's keep it."

She beamed, "All the convalescing soldiers love to stand around this table to admire the trophies and exchange war stories. It provides them comfort to think that they are helping to win the war. Every object means one less Japanese soldier for them to fight."

"Yes," I agreed. "And the laughter and camaraderie will help in their recovery." I patted her shoulder.

I left to check on the Japanese patients in the prisoner compound. My heart beat faster the closer I got and I heard moaning and cries from the wounded. There was not one medic or nurse in there. I glanced around and knew most of the Japanese patients needed to be brought to the operating rooms or given food.

I went to talk with a few of the nurses about the situation.

Annie spoke up first with fire in her eyes. "No way will I nurse the enemy. The Japs killed my fiancé. Now I have nobody!"

No one said a word after that outburst.

I gathered my thoughts and after a few moments, said, "Nurses, it is our job to heal. Who here took the Army Nurse Corps pledge to join up?"

Everyone raised their hands, including Annie.

"If you remember the pledge, there is one line you all promised to obey: *With loyalty will I endeavor to aid the physician in his work, and devote myself to the welfare of those committed to my care.*" I took a deep breath. "Your government, the United States of America, agreed with Britain in August 1942 to take in 50,000 prisoners of war. Our government also signed the terms of the Geneva Convention of 1929 to protect captured soldiers from inhumane treatment. It is part of our job to nurse the enemy after they are captured and put in our care. Keep in mind that most of our men have joined the service and we have a severe labor shortage. These prisoners of war work and help our economy while they're in our country."

The entire room was silent. Most of the nurses stared at the floor or fiddled with their fingernails.

I broke the silence. "Suffering knows no uniform. We must all take a turn in the Japanese ward. It is part of our duty. Who will attend to them first?"

No one raised a hand.

Molly spoke up. "I went in there, Chief, and those Japanese would not let me touch them to clean or dress their wounds. They slapped my hands away."

Susie added, "I tried to help one in the operating room and the wild-eyed Jap rolled off the table with a bullet wound still in his leg and tried to hobble back outside. Medic Johnny brought him back and held him down on the table so I could give him a shot. After he fell asleep, Dr. Ericson fixed him up. They are an unruly race."

I pursed my lips in determination. "I will attend to the Japanese first with a medic interpreter to discover any problems we may not understand. Then we'll meet again and I will expect everyone to do their duty and sign up on a rotating list."

One of the Filipino medics knew how to speak Japanese.

"Chief, this is the problem. Their officers tell them that Americans torture and kill all prisoners. The Japanese are trained from infancy to follow the orders of their superiors with total obedience, and are told that if captured, their families back home will be tortured by their own army."

With this new understanding, and with Angelo to interpret, I went to the prisoner compound to gather some information. I asked one prisoner, "Why are you fighting?"

He answered, "Because we are ordered to."

Another prisoner with a wounded arm added, "We are told that Americans never cure us. We wait in here to be shot or hung."

A Japanese soldier with a gaping shrapnel wound on his thigh said, "Our commander told us is better to die in combat than to be captured."

I answered in a calm whisper, "We want to take care of your wounds and keep you here until the war is over, then you will be released. We are healers here—nurses, medics, and physicians—and have taken an oath to do no harm to any human being."

After Angelo interpreted, all the captives remained silent.

I continued, sensing their apprehension. "Soldiers, we'll have a nurse come in each day to wash, feed, and take care of all of you. Then a medic will take anyone that needs an operation to surgery. I hope all of you will allow this. Please, we want to help you." I then said to Angelo, "Thanks. I may need you later to assist our nurses in here."

"Glad to help," Angelo grinned.

I gave the Japanese captives a sincere smile, then touched one of the soldier's hands. I left and returned with Molly, who I was confident would help me with this sticky situation. I introduced her and a few of the soldiers tried to say her name. She managed to say one of theirs.

The next day, we both attempted to figure out how to deal with a few of the ornery Japanese patients with Angelo's help. When I tried to spoon-feed an emaciated soldier, he pushed the spoon away. Molly tried to feed another one and had the same experience, but this one shouted in Japanese in her face.

We had the medics bring in small tables to put beside the patients, and we placed meals on the tables and left. When we came back, we saw that this method was successful. We took the empty trays and left a pack of cigarettes as a reward.

"Oh my, I can see that these patients need to be treated in a special way," Molly remarked to me in confidence.

I went back to the barracks to make a schedule for every nurse to go to the Japanese ward, and asked Molly to explain to the nurses how the prisoners were to be fed. And, as time went by, our Japanese prisoners were grateful for the decent treatment we gave them, which was rewarding for all involved.

Chapter Fourteen
Dottie
Camp Livingston, Louisiana – Tagap, Burma
September – October 1944

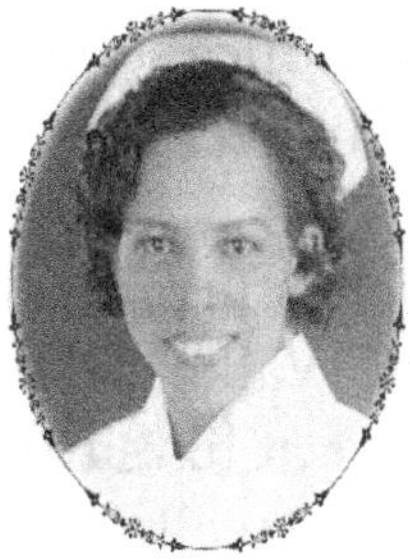

Our 16 nurses waited on the platform to board the train from Louisiana to New York City for 10 days of processing before we went overseas. I could not tell my nurses where we were being deployed, just that it would be overseas.

Out of the corner of my eye, I saw Dr. Walker in the window seat inside the train. I pushed ahead of everyone and knew that with my rank, I could gain the privilege of sitting with the doctor for the two-day journey ahead. My heart pounded so loud, I wondered if anyone could hear it. But I calmed down as I approached the doctor and asked, "Mind if I sit here?" I smoothed my hair back into my nurses' cap.

Dr. Walker closed the medical book he was reading on his lap. "Of course. Where are you assigned, Chief Williams?"

My heart fluttered again as he said my name and his attentive eyes drew into mine. "Tagap, Burma," I said in a practiced, smooth tone. "And you?"

"The same. It'll be nice to work with you. I know from your sharp skills in class and competent ability to lead that you'll be a great asset to the 335th Station Hospital."

My face flushed at the compliment. "I'm happy to serve my country overseas and care for our fighting soldiers to help win this nasty war."

"You and me both. Tell me, where are you from?"

"Near Atlanta, Georgia."

"Did you train at Grady?"

"Yes, I received a fine education there."

"Do you know if Grady ever allowed Negro physicians to practice there?"

"When I left, there were still only White physicians. Where did you go to school, Dr. Walker? Do I detect an accent from Back East?" I glanced over at his surgeon's hands. They were quite fair in color, clean, and well-manicured. I was still trying to ascertain whether he was Negro or White.

"Right you are. I graduated from Lincoln University in Pennsylvania, then received my medical degree from the Howard Institute of Medicine in Washington, DC."

A smile formed on my face and I was satisfied at last to be sure that he was a Negro physician. Both colleges he mentioned were Negro schools.

Dr. Walker took off his cap. His hair was closely shaved and did not have a nappy texture. Because of his light skin, I surmised that he must have come from a mix of White and Negro parents.

"I wonder what Burma will be like?" I fluttered my eyelashes and looked at his clean-shaven, light-beige face. Behind his spectacles, his eyes were green with brown specks.

"As soon as I found out where I would be sent, I went to the library in Huachuca and looked up as much information as I could about Burma. I'm happy to share with you what I've researched. After all, it will take a couple of days to get to New York City."

"That would be very helpful for me as chief, thank you."

While the doctor looked through his notes, my mind

drifted back to Fort Huachuca. I knew there was no Negro library in that town. I suspected that Dr. Walker must have passed for White to gain access to the library he mentioned. But I didn't dare ask for fear of being rude.

"Would you be interested to see a map of the world? I'll show you where Burma is," he said.

"That would be informative, thanks." I crossed and re-crossed my legs. I noticed that the doctor watched out of the corner of his eye.

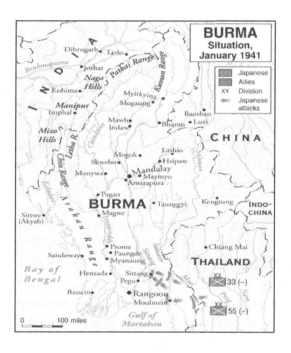

Dr. Walker unfolded the map. "Tagap is in the British colony of Northern Burma, part of the continent of Asia. Right here." He pointed. "Its neighbor is India on the northeastern border, also a British colony. China is on the other side. They're our allies in the war. The Chinese help us fight the Japanese, who have taken over Eastern China and are aligned with Nazi Germany and Fascist Italy."

"I see that it's farther than Liberia, where we were

stationed previously," I observed as I looked over the map.

"Yes, it's way on the other side of the world from the States. What was it like in Liberia?"

"It was wonderful to travel on a troop ship to get there. I was quite fascinated to meet and care for some of the native Liberians. But we were recalled back to the States after most of the nurses got malaria."

"That's a shame."

"The other problem was that the hospital did not have many patients and we were overstaffed with medical corpsmen, who were there before we arrived."

"I wonder why they sent your group there in the first place?" Dr. Walker mused.

"That's what I'd like to know. Do you think it was because the quota for Negro nurses was raised by the Army, and the War Department wanted to make a showing?"

He nodded. "Yes, that sounds about right because there is plenty of racial politics going on all the time. I read that the National Association for the Advancement of Colored People is a civil rights organization that campaigns for equal rights for our people and does everything it can to end segregation."

"I pray my nurses will be valued as well as needed in Burma—both for their sake and to show that we can do a successful job."

"I have a good sense that your prayer will come through. After all, we will be near the war, unlike where you were in Liberia." He folded up the map.

"Thanks for the information about Burma. You are a wealth of information. I wonder what the 335th Station Hospital will look like and what type of patient care there will be…" I displayed an enthusiastic smile.

"We'll be taking care of our American Negro troops as well as our allied Chinese soldiers. Sixty-five percent of the patients are colored, which is why the 335th Station Negro Hospital was built. The Chinese soldiers fight the Japanese to keep Ledo Road open, and the Negro soldiers help build the road and drive the trucks to transport supplies to China. All the engineers are White."

"How interesting. I've never seen a Chinese person before."

The conductor announced that we were about to get underway.

After a few fun-filled days on the train, we arrived in the big city of New York. We piled off the train with our barracks bags and waited for a bus to take us to a U.S. Army medical hospital for processing.

At the bus stop, our eyes were drawn upward. Mesmerized, we searched for small patches of the cloudy sky between the tall city buildings and towering skyscrapers.

Clara stared at the ground and said with a sad face, "I wish I could see my family. They're not too far from here."

I put my arm around her. "I'm sorry we don't have time to visit them. Try to keep your mind on our upcoming trip overseas."

I hugged my insufficient jacket and felt the chill of fall in the air.

The bus arrived and we were taken to a huge U.S. Army hospital. Once there, we were taken to the basement to sleep on small, crowded cots. It reminded me of the Negro nurses' quarters at Grady.

Our 10 days in the New York hospital were filled with taking physicals, and many immunizations like typhus and cholera. We were sworn to secrecy and signed paperwork declaring that we would never discuss military information with anyone.

On the last day, boxes of all sizes were delivered to our

basement room. It was like an extravagant birthday party. We were issued brand-new fatigues, field jackets, shoes, and cotton socks. We sorted through the clothes to find the right sizes. It was a joyous occasion that made the trip more of a reality.

I reached inside another box and pulled out an Army Nurse Corps garrison wide-brimmed peak cap with the gold seal of the United States displayed in the center. I put it on my head with a grin and everyone clapped. Then I handed out the official caps as the smell of new clothing wafted in the air.

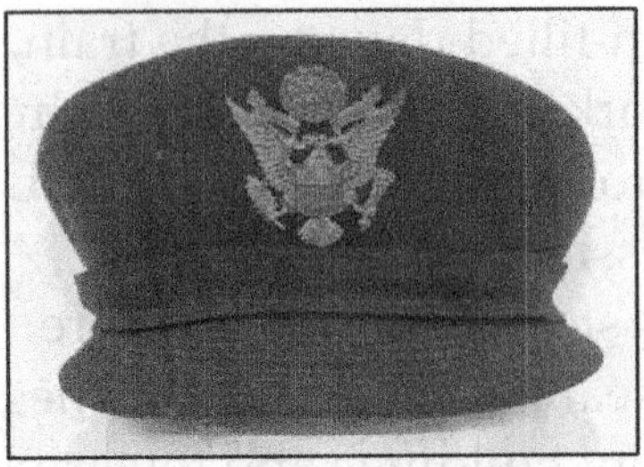

Everyone put on their caps. Clara walked around the room and saluted all the gals and they returned the gesture with chuckles.

Hazel burst out, "Chief, does this mean we'll have the full Army Nurse Corps uniform to wear?"

"Yes!" I pushed the last boxes toward the group, which contained brand-new service jackets with matching skirts and khaki shirts. "Here you go, gals, pick out a set and put them on. They're the real deal and boy, do we deserve them!"

Hazel inhaled the scent of the new jacket. "Ah…I love the smell of fresh fabric!"

We changed out of our old fatigues and put the tailored service jackets on over our new U.S. Army shirts. When everyone had their uniforms on, I retrieved a small box of insignia pins and showed everyone the accompanying diagram that indicated how they should be worn.

Demonstrating on Mary, I put two gold "U.S." pins on each collar of her jacket as the nurses squealed in delight. Next, I placed the two gold pins of serpents entwined on a staff. Everyone was enchanted by those as I read the explanation of what they meant.

Prudence hollered through the exuberant chatter, "That sparkling snake is stunning!"

After everyone attached the pins to the proper place on their jackets, I took out the ties. A few of the gals knew how to fix ties after helping younger brothers, and they assisted anyone who needed help.

Lorna found the mosquito netting for our caps and pulled one over hers. "Don't I look cute!" She paraded around the room and showed off as everyone exploded with laughter.

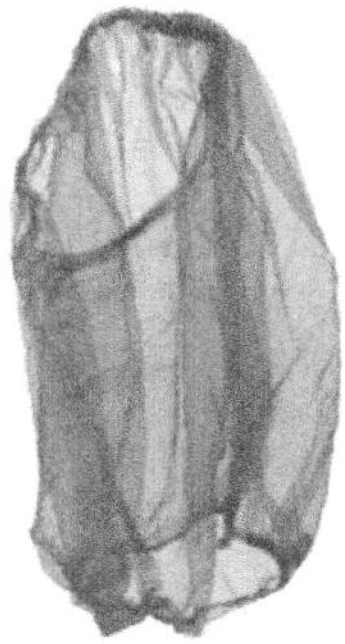

I wished I could have taken a photograph of our entire group wearing mosquito netting, which disguised their faces and made them look quite funny and strange.

Mary had tears in her eyes from laughing so hard. "We could have used those head nets in Liberia!"

I announced, "Now we can march into our new headquarters with our heads held high." Once the laughter subsided, I finally revealed to my nurses where we were headed. "We'll be leaving for the tropics of Burma on the continent of Asia. It will take several airplanes to get there. We have been assigned to the Negro 335th Station Hospital in Tagap, Burma."

Betty exclaimed, "Asia! How exotic!"

Lorna said, "I have no clue where that is."

I shared what little I knew. "Dr. Walker told me the hospital is up a very high mountain in the jungle. And don't forget, there's a war going on and we might be near the battlefield. I doubt we'll have any free time."

The raucous laughter that had filled the room moments earlier was now replaced by a somber silence as we all considered the reality of what we were headed for.

We boarded a bus to La Guardia Airport wearing our super-smart nurse uniforms. As we piled in and took our seats, Dr. Walker whistled at us.

I sat next to him.

He exclaimed, "You were finally issued uniforms! Congratulations!"

"Thank you. I'm happy for our nurses, who certainly deserve them." I smiled with pride.

The bus stopped on the tarmac and a guard directed us toward a colossal U.S. Army transport plane. None of us, including the doctor, had ever been on a plane. I saw fear and nervous anticipation on the faces of my nurses.

To make matters worse, Hilary asked, "How's that giant piece of metal going to get up into the sky and stay there without crashing down?"

Lorna added, "No way am I going up there."

Dr. Walker gave me a look that said, *Better do something to squelch those comments.*

"Girls," I said, "we are fortunate to be flying in an airplane instead of being stuck on a ship and seasick for days, like several of you were when we went to Liberia. An airplane is a marvelous invention to be able to deliver important people like us, fast! Let's focus on the majestic mountains and gentle elephants who roam where we're going. Most of all, remember that we are badly needed to help win this war. Let's get to the hospital to prove our worth, both for our profession and for Negroes!"

Dr. Walker gave me a wink. I grinned as a shiver shot through me.

The doctor boarded first. I went to the back of our group and stood behind Lorna and Hilary to make sure they got on the plane. I had them sit with Polly since she was such a cheerful gal.

Dr. Walker patted the window seat next to him for me to sit on. As we flew, despite all the airplane changes and layovers, the journey went by fast for me, thanks to Dr. Walker and his stimulating intellectual conversation. He kept his map out and showed me where we were and where we were headed as we traveled.

"Tell me about Ledo Road, it sounds important." I smoothed my new uniform skirt.

"It's a vital supply route that begins in Ledo, India that connects the countries of India, Burma, and China. This road will serve as an alternative to Burma Road, which was cut off by the Japanese a few months ago. Ledo Road will enable the Allied Forces to deliver necessary wartime supplies to China and aid them in their fight against the Japanese."

"Why does Japan want Burma?"

"Burma has natural resources, like oil and metals for warfare. There are thousands of Negro troops reconstructing this highway to get food and materials through to the Chinese troops that are fighting the Japanese."

"Doctor Walker, have you researched what it looks like where we'll be stationed?"

"I only know that it's near the top of a 4,500-foot peak of the Patkai Mountain Range in a jungle."

"I wonder what our job will be like in Tagap…" I took off my cap and smoothed down my hair. It was becoming warm inside the plane.

"I've been told that our work is to treat the American and Chinese troops who are fighting the Japanese. We'll repair battlefield wounds and accident injuries that occur to those building the road."

We flew to Karachi, Pakistan with stops in Newfoundland, Casablanca, and Egypt. As we flew over the Holy Land, I reflected on the bible stories I learned as a child in Sunday school and mentioned this to the doctor. He said he had the same thoughts. We found out we shared the Baptist religion, which further spurred the affection I felt for him.

I overheard Lorna say she was glad when we had overcast skies so she couldn't see the ocean below. I felt the opposite and was happy when there was clear weather so I wouldn't miss all the wondrous sights out of my small window. I turned my head toward Polly and flashed her a big, thankful smile when she distracted Hilary with a funny story about one of our favorite patients.

Most of the nurses got used to all the plane flights but I could tell by the occasional retching sounds that not everyone was handling things well. I took the lead to pass the time and we played guessing games like "I Spy," sang limericks, and tried tongue-twisters.

Dr. Walker added his favorite, "Fuzzy Wuzzy was a bear, Fuzzy Wuzzy had no hair, Fuzzy Wuzzy wasn't fuzzy, was he?"

I added, "Whoever says it three times without a mistake wins."

Lorna frowned, "Wins what?"

Polly saved me. "Wins a fun time and cheers!"

I turned around in my seat to look behind me. "That's great! Thanks, Polly."

Clever Hazel made up her own silly ditties, which we all copied, then roared with laughter.

Our last plane landed in Assam, India, which was the start of Ledo Road. We exited the plane and the temperature of 120 degrees hit me with a powerful blast. It was extreme weather.

We stayed at a cheap hotel. The next day, we explored the crowded city. The shops were full of colorful trinkets and clothes. There were tables full of spices piled into pyramids of many colors, and their heady smells wafted into the air. I felt free to browse and mingle among the brown natives who welcomed our business. There were no "Whites Only" signs in this country.

But after a while, the conditions that the Indian people lived in were frightful for all of us to view. There were many malnourished people dressed in rags and children with distended stomachs who begged for food or coins. I had never seen anything this heartbreaking. It shook my faith and made me wonder, *Where are you, God?*

Drained and exhausted from the severe heat, we left the market.

The next day, we traveled in two trucks up and over Ledo Road for 80 miles into Northern Burma. It made for a long ride what with the humidity, dust, and bumps on the narrow dirt road. There were deep ditches on each side of it and we bounced and rocked back and forth in our seats. We had to make several stops due to upset stomachs as the trucks snaked through the mountainous jungle.

Finally, our Indian-garbed driver announced, "Tagap!"

Each driver got out and helped us retrieve our barracks bags.

Dr. Walker asked one of the drivers, "Where's the hospital?"

The driver pointed to a path that disappeared into the immense jungle and announced in his thick accent, "Hospital."

Both drivers jumped back into their trucks and drove away with incredible speed, blowing dust all over our new Army Nurse Corps uniforms.

Dr. Walker brushed off his uniform, pushed up his glasses, and mopped the sweat off his face with his sleeve. Then he took off his jacket, undid his tie, and put them in his duffle bag.

We followed his example and took off our jackets and ties, then dragged our oversized duffle bags and followed single file behind him up the jungle path. The bushes caught on our clothes and stockings. The jungle was not the place to wear a uniform, but we all wanted to properly present ourselves and kept our professional caps on. *Slap, slap* was the sound from the nurses as they swatted at their legs to keep the insects away amid the tropical bird calls and occasional wild-animal noises as we wound our way upward through the mesh of tangled, twisted undergrowth.

Giant, graceful, densely packed trees towered over us and dwarfed our group as we plodded among them. I cupped my hand above my eyes and couldn't see the tops. These strange trees had dark-green, pole-like trunks. Clara dropped her bag and hugged one to feel its width. Hazel did the same. Each tree had a tan ring at even increments on its trunk. Delicate, teardrop-shaped lime-green leaves situated up high sprouted from thin branches. The further we climbed, the darker it became as the canopy thickened and blocked out the light. We continued upward on a reddish-brown dirt path and soon heard a hammering noise off in the distance. We hiked toward the sound.

It was an hour later when Dr. Walker declared, "I see someone."

"Praise the Lord," exclaimed Polly.

Thank goodness, just in time, I thought. The tropical heat was intense.

Sure enough, there was a small clearing up ahead, and from it emanated a frantic banging noise that reverberated throughout the overgrown jungle. A bare-chested, muscular, deep-russet Negro man stopped hammering two large green poles together. I heard a few of the nurses gasp. He was quite attractive.

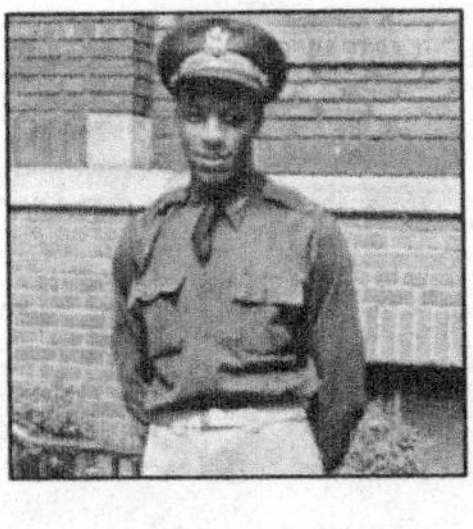

"Greetings!" he said. "I've been expecting nurses and I see you brought a bonus doctor. I'm Major John Harris, commanding officer of the future site of the Negro 335th Station Hospital. Call me Major John."

We were speechless when we heard the word "future."

"I'm glad to have another physician, in addition to all these *lovely* nurses." He smiled and raised his eyebrows when he said "lovely."

"What do you mean by *future* site?" I gulped. A flush crept onto my face and I noticed that all the nurses stared at the major. He was over-the-top good looking, and those muscles did not come from being a surgeon.

The major explained, "The hospital is not finished. It's built from an abandoned quartermaster road station that used to store supplies when Burma Road was first built. Our section here is called Ledo Road, which starts in India."

"Tell me, Doctor, what type of patient care will we expect to do here?" Doctor Walker asked. He pushed up his glasses, which continually slid down his sweaty nose.

"First, we need you all to help build the hospital—"

Before he could finish his sentence, most of the nurses groaned.

Clara shouted, "We *don't* do that kind of work!"

Major John chuckled. "Don't worry, we just need you all to supervise the workers to build the permanent hospital. It's built mostly by Burmese natives who need the work as well as the pay. Your supervision will help keep the pace and get it done, then we'll have a brand-new hospital in no time." He puffed out his bare chest. "What's your first name, Chief?"

"Dora…or Dottie..."

Dr. Walker spoke up. "Dr. Samuel will do just fine for me." He pulled out a handkerchief and wiped a drip from under his glasses.

"Do you have more appropriate clothes to wear in the jungle here?" Major John asked.

I spoke up, "We do have fatigues but didn't want to wear them to greet you." I stared at his bare chest and felt silly in my formal, hot clothes. "Most of us have never been in a jungle before. I can see that we should keep our uniforms packed up."

"Yes, obviously it's an informal atmosphere here. Follow me. I'll show you to your quarters so you can change," Major John said.

We tramped up the jungle path in the intense heat. The forest around us was filled with emerald-green ferns and a riot of colorful flowers on tangled vines. It had been a long day and I hoped for my nurses' sake that we would get to our quarters soon to change into our cooler fatigues.

Chapter Fifteen
Bea
Baguio, Philippines 1942

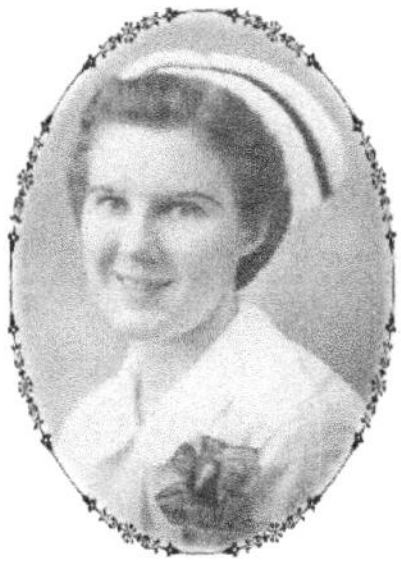

I was assisting in surgery when a small Japanese soldier was brought in with a broken leg. Dr. Charlie decided to break it and reset it and called for an anesthetist. But when the doctor tried to anesthetize the soldier, the man rolled off the table, then hobbled around the room screaming something in Japanese. A Filipino man on the next table was able to interpret that he was begging us not to kill him.

"Soldier," I said, "tell him we need to fix his leg and do not want to harm him."

The man settled down and the anesthesia took effect. When he woke up, he shook the doctor's hand, glad to find that he was still alive.

After that incident, I assigned a strong medic to bring in the Japanese patients and put them on the operating tables, and if necessary, to hold them down until the anesthetic put them under.

As the days went by, we found that with the reward of cigarettes or chocolate, some of the patients allowed us to wash and bandage them. Molly and I attended to the Japanese soldiers as more captives were brought into the compound by the medics.

I noticed that one of the Japanese men wore several American wristwatches lined up on one arm, and asked Davy, "Why is he wearing that many watches?"

Davy said, "Just like our men, they take trophies when they kill someone. Each of these watches means one of our soldiers was killed."

I gasped and began to tear the watches off the soldier's arm. But this was a stupid thing to do. The Japanese patient slapped me across the face. Davy grabbed his wrist just as he was about to try it again.

I moved away with a fistful of watches. My cheek stung as I crouched in a corner of the room and flipped over each watch to look for an inscription. My heart nearly stopped when I turned over the last one. "Oh my god, it's here..." I threw the other watches down and held it to my chest, then ran out into the jungle. Sobs heaved out of me as I leaned against a papaya tree, my head swimming.

Molly followed me out. "What's wrong, Chief?"

I showed her the inscription on the gold watch: *Airman Robert L. Johnson, Love Dad and Mom.*

"Oh, no!" Molly screeched. "I'm so sorry, Chief Bea. What a horrible way for you to find out about his death!"

I took a day off and lay in my bed with a sheet over my head, only getting up now and then to go to the toilet area, where I could cry in privacy. But the patient population was growing as the war escalated and it left me no time to grieve. I continued to do my job in a state of shock.

The Japanese bombing near the battlefield became an everyday occurrence. One day, I wandered out into the jungle and saw sheet-covered bodies all over the ground. The corpsmen left them there as there was no time to bury all the dead—their main job was to find soldiers who were alive and needed treatment. I walked farther and saw the mass gravesites ready for the dead. I tried to mute my cries but morbid questions flooded my mind. *Will one of my nurses be next…or will I be next? Will the war ever be over? When will our American ships rescue us? Have they forgotten about us on this faraway island?*

I stayed in the hospital and worked long hours to cope with the flood of casualties from the incessant fighting and to distract myself from images of Rob being shot down. Most of the wounded soldiers couldn't have cared less about their wounds and just wanted food because they starved on the battlefield while they fought.

One soldier said to me, "I'm so hungry, I could eat barbed wire. I haven't eaten for days. Nurse, please get me something—*anything*—to eat!"

Another patient told me that his unit had been led by a commanding officer on horseback, and they had been without food for days. The leader dismounted and shot his horse, then they made a fire and the horse was cooked over it for supper.

When we first arrived, there were 500 cots. Now, as the battle escalated, the nurses set up cot after cot, and the corpsmen followed behind with stretchers and filled the cots with soldiers. Amid the chaos, we performed our jobs as nurses and were glad to be away from the frontlines in the protected mountains.

New wards had to be added to the hospital and were set up in the jungle along paths cleared under the tall trees. Filipino workmen were hired from the surrounding countryside and built hundreds of bamboo beds that soon became triple-decker bunks. They worked for army chow and the American dollar. These hard-working men used bamboo for everything and made us brooms and much-needed crutches. They even made wooden ladders so the nurses could get to the top row of bunks to tend to their patients.

I went to the kitchen to see if there was anything new for breakfast besides rice. After getting a plate, I found Major Arnie at a picnic table eating a small amount of carabao meat with rice. I sat down next to him. A gust of wind blew in from the mountains and dust settled on our meals. We ignored it and ate our food anyway. I laughed wryly to myself. We used to dust off our meals. Now we didn't care.

Sergeant Moreno, our head cook and a retired member of the 27th Philippine Scout Cavalry, walked by.

Major Arnie said, "Where are the canned vegetables?"

"I've been meaning to talk to you about that, Doc. We are out of canned food." He wiped his big hands on his apron.

"What do we have left to eat?"

"Come with me to the corral and I'll show you."

I went with them and in the corral saw just a few carabaos with some horses and mules.

"Where are all the carabaos?" Major Arnie asked. "They're the most plentiful animal on the island."

"They're harder to find here and we have over 3,000 patients and a staff to feed," Sergeant Moreno said.

I looked over at two brown horses, who looked back at me with large, adorable, melting eyes. "Why are there horses in the corral?"

"They're the old horses. I'll have to butcher them to feed everyone." Sgt. Moreno's face fell.

Major Arnie raised his eyebrows, then thought for a moment. "I think I'll ask some of the workmen to find us some wild pigs. Meanwhile, everyone is allowed to eat only two meals a day."

When the sergeant took up his butchering tools and stroked one of the gentle horses, I teared up and left. That night, I sat with Annie at chow. I pushed aside the meat on my plate and just ate rice.

Jane took one bite of her meat and spit it out. "This tastes like leather shoes. I can't chew it and the smell is repulsive. I wonder what it is?"

"It's horse." I looked out at the mountains to avoid her gaze.

She was silent for a moment. "No way am I eating horse. I

used to have a horse I'd ride every day in the woods back home. Oatie was my friend and companion." Jane pushed her plate away.

I informed my staff that we were to be rationed to two meals a day. Our patients were the top priority to feed to help them get better to win this god-awful war.

A heavy gust blew into our nostrils and mouths. We gave up sitting outside and took our food back to our barracks.

It was bad enough that we were about to run out of food, but we were now out of cigarettes as well. Cigarettes relaxed the soldiers and kept them busy until they could return to the battlefield. The ambulatory men walked around and picked up butts off the floor. Two of the nurses laughed and watched as they smoked these small stubs in little holders made of bamboo twigs or wrapped them in newspaper.

When all the animals in the corral had been butchered, the workmen brought in anything that moved. A wild pig was the best find, but when the nurses saw our pet monkeys disappear, some refused to eat any type of meat. Snakes and lizards were in abundance but the sight and taste of them was not for everyone.

Molly scouted around and found a big can of peanut butter in what was thought to be an empty box in the kitchen. Any available nurse on break was invited to the peanut butter party. We acted like it was Thanksgiving when the can was opened. The smell was exhilarating. Four of us gathered around the can at the picnic table and dipped in a spoon. The peanut butter filled our shrunken bellies but it was a short-lived celebration, as the rich food upset our stomachs and gave most of us the runs.

One morning, a medic brought in a difficult patient. Annie tried to examine his wound, but he pushed her away.

Annie asked, "Why won't you let us heal you? This is a bad injury on your leg." She washed his forehead in an attempt to soothe him.

The soldier shouted, "I want out of here to go help fight! My best combat buddy was shot, then knifed. And I saw him hung in a tree after he was dead."

"Soldier, I'm sorry you had to see that. It must have been terrifying. But please, let me fix you up so you can go back to the battlefield and help us win."

I watched Annie's patience and compassion, and it gave me more courage to carry on despite my troubles.

Later that day, Nurse Annie confided in me, "Chief Bea, I'm gaining strength from these brave soldiers and I'm feeling less sorry for myself. My Frank gave his life for our country, and I know in my heart that he would want me to help all these wounded men."

I touched Annie's shoulder. "I'm proud of you, Annie. You go the extra mile when you care for difficult patients."

When I saw Annie's eyes twinkle in delight over the compliment, I took the opportunity to ask, "Do you think you're ready to take your turn in the Japanese prisoner ward now? The other nurses notice that you don't take your shift there and I must enforce equal treatment."

Annie waved her hands at me. "I will *not!* Those people killed my one true love." She rushed off.

I knew I would have to wait longer before I asked her again.

Later in the day, Annie came to speak with me. "I will not heal the enemy, but I would work in the gangrene ward," she offered.

"Thank you, Annie, that would fulfill your obligation and all the nurses I'm sure would feel that would be fair."

Not many of the nurses wanted to work in the separate outdoor gangrene ward. The wounds had to be cut open and if it was an arm or a leg, the entire limb had to be laid open to the bone, which was necessary to remove all the infected tissue. Then it was swabbed with peroxide and the wound was left uncovered except for mosquito netting. The exposure to sun and oxygen destroyed the bacteria. Along with the putrid odor emanating from the hideous exposed wounds, the patient was in constant agony. Deadly gas gangrene ravaged the soldiers who got it from the dirt, especially if it was contaminated by animal manure. Bataan's earth was infected by anaerobic bacteria, which caused gangrene in wounds. The germ infected open wounds and caused tiny gas bubbles. If the limbs were not tended to, they swelled to such large sizes that the surgeons had to amputate or systemic shock occurred, followed by death. Incisions had to be made to expose the soggy, swollen tissue, which released the gas, hence the separate ward. We had many cases and because of the agony of the patients, exposed wounds, and the toxins that caused a foul-smelling gas from the brownish pus and rotting tissue, the gas gangrene ward was outside.

I went to the ward the next day to check up on Annie and heard the usual cries and moans from the soldiers.

One of them wailed, "Cut it off, I beg you! Just take my goddamn leg off!"

I spotted Annie, who sat next to a patient's cot and consoled him. She wore two surgical masks to help her tolerate the repugnant stench as she swabbed the gangrene with peroxide, then covered the morbid area with mosquito netting.

"Hi, Annie. You are doing a fine job here," I said after she finished with her patient and approached me.

"Yes, Chief. These helpless soldiers sure need it." She pointed at the sky. "It's smart that there's no roof. This way the sun can help destroy the bacteria."

One of our medics, Sammy, used his long nose and delicate nostrils as a diagnostic tool to sniff out gangrene cases on the general ward. We called him "the sniffer." Sammy could smell gangrene before we knew it was gangrene. The nurses were quite impressed by his ability because no one had the time to examine swabs or samples under a microscope.

The next month, I was hard at work with patient charts, sitting on a bamboo chair in the ward, when Dr. Harold came to talk to me. He was egghead bald. He used to be rather fat but had slimmed down and caught my glance at his flat belly when he approached.

"Hi Chief," he said. "I see you like my boyish figure now." The physician rubbed his stomach while he leered at me.

"What do you want, Doctor?" I snarled. I was glued to the charts and wondered whether he was flirting with me or I was delusional from hunger.

"I'm sure you know this, Chief, but we only have enough food for just one meal a day now. Inform your staff." He winked at me.

"I'll let all the nurses know." I gathered my charts and left to get away from the nasty man. I'd always been a big gal all my life and was not used to men flirting with me. But now that I was lanky, maybe I looked more attractive. Back in the barracks, I noticed petite Molly and the poor girl looked emaciated.

In the morning, Sergeant Moreno gave me a big bowl of oatmeal—a welcome change from rice—for my one meal. When I found worms in it, I didn't even care and took a big spoonful. I figured they were cooked and besides, the worms added protein. Most of us drank hot or cold tea the rest of the day to fool our stomachs and make us feel full.

The wounded came in by the hundreds on buses, trucks, and mules as the war continued to rage on. Luckily, we were still far enough away from the frontlines that we did not see exploding shells or hear machine-gun or rifle fire. Many of our combat soldiers had to sleep in the mosquito-infested jungle without nets or Atabrine. Eighty percent of our patients were racked with malaria, and we treated them with Atabrine and bed rest. We had more cases of cerebral malaria, which was fatal, and these sick soldiers were brought in convulsing, then became unconscious. Treatment was quinine intravenously. When they died, we sent them to the autopsy tent.

Most of the soldiers were dehydrated from the tropical heat or had blood that oozed from massive wounds. Our operating room was flooded and patients on litters covered every inch of the floor. Some soldiers had faces that were puffy from beriberi or gums bleeding from scurvy.

Water trucks were few and far between in the combat zone. The soldiers were brought into the hospital with a fierce thirst. Some told us they had to suck morning dew off of plants just to get a few drops of water. The lister bags first issued to the soldiers were not plentiful enough, plus we ran out of chlorine tablets to make the water safe. The thirst-crazed men in battle drank polluted water that animals had been in, or from stagnant mountain pools. No wonder 30 percent of our patients had bacillary dysentery, and 10 percent had amoebic dysentery. A man could go a long time without food in the tropics but only a couple of days without water. Medicines used to be brought over by boats at night from Corregidor Island but now it was too dangerous, and supplies were running low.

As our patient population grew, Major Arnie gave orders to all the doctors in the operating room while he performed surgery on a patient.

"You take the belly case, Doc Harry. I'll take the brain." He unwrapped a bandage that exposed a mess of soggy mush caused by a bomb fragment that had sheared away the posterior half of a soldier's skull. The surgeon wrapped the soldier back up and shook his head. "Why's this guy still alive? It's hopeless. Davy, get him out of here. We need to make room for someone who has a chance of being saved. Dr. Charlie, you take that spinal bullet wound."

Major Arnie examined the next patient, who had sunken cheeks and mottled skin. The man's mouth was open and filled with a bloody froth. Major Arnie threw a sheet on him and screamed at Davy, "Bury this one!"

The horrors came one after another, nonstop. And everyone had to carry on.

The nurses would often debate whether they should tell a dying soldier that he wasn't going to make it.

I joined in on one such discussion. "I think he should be told the truth."

Nurse Molly agreed. "Yes, it will give him time to write home to his family."

Susie disagreed. "Let a soldier die in peace. Why make them live their last few hours in misery when they just want to be reassured that they'll live?"

Nurse Agnes added with conviction, "I say slug 'em with morphine and let 'em drift away without pain."

Consuela held her cross. "I think Father Garcia should be consulted on this matter and let him decide what's best to do. He's trained in how to comfort a patient."

I interjected, "That decision is up to the physician."

Arguments raged back and forth on this delicate subject until it was time to get back to work.

Outside the hospital, I passed rows of injured soldiers. Some were well-behaved and most didn't cry out or scream. I could see on their faces that they fought back their pain with clenched teeth as they waited patiently for one of our "angel" nurses to help them with shots of morphine.

As the month dragged on, the hotter weather brought rats and snakes, which multiplied. And flies swarmed inside in droves. Patients were brought in from the battle lines and the hospital was short of the precious Atabrine used to cure malaria. In one month alone, the epidemic rose to 290 cases.

Food had stopped arriving by boat or parachute drops from planes.

One afternoon, Nurse Agnes and I walked through the jungle to the hospital for our shift. When we heard an airplane overhead, we instinctively looked up to see if any food was being dropped. It was a Japanese observation aircraft and we hit the ground and covered our heads only to have pieces of paper flutter down and litter the jungle floor. After the plane left, we got up and I grabbed one.

We read it together. *Surrender now! Then you'll be fed and clothed!*

Agnes crumpled it up and shook her fist in the air. "What a bunch of baloney! We're not that stupid to fall for a false promise like that!"

"Come on, let's check on our men." I put my arm through hers and felt her body quivering with anger as we hiked toward the wards.

I moved through the long corridors of cots and came to Tex, an all-American boy, 18 years old with wide, football-player shoulders. This unfortunate lad had to have both of his legs amputated above his knees.

He asked me in his delightful Texas twang, "How are you today, Chief Bea?"

"I'm fine but how about you? Are the legs healing?"

"Just fine, thank you, ma'am."

I noticed the patients around him were startled to hear his lighthearted voice after seeing his bandaged stumps.

Ronny, who had a shrapnel wound, spoke out, "Tex, would you like me to read a chapter from this Western book?"

Tex said, "Sure thing! You read the first chapter and then I'll read the second one."

"Deal!" Ronny exclaimed.

Tex had an instant glow of cheer for anyone who came by to visit, and he received many spontaneous little presents from the nurses, like homemade cards. The other wounded soldiers gave him re-rolled cigarette butts. Nurse Maria, our innovative puzzle maker, made him a puzzle in the shape of Texas, and he drew in as many cities as possible on it. No pity was bestowed upon him because of his exceptional optimism. At first, he was depressed and seldom spoke, though he was always well-mannered when we bathed him or brought him a meal, but with inner strength, he improved and spread hope and joy to everyone.

Another star patient was a young Filipino boy, Carlos, who lost both of his eyes after a severe head wound. At first, he remained silent. Then as time went by, he improved. Each nurse gave him special care. They would sit on his bed, speak soothing words, and hold his hand. Everyone took turns visiting him – doctors, nurses, corpsmen, even other patients. Someone was always near his bed and spoke in light conversation, and his spirits began to rise. Carlos's hearing perked up and he knew every visitor by their voice. Pastor Miller would walk him around one day and Father Garcia would read to him the next.

These brave soldiers kept our faith alive and reminded us of our importance in their healing process. And they caused us to count our blessings.

One day, I went into the operating room and noticed Dr. Ericson with a scalpel in his hand standing over a patient. He began to shake with obvious malarial chills and held onto the table with his other hand to keep from falling. I found Major Arnie to take over for him, and Dr. Ericson was sent to his quarters for bed rest. Those damn mosquitoes were the cause and there was little to be done about it since we had run out of Atabrine.

Back in the ward, I went to examine my nurses. I saw Nurse Joan dressing a wound. She almost fainted with weakness from the fever, and I took over for her and sent her to bed. When I came down with malaria and was dizzy and weak, I set up my cot in the middle of all the patients and whispered out orders to the staff. That way they could keep working.

Dysentery patients had to make many visits to the latrines, which were too close to the wards. The smell was difficult for everyone to bear. It was hard to even eat. We ate our rice with one hand and shooed the mosquitoes away with the other, and saved our cup of tea for last. Malnutrition made everyone weak and susceptible to catching anything. Dust blew into the wards and made it difficult for the nurses to keep a clean environment.

Patients continued to be brought in by the medics from the frontlines and arrived by the hundreds. We now had a total of 4,500 soldiers, all weak from trying to fight in the mountainous jungle terrain with little or no food. With no room inside, the medics left new patients under trees to wait for treatment. Our nurses and doctors worked overtime until Major Arnie or I sent them off to get some sleep.

One evening, on the way to the barracks, a tin can dropped on my head. I screamed, "Ouch, what the hell was that?"

Littered all over the ground were hundreds of little tin cans decorated in the Japanese colors of red and white. Inside each can was a letter addressed to Lieutenant General Wainwright: *You are outnumbered. Surrender by March 22 or we will bomb you for 15 consecutive days and nights.*

I went back to show Major Arnie, who said, "Ignore it. It's the usual propaganda bullshit. Go get some sleep, we need you." He hollered at the nurse at his table, "Scalpel!"

March 22 came and went, and I calmed myself down and worked as much as I could. Our hospital was now smack in the middle of a zone of action and we were subjected to being bombed. The battle line was closer. It was unsettling. The enemy might not bomb our hospital, but our own anti-aircraft guns left fragments of shells that fell near us. Could an enemy bomb fall by accident? These were among the many worries that interrupted our nursing duties. With a sigh, I knew we'd just have to stick it out no matter what came our way.

Chapter Sixteen
Dottie
Tagap, Burma 1944

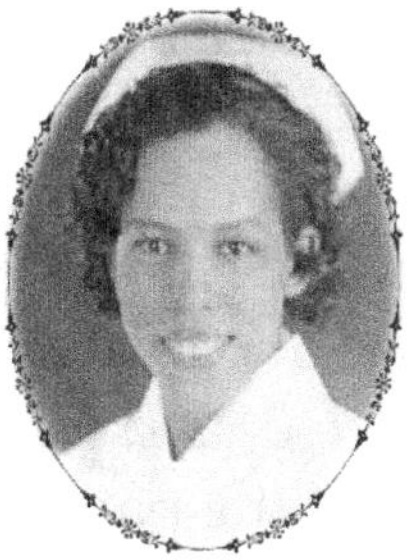

This is Burma, and it is quite unlike
any land you know about.

—Rudyard Kipling

We followed Major John up a higher hill to another area where a pile of tan canvas tents lay. I hid the anxiety that flew around in my brain and thought, *I joined the Army Nurse Corps to see the world, but this primitive place was not what I expected.* I snapped out of it and listened to the major.

"You'll have to sleep two to a tent until your bashas are built, then you'll have a nice hut. The cots are over there." He pointed to a tangle of canvas cots that lay in the red dirt.

"What exactly are bashas?" I tried to flash him a smile as I looked at his magnificent body and attempted to project a positive attitude.

"A basha is a native hut and means makeshift shelter. It is constructed entirely of bamboo except for the roof, which is made from palm leaves. Bamboo is a versatile woody plant that grows like a tree. It's a member of the grass family and lucky for us, is the fastest-growing plant in the world. It can grow 36 inches in 24 hours! Giant bamboo can grow over 65 feet tall. Most of the trees you see around here are bamboo. Large green bamboo poles are hammered until they soften and become pliable, then are split lengthwise and laid flat. Rafters, corner poles, and joists are made of whole bamboo poles. And pieces of bamboo are used in strips to hold the palm leaves in place," Major John explained.

After Lorna yawned, he turned to Doc Samuel. "I have room in my basha. Come, I'll show it to you." Before they left, Major John said in a warm, welcoming voice, "Thank you, ladies. You're sorely needed, and all the doctors will be glad to have you taking care of the patients. I'll leave you gals to set up your sleeping quarters. Then hike up that path over there to get some chow."

None of us had ever slept in tents before. We sorted through the poles and figured out how to erect them. I marveled at how basic training had toughened most of us up and I heard only minor complaints.

After everyone had changed into the more appropriate garb of fatigues, I announced, "Great job, everyone. Let's head up to chow."

To get food, we had to climb the highest hill in the entire encampment.

Betty let out a bone-tired groan. "Lordy, Chief, every place around here is up and over hills. My feet are swelling. Do you think we're almost there?"

Mary joined in, "It's too far. I think I'd rather turn back and go to sleep."

"We're close," I lied.

Betty was still quite overweight, even after basic training, and it was no wonder her feet were swollen. I was tired of the complaints, but it had been a very long and arduous day, so I let them slide. I tried to raise everyone's spirits. "Remember, gals, focus your thoughts on the positive. I bet the view from the top will be spectacular." I sang an Army song to boost morale:

When she was needed, she was there.
When the call went out for freedom, she was there.
Well, it wasn't always easy, and it wasn't always fair,
but when freedom called, she answered, she was there.

As the nurses joined in on the refrain, I knew we would make it.

Hazel pointed "Look, I see huge mountains."

"Hey, Lorna, did you get a load of Major John's muscles? I couldn't take my eyes off him!" Clara gushed.

"He's a knockout—almost as handsome as my Tommy," Lorna agreed.

"Well, you're a taken woman so I get first dibs on flirtin' him up," Clara laughed.

"No, it doesn't work that way. Whoever gets the most opportunity to bat their eyelashes wins." Prudence fluffed up her hair and tucked it behind her ears.

I was glad all the complaints had been replaced by swooning, even though I was secretly pining after Major John myself.

We made it to the top and everyone was breathless not only from the climb and altitude, but from the spectacular view. There before us was a tall, multi-peaked mountain range, and farther behind it we could see snow. In complete silence, the nurses stood in awe at the picturesque view.

"We are blessed to be here..." I said in a quiet, breathless voice.

A couple of the girls pulled up bamboo benches and chairs and sat down, mesmerized by the landscape.

Clara remarked, "It's astounding to sit here in the jungle heat and look out at the snowy mountains."

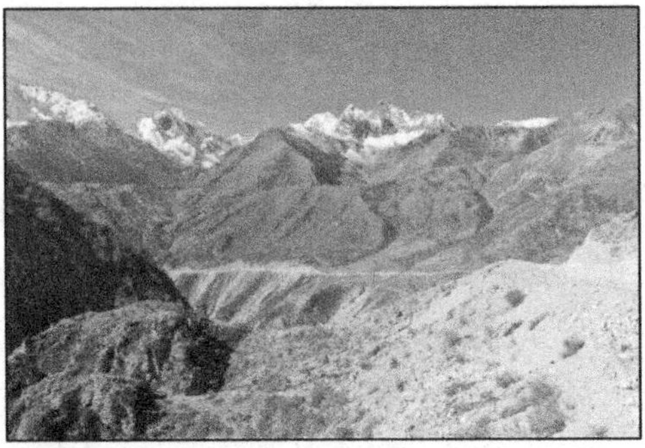

Nearby, I spied dinner, which meant sorting through boxes of canned goods and supplies. I opened a few cans of Spam, Vienna sausage, chili, and a box of dehydrated potatoes. There were powdered drinks like sweetened cocoa, lemonade, or bullion. Hershey bars were available for dessert. A fire pit and a pile of wood were nearby for those who wanted to heat something, but no one did after that strenuous climb. At least there was a water pipe up there, and we all couldn't drink enough water in the tin cups we found in a box of mess kits.

The two doctors arrived just as we finished our food and sat with us. Major John ate a can of cold beans with a spoon and Doc Samuel ate a can of Spam with a fork. The attention from the doctors squelched the girls' complaints about the food. Now, entertaining conversation and laughter filled our dining area.

Major John explained that chow was located way up there because the airplanes dropped surplus food as well as medical supplies by parachute. I noticed a silk parachute balled up near a rock. Some of the gals hunted through the boxes and found packs of Chesterfield cigarettes. They formed a circle and a few of them had a good smoke. Boy, did that boost morale. A short time later, we hiked back down to our tents and fell asleep with ease.

In the middle of the night, I woke to a strange howling

noise. We were surrounded by a jungle and heard elephants, tigers, and all sorts of wild-animal calls. I later found out the howls were from jackals.

After dawn broke, I woke again to the alarm-clock sound of monkeys climbing trees and an orchestra of insects chirping. At first, I lay there in my underwear and scratched the insect bites all over my body from yesterday's jungle hike. Then I pulled on my fatigues and ducked out of my tent quietly so as not to disturb Clara.

It wasn't long before everyone came out of their tents itching and moaning about the bites. I inspected the tents to figure out how the insects had gotten in, and found that they had poorly sewn, worn-out seams.

I was just as upset as everyone but didn't know what to do. "Let's go to breakfast."

Up we all went to the top of the hill, where several doctors sat and drank hot coffee.

Major John gave us a hearty welcome. "Good morning, ladies! I hope you all had a good sleep. Help yourself to the kettle of coffee on the fire."

We drank our coffee with one hand and scratched our legs with the other.

Major John said, "I'll have the laborers make you up some mosquito bars for tonight, so you all don't get bit again."

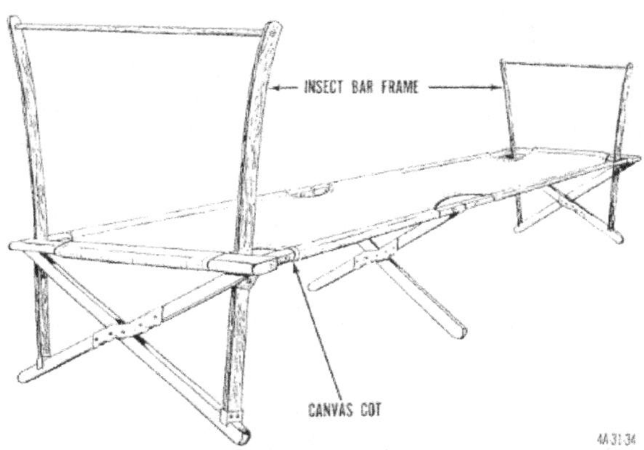

We scrounged through the boxes to find breakfast. After we ate, the group that smoked gathered with a few of the physicians, who offered them Chesterfields.

Major John, the commander of the hospital personnel, said, "Break time's over. I'll show your group the surgery."

The other physicians left first.

"Follow me to the ward. It will be situated on the side of this 4,500-foot peak at an elevation of 3,000 feet," Major John said.

Doc Samuel and our 16 nurses followed behind Major John. As we walked, we heard hundreds of supply-laden trucks roaring up the Patkai Range on Ledo Road on their way to China. We all stood on a hairpin curve on Ledo Road and saw another spectacular view of the mountain range.

Major John said, "We are on Ledo Road, which begins in Assam, India and goes to where we are here, in Northern Burma, then ends in Kunming, China. It's 1,072 miles long."

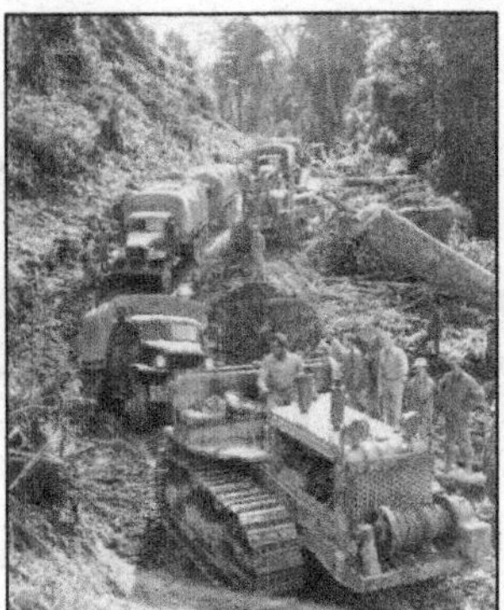

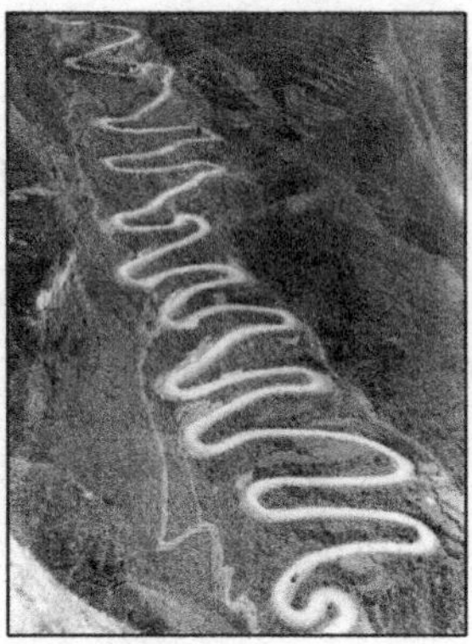

First convoy on Ledo Road (left)
Aerial view of Ledo Road (right)

"It's glorious here," I said to Major John as I took in the view.

"Indeed, it is. Over that way are the mountain ranges of Tibet." He motioned with his hand.

The nurses followed the doctors down a narrow pathway and pushed the jungle growth out of the way to get by. On my left side, the path disappeared altogether. The thick jungle mist half obscured a steep drop that concealed unexplored valleys, waterfalls, and tiny collections of huts.

"Who lives in the huts?" I asked.

"The Naga tribe. They are the natives that work for us. I've been inside one of their huts and they keep skulls of their enemies as souvenirs, passed down through the generations from when they used to be headhunters."

I noticed Lorna had a shocked look on her face.

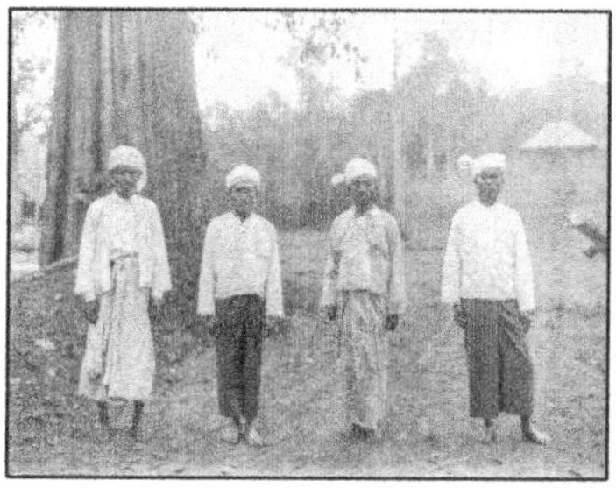

At the so-called hospital, Major John showed us a shack-like bamboo building with dirt floors and open sides.

We walked into one of the primitive huts and watched a physician who performed surgery on a soldier's arm with the help of a medical corpsman. Doc Samuel observed for a moment, then we walked to another hut.

"Chief Dottie, this will be your staff's wound-dressing room until a larger one is built."

I stuck my head into the tiny space we would have to use to fold and sterilize cotton bandages. There was just one large shelving unit made of bamboo that held syringes, sterile gloves, cotton dressings, tubes, needles, and Novocain.

Thank goodness my nurses remained quiet.

Major John said, "I would like to suggest that since we

only have your 16 nurses here, half can supervise construction and half can work on the ward with the patients or assist the doctors, then rotate each week."

Doctor Samuel inquired, "What would be the best job for me?"

"Because we are short on physicians, we'll need you in one of the operating rooms but when there's no surgery, you could supervise the building of the hospital."

"Glad to help. How many physicians do you have here?

"Seventeen, including you. But we do have five medical corpsmen."

Doc Samuel made a nervous gulp, then asked, "What type of surgeries are performed?"

"Mostly amputations."

I could tell by Dr. Samuel's raised eyebrows that this was not one of his favorite surgical procedures.

"What kind of patient care should the nurses expect?" I asked.

"The majority of the troops here are Negroes who build and maintain Ledo Road and supervise the natives. The soldiers also drive supplies into China for the American-trained Chinese to fight the Japanese. Our army is rebuilding Ledo Road, which the Japanese destroyed."

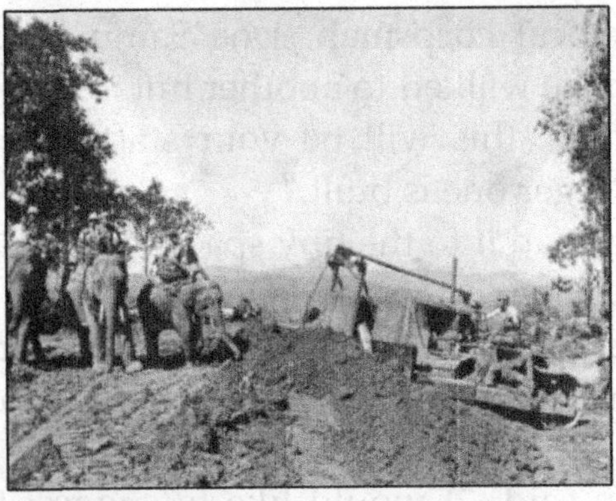

Bulldozers meet elephants

He continued, "The nurses will deal with wounds from truck accidents on the treacherous mountain road and battlefield wounds of the Chinese. There are plane crashes as well. Our Chinese Allies have been taught by the U.S. to fly and combat the Japanese airplanes."

Next, we followed Major John back through the dense brush, which opened into a clearing that housed an endless ward smack in the middle of the jungle. It was made of bamboo poles and had a thatched palm roof with open sides and a dirt floor. In front of the ward outside was a native Burmese man wearing a head wrap and loincloth. He sat on top of an elephant that had bright-white ivory tusks.

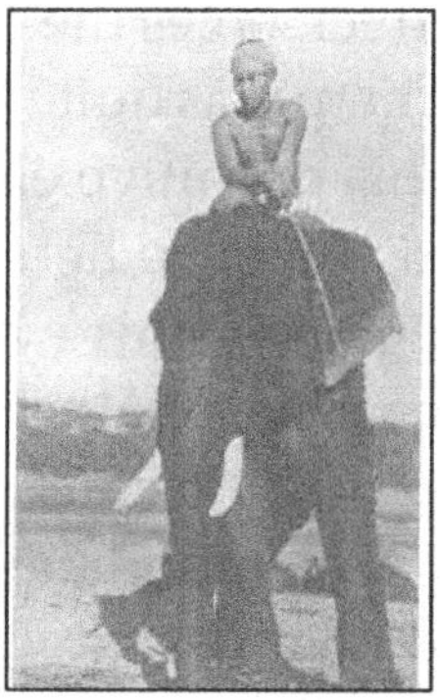

The nurses gawked in disbelief. The elephant was huge—nothing like the pictures some of us had seen. Not only was the elephant's height and width enormous but its floppy ears and trunk were huge as well. Major John patted the gentle giant on its thick leg and chuckled, then told us that elephants were used for labor there.

We followed the doctor into the vast ward, which was filled with a culturally diverse group of patients who chatted away nonstop in a variety of languages. Their voices blended into an amalgam of high and low tones. The ward was as large as a football field. There were a few medical corpsmen who attended to the patients.

Major John shook one of the sturdy poles. "Thank God for bamboo. Everything here is made from it. We learned about bamboo from the Burmese natives and it's as strong as hardwood timber."

Doc Samuel whistled and marveled at Major John's description as he felt one of the ringed poles. I noticed that the beds, tables, and chairs were all made from this practical tree.

"The native workers will make bamboo huts for all the nurses," Major John added.

"Girls, won't it be wonderful to have our own huts?" I asked. It wasn't easy to get their enthusiasm aroused and there were only a few nods from the group.

I thought about the thick poles the doctor was hammering when we first arrived. There was quite an ingenious use of the abundant materials in this primitive environment.

"How many beds do you have here for the patients?" Doc Samuel questioned. He pushed his eyeglasses back up onto his nose. The tropical heat was hotter as the day progressed and perspiration caused them to continually slide down.

"Presently, we can accommodate 75 patients. This war does not seem to be ending anytime soon and more beds will have to be made by our natives," Major John answered.

I almost gasped when I heard him say 75—and we would be the only nurses on staff! I covered my mouth and pretended to cough, then composed myself. "What type of illnesses will the nurses have to deal with?"

Major John counted on his fingers as he rattled off a list. "Malaria, pneumonia, scrub typhus, fly fever, gangrene, and dengue fever. Venereal disease, of course, and many mystery sicknesses as well."

I remember Doc Samuel's lecture on jungle diseases and was happy he knew most of them.

"Well, ladies, why don't half of you work on the ward and

I'll take the rest to supervise the bashas and mosquito bars. Doc Samuel, I'll introduce you to the other surgeons and see where you're needed."

Just the mention of the word "mosquito" got the nurses scratching again. We had learned at the Fort Huachuca hospital that it was difficult to tell the difference between ordinary, non-infectious mosquitoes and ones that caused malaria. In Liberia, we learned firsthand how this disease produced high fevers and shaking chills. Thank goodness it was not usually a fatal illness.

I stayed in the ward with half of my nurses and introduced myself to one of the medics. Corpsman Stevie was young, friendly, and adorable. I noticed that he wore a small silver cross with his dog tags. He took us through the loud ward, which was filled with conversation as well as groans from patients recovering from surgery.

"Tell me, Stevie, what training does a medical corpsman have to have? I always wanted to know."

He answered with pride, "We are trained by the Navy in first aid. I got sent here a while ago because of the shortage of Negro nurses available." Stevie was only a little taller than me, with a soft voice and sweet dimples that winked when he spoke.

With Stevie by my side and seven nurses, we roamed the length of the ward. I assigned each nurse to a section and prioritized what patients needed care first.

Stevie stuck with me like a hungry puppy dog looking for something to eat. But I was grateful as he was quite knowledgeable and knew most of the patients.

A soldier was carried in on a stretcher by two Burmese workers. I was quite shocked by the amount of blood that spilled out of all the wounds on his body.

"Stevie, please round up bandages and a bowl of water so we can assess what injuries this young man has," I directed. "What happened to you, soldier?"

"It was my first assignment, and I was highly nervous as nightfall came. Suddenly, the cargo carrier fell into a ditch, which caused the truck to roll on its side and I was trapped and injured."

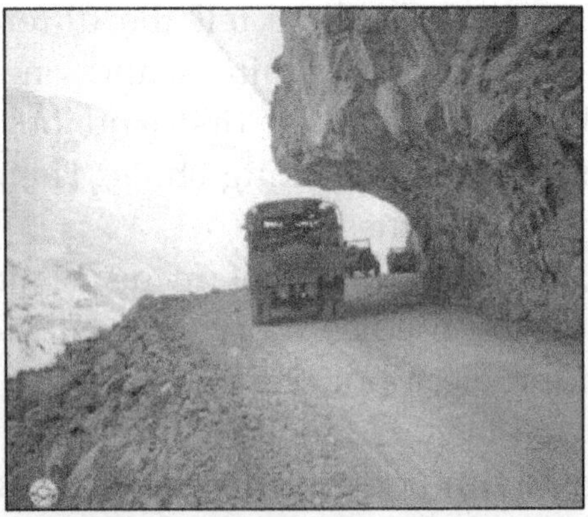

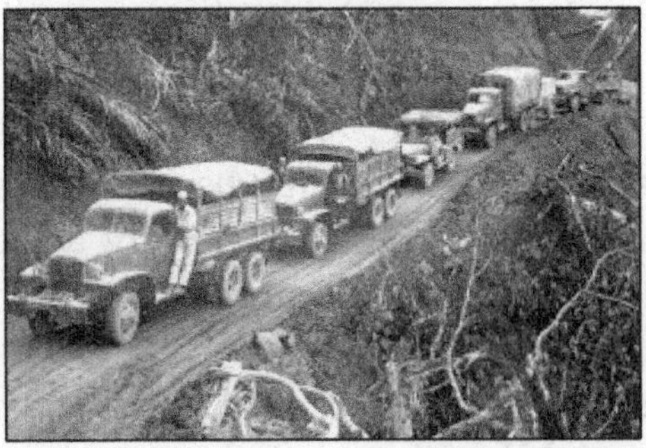

A section of Ledo Road where part of a mountain was hacked away to form the roadway.

He was quite young and would have been an attractive colored guy if he hadn't been covered in blood.

The soldier continued his story between gulps and grimaces from the tremendous pain he was in. "Lucky for me, the local native workers found me."

"Don't worry, soldier, we'll take good care of you," I sympathized.

After Stevie and I cleaned him up, I said, "Looks like you have a fractured leg and broken ribs. Better take him to one of the physicians, Stevie."

The soldier flashed a painful smile. "Thanks for saving me."

"You owe more thanks to those natives who rescued you and brought you here just in time. You're a lucky man that they were able to get you up and out of that truck from what you described." I gently held his hand.

Later that day, Major John came by with a big bottle of Atabrine tablets and told me it was imperative that all the nurses take a pill every day to prevent the ever-present malaria. I touched his arm to thank him, and he smiled at me, then winked.

I handed Stevie the container of Atabrine, told him to dispense them to the nurses and to take one himself, and to make sure he distributed them daily to everyone.

Chapter Seventeen
Bea
Baguio – Corregidor
March – April 1942

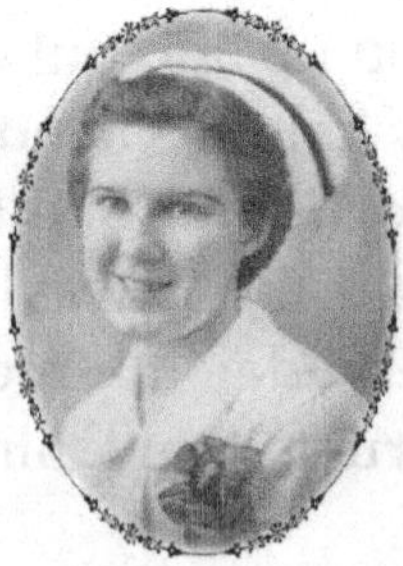

At the end of March, a 50-caliber bullet blasted through a lone, empty bed and frightened the hell out of all of us. Our cook, Sgt. Moreno, tried to avoid a spray of bullets by lying flat on the ground but a three-inch shell went through his chest, then several feet into the ground. Luckily, it never exploded and thank the Good Lord he survived.

The same day, constant shrapnel and shell fragments fell all around us outside the ward. Hundreds of shells fell on the picnic area, killing several medics and injuring 12. The patients who suffered from shellshock cried out and were traumatized every time a bomb was heard. Some would roll under their beds when they heard the explosive bursts. Even the sound of a truck driving by could cause violent trembles for the soldiers. It had been almost three months since the war broke out and we were desperate to hear the words, "The war is over!"

On March 30, a bomb hit near a wing of the officers' quarters, waking Dr. Arnie, who was sound asleep after a long shift. The next day, after the Japanese attack, arguments broke out among the nurses as to whether it was a deliberate bombing or not. When an enemy bomb made a direct hit on one of our trucks that was loaded with artillery ammunition and parked at the front of the hospital, the explosion killed 23 patients. The entire staff was devastated and we were no longer under the pretense that the hospital was a protected zone. Our hospital in Limay certainly hadn't been.

The next day was not any better. The Japanese dropped incendiaries in the rear area of our compound. The enlisted men's barracks caught on fire and almost burned down. Private First Class Andersen had his upper jaw blown off. We knew we were living on borrowed time.

More whistling bombs dropped down on over 150 already wounded patients who had been waiting outside to be treated. Some of the unfortunate men were blown into the branches of the massive mango and avocado trees. The smell of battle was in the air—an acrid mix of heavy smoke and burnt gunpowder. There was a constant ringing in our ears from the blasts. My nurses and I were now in the battlefield. Everyone was frantic and sporadic conversations were heard between explosions.

"When will help come?"

"When will the war end?"

The worst question was, "What will happen if the Japanese take over?"

Of course, no one could answer these questions, but they were always swimming in our minds every time we heard the frightening sound of a bomb.

In the new month of April, we had 1,000 cases a day to care for. We ran out of plasma and all the nurses who were not sick donated their blood to help the patients. On one eight-hour shift, 285 American and Filipino patients were treated, along with Japanese prisoners.

One morning, a bomb exploded directly outside our ward. I ran out to survey the rubble and saw mangled bodies under it all. There were legs and arms all over the jungle, and torn-up torsos impossible to identify. I stood in the middle of it all and wept like a child. Davy put his arm around me and led me back inside.

The medical corpsmen climbed up the trees to bring down bodies, blankets, mattresses, and pajama bottoms that had been blown into the branches. The medics moved into action and worked at a wild pace to unbury patients who might still be alive under the massive wreckage from the bombing. As the bombing ceased, the screams of the wounded and dying replaced the noise of the bombs. After one bombing, over 100 patients died in an instant and over 150 were wounded.

Angelica rushed into the hospital ward with blood streaming down her face.

"Are you all right?" I screamed.

She waved me away. "It's just a nosebleed," she said, then went to wash up.

Doc Arnie ran into the ward and ordered all the nurses to sleep in the foxholes outside, and to keep their helmets on.

That night, I tried to sleep in the dirt hole but couldn't for fear of getting bombed again. I felt like a hunted animal waiting to be killed, and huddled in the long, grave-like hole with a blanket. My anger prevented me from falling asleep. How could any human being bomb a hospital, even if we were the enemy? After all, we had a ward full of *their* people! The Red Cross signs were visible and the Japanese knew it was a hospital from the air.

At first light, I crawled out of my hole, head aching, back stiff, and legs cramping. I watched my nurses clamber out of their foxholes and we dragged ourselves into the ward. In a depressed state, we gave the morning medications, checked for any medical emergencies, then threw our helmets on and jumped back into our dirt homes. The sound of bombs continued to rage everywhere.

In the foxhole next to me, I heard Nurse Carmelita

repeating a chant over and over, "Lord, protect us and send them away…Lord, protect us and send them away…" When it was quiet for a moment, she jumped out of her foxhole and shook her fist at the sky. "Don't you dare come back!"

She scrambled back into her hole before I could chastise her. But I understood her anger. Annie made pitiful whimpering sounds after Carmelita's outburst.

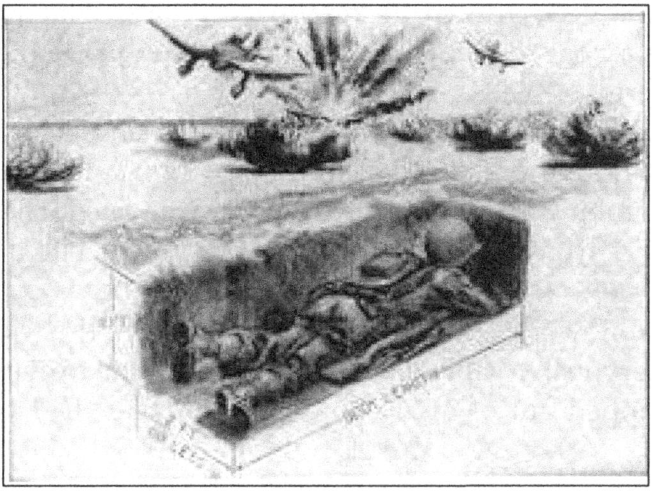

On April 6, the day after Easter, our hospital commander got word that the Japanese army was advancing and was within a few miles of the hospital. Our patient population increased to over 7,000. The next night, a massive bomb exploded in the middle of the ward and killed or re-wounded many of the patients. Two of our nurses, Rosemary and Rita, were hit by shrapnel on their chests and legs while they sheltered in foxholes nearby. They came into the hospital moaning and clutching their wounds. When I saw them, tears streamed down my face as I tried to endure another blow to my weakened nervous system.

Dr. Charlie and Dr. Arnie each took one of our wounded nurses and removed the shrapnel, then they were placed in the bombed-out ward.

In my mind floated the reality, *I can't believe this has happened! The Japanese made a direct hit on our hospital and re-wounded our patients. Plus, our own nurses!*

Lieutenant Colonel James Duckworth, our resident hospital commander, stormed into the hospital, walked around the bomb crater, then took one look at our two wounded nurses who lay on cots nearby. He ordered, "Someone pack up their belongings! I'll have a medic drive them to a boat to recover at the hospital on Corregidor. It's safer there."

A group of medics dug through the immense crater in the ward to find any patients who might still be alive. It was a mind-numbing experience for the nurses to watch. The rest of the medics went outside to dig deep pits in which to bury the dead.

The following day, Doc Arnie found me in the ward and paced nervously. "Chief Bea, all the nurses need to evacuate."

I snapped out of my sleep-deprived daze. "Did you say *all?*"

"Believe me, I don't want any of you to leave. But I received a direct order from Lt. Colonel Duckworth to evacuate all nurses. He informed me that the American Bataan commander is surrendering to the Japanese tomorrow."

I said again, "Every single nurse?"

He stared at me. "Yes. You don't want any of your nurses imprisoned or tortured, do you?"

"No, sir." I turned my head away to prevent my tears from showing, and stood in the ward looking at the wreckage.

Major Arnie barked, "Captain Bea, Bataan has fallen! All the nurses must evacuate. Pack up, now! You'll leave on a boat to work in a hospital on Corregidor Island. It's safer there. You've got 20 minutes until transportation shows up. This is an Army order." He pulled at his beard and cracked his chewing gum. I saw tears gleaming in his eyes as I turned and left to tell my nurses.

I gathered my thoughts and reminded myself that we were U.S. Army nurses, and were not free to quit or disobey orders. I relaxed my face and hurried into the operating room to inform all the nurses assisting the surgeons. "Nurses, we've been ordered to leave and go to the hospital on Corregidor."

Molly said, "But Chief—"

I interrupted her with a stern tone. "This is a direct order from Lt. Colonel Duckworth. We must leave immediately!"

All the operating room nurses took off their gloves and gowns and walked out in the middle of the operations. There were still hundreds of wounded soldiers lined up outside under trees waiting for surgery. I was devastated as I watched the nurses pull themselves away to pack up. We had been in Baguio for two months but it felt like a year. I sighed. Battlefield nursing certainly altered one's sense of time.

Next, I went into the wards and told all the nurses there to report to our barracks on the double. Once in the barracks, I repeated the order.

"Who will care for all the wounded soldiers?" Annie said and stomped her feet.

Other nurses protested until I stated, "Bataan has fallen. Our army surrenders tomorrow, then the Japanese will arrive. It's dangerous for us to stay here and be imprisoned or whatever else they could do to women."

This silenced the nurses and they all stood there in disbelief.

I raised my voice. "Pack your bags now and meet in the front of the hospital for transportation!"

I went to my cot and started shoving my meager items into my musette bag. Besides a few clothes, I included the cracked photograph of my parents, my beloved's watch, and my worn-out picture hat, and I put my diamond watch on my wrist. Then I shoved the Colt .45 and sock of bullets into the big pockets of my coveralls. I trudged into the jungle to vent my anger. *Uncle Sam, when will this god-awful war end?* I fumed to myself. I shook both fists in the air at a Japanese fighter spying overhead.

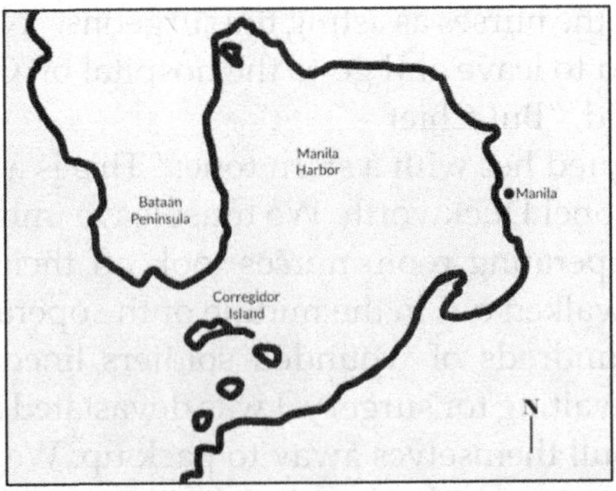

Two ancient, rickety buses rumbled in the twilight toward our hospital. The Filipina nurses boarded the first bus. We had been through this twice before. We knew the drill. Most of the nurses wanted to say goodbye to the patients and disburse instructions to the physicians and medical corpsmen on how to care for them, but time had run out. *How can we abandon this many patients?* I thought as I squeezed my hands together to keep them from shaking.

"How can I leave Ronny in his full body cast?" Caroline cried out.

"Wh-what about our blind patient, Carlos? Who will give him enough attention?" Carmelita stuttered.

One of the medics walked by and I asked, "Where's Davy? I want to thank him for all his help in the hospital."

Medic Fred whispered to me, "Davy left. He told me he did not want to be captured or tortured by the Japs. A few medics snuck out into the jungle. Please don't mention it to the doctors."

"Do you know where he went?"

"He said he'd walk to the dock and swim to Corregidor."

"It will be dark by then, How far is it?"

"It's eight miles swimming through shark-infested waters."

"Oh my god, this is atrocious. Do you think he'll make it?"

Fred hung his head. "Don't know. I've got to get back to the patients. Tell all the nurses Godspeed, Chief."

I murmured a quick prayer for poor Davy.

One of the bus drivers honked his horn and yelled, "Everyone get in, now! The road is crowded. Make it snappy before the Japs come!"

Many of the medics and physicians came out and waved to us, which produced many tears from the nurses. I glanced over at all my nurses. They looked thin and worn out. I counted as they boarded the bus with downturned faces, then followed behind and slid into a seat.

"Wait—where's Molly?" My voice cracked as I turned around in my seat and looked for her.

The driver honked again. Then I spied Doc Charlie out of the window. He got on the bus carrying Molly in his arms. She clung to him and sobbed. Charlie kissed her cheek as he set her tiny body down next to me. I put my arm around her shoulders. Molly wailed, "Come with me! I can't leave you. What if you go to prison? What if they kill you? I'm too young to be a widow." Molly heaved great sobs as she held on to her husband's neck.

"Darling, I need you to go. It will be safer for you under the rock in Corregidor." He whispered, "I'll come to Corregidor later."

Knowing there was nothing she could do, she leaned on my shoulder and continued crying. All the nurses were heartbroken and teary-eyed as I stroked her hair and soothed her the best I could.

We traveled 18 miles to the Mariveles dock up and over

steep mountains on the congested roads. The old bus creaked and groaned. I kept my arm around Molly and held her until her sobs turned to sniffles as the bus took us down the windy road toward the bay. We were all in a state of shock and refused to believe that Bataan had fallen, even though all the bombs that fell made it obvious we were losing. In silence, we worried about what was to become of our hospital, our needy patients, the medics, and the physicians we had left behind.

The heavy dust rose and gave a ghost-like appearance to the early evening as the evacuation of Bataan bordered on the insane. The jungle was thick on the sides of the roads, making them almost impassable. Nighttime was the safest time to travel on the bumpy road, but also difficult because we had to have partially blacked-out headlights.

The night became darker and we were stuck behind lines of soldiers many miles long. Any time we had to stop, soldiers would fist-pound the bus, crying, "Let us in! Help us before the Japs pick us off!"

Frantic natives clogged the road. All the poor refugees dragged carts filled with their meager life possessions, and their children either rode on them or were pulled along by their arms. We witnessed Filipino civilians fleeing while the Japanese pommeled them with shells from overhead. The pleas of the hikers were unbearable and we were helpless to assist them.

Nurse Angelica cried out the window, "Sorry, we have no room!"

Some of the nurses held their hands over their mouths to silence their cries. Where were all these poor people headed?

Our buses inched along the crooked, narrow road to the port of Mariveles. The night sky glowed with fire from the bombs. The short ride from our hospital to the boat turned into hours as our bus jolted and bucked along the road. The sound of shellfire made us feel vulnerable. I shouted behind my seat on the bus, "Put on your helmets and hold on to your gas masks!"

At last, we reached the naval base at Mariveles. We almost jumped out of our seats when we heard explosives that made a tremendous boom. There was a stall in traffic, and I called to the driver, "Are we being bombed?"

"No, lady, our ammunition dumps on the hill are being set off. That way the Japs can't steal the ammunition and use it against us."

The nurses held their ears with their hands as the ordnance stockpiles were detonated.

We arrived at the crowded dock behind massive groups of soldiers who waited to embark while officers snapped out orders in the dark of night. The nurses found a small space on the wooden dock where they huddled together and rested their heads on their bags, exhausted from the heartbreak of the journey. I felt hunger pangs and rubbed my shrunken stomach. It had never been so flat. At least I had the fat to lose, unlike most of the gals.

The water lapped at the pilings as boats pulled in and took soldiers away. I watched the shadowy forms of the native boats and rafts that tried to escape. Were we too exposed on this dock? I patted my pocket to feel for my gun and sock of bullets. The well-traveled Colt .45 had become more of a good luck charm than a weapon. The suicide pills were lost long ago, probably eaten by a rat looking for a meal.

At the harbor, I could make out the disguised surface submarine where we had dined and danced into the night. It seemed like a long-ago, faded memory and I sniffed back some tears. Above us, enemy planes strafed as many boats as possible on the bay. The weak gurgle of, "Help me! Help me!" rang out as several boats were hit by Japanese artillery fire.

Would there be a boat for us, and would we be safe? I held my pounding forehead.

Molly hollered out into the darkness, "There's a sailboat but we can't all fit on that!"

Enemy planes hovered overhead like lions ready to pounce on their prey. We waited for two anxious hours before a harbor boat appeared and we were called to board, but after a blanket of Japanese planes swarmed in the sky and let loose their bombs, the boat blew up in flames.

A military officer boomed, "Girls, run into the jungle for cover!"

We dashed off the dock and headed for the trees. In the jungle, we found a few foxholes and bushes. The rest of the nurses lay flat on the ground.

A short time later, the officer found us. "There should be a boat anytime now that might fit all of you. Stay where you are, and I'll call you when one arrives."

More time went by as we lay there and shivered with fear in the dark. We continued to hear the deafening noise of our own ammunition dumps as they blew up and made the night sky glow with fierce fires. It was the opposite of a cheerful Fourth of July celebration.

After a complete hour of silence from the skies, we heard, "Here comes your boat, nurses! Hurry up!"

We tramped back down to the dock.

A sailor on the boat called out, "Nurses only. Hurry!" He pointed to a rickety rope ladder we had to climb to get into the boat. It was difficult because we were all weak from hunger.

The sailors on board whistled and smiled, overjoyed to see a "skirt" even though we wore fatigues. We squished onto the deck and sat on our bags, shoulder to shoulder, with a few of us on the boat's gunwales.

As we headed away from shore, we watched the fireworks that continued to explode on Bataan. Flames streaked through the black sky and the ammunitions echoed from the cliffs that surrounded the harbor.

The boat ride was fun at first as flirtations between the sexes ignited. Several sailors brought our group opened cans of hash, peaches, and beans with spoons for all. We gobbled the food like primitive savages, and drank the juice from the peaches for dessert.

Halfway to Corregidor, we got caught in a crossfire and hugged ourselves in fear. It should have taken less than an hour for the boat to get to Corregidor but the captain steered in a zigzag pattern to avoid being targeted, so it took longer. When the ship finally began to go full speed, Nurse Annie was the first to throw up, followed by Carmelita, who retched over the opposite rail. Her large helmet wobbled on her head as she heaved over the side.

After all of us had vomited our meager dinner overboard, I wound my way through the crowd to find the captain at the wheel of the vessel. "Captain, could we please go straighter? My nurses have gotten sick."

The big, rugged captain gave me the once-over and snapped, "Listen, miss, we've got to zigzag to avoid getting hit. Just empty your stomachs and hold on. We'll have to dodge the enemy aircraft the entire way."

The two-mile boat ride from the Limay dock took three-and-a-half hours. Japanese planes flew overhead the entire time, setting our nerves on edge. Soldiers and Filipino islanders swam into the night, away from fallen Bataan, and tried to get boats to pick them up. Some found leaky, abandoned rafts to ride on. We continued to hear the cries of people who were drowning.

Carmelita recited a prayer for our medic, Davy, who was swimming out there somewhere among the sharks. We passed many stragglers calling, "Save me, save me!" But we had no room.

The captain of the ship told me about Corregidor. "Up ahead is what we all call The Rock. It has a strategic location at the entrance to Manila Bay and is an underground, impregnable fortress with a vast network of tunnels. Corregidor island is four miles long, and is a fortified outpost that guards the entrance to the bay."

I paid attention to him the best I could, but I was quite nauseated from the ride and couldn't reply to anything he said.

Dawn was breaking when I saw the fascinating, pollywog-shaped island. All our weary, seasick nurses gathered their musette bags and we climbed down onto the dock. The sweet scent from the gardenias that bloomed throughout the island invigorated our senses.

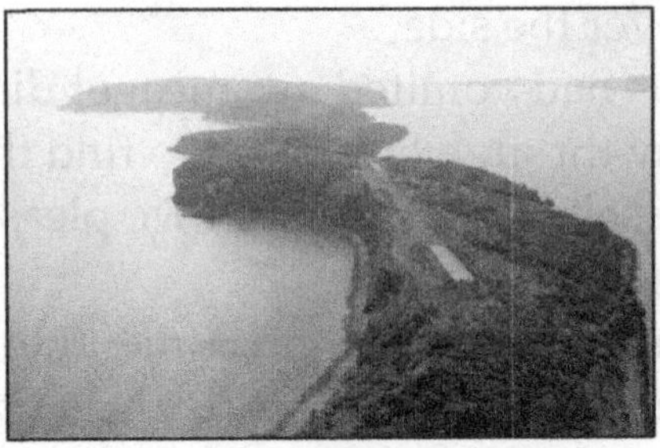

The well-muscled, serious Sergeant Hallahan met us as we disembarked and gave us a tour of the island. "We're on the Topside of the island of Corregidor. Over there is the abandoned Fort Mills with a two-story stone barracks building, military headquarters, and an empty hospital. Also on Topside are modern officers' quarters for General MacArthur, but he left for safety on March 18 and went to Australia. Lt. General Wainwright is the Commander of Allied forces in the Philippines and resides here. That level is off-limits for everyone. Over there are the many major gun batteries, plus two concrete pits holding mortars. It's all camouflaged by trees and scrub with soldiers at the ready. Before the war, Fort Mills had a 90-bed hospital, an officers' club, golf course, tennis courts, bowling alley, and swimming pool. We have here over 12,000 Allied American and Filipino combat troops with over a thousand U.S. Marines in dugouts along the beach, and U.S. Army soldiers who man the big guns."

Several of the nurses yawned. After all, it was 6:30 a.m. and none of us had slept during this frightful night.

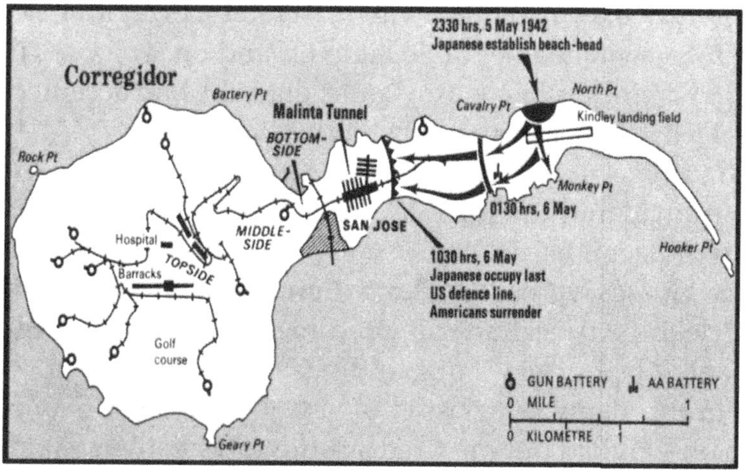

Sergeant Hallahan said, "It's just a short walk to Bottomside and the Malinta Tunnel, where the nurses' quarters are."

I heard someone sigh with relief.

We went through a concrete entrance that had "1932" carved above it. Our dirty, disheveled, worn-out group followed the sergeant through the elaborate labyrinth into one of 20 tunnels to the nurses' quarters. I noticed that the well-lit tunnels were all numbered on the clean, shiny-white walls.

Before we entered the dormitory, the sergeant said, "Girls, choose an empty bed and get some sleep. I'll come back later to take you to chow."

We tiptoed around the Corregidor nurses, who were sound asleep, found a group of sturdy iron beds, and dropped onto them, exhausted.

I was the first to wake up and saw that each bed had a

shiny enamel table with a lamp and a small dresser with several clean towels on it. The resident nurses were at work in the hospital.

Susie saw me stir and said, "This is like the Ritz Hotel compared to our jungle hospitals."

Molly woke up with a yawn. "Hotel Corregidor, I love you!" She switched her table lamp off and on.

I gave Molly a big, warm smile, glad she had accepted her fate of leaving her husband behind.

Annie exclaimed, "Let there be light! Halleluiah."

I grinned and thought, *No need for forced blackouts here like we had in Baguio a few times.*

The nurses were all smiles within the safety of the tunnel, with clean beds and after a good night's sleep. We were all enchanted by our new surroundings.

I grabbed my eyeglasses off my bedside table and put them on. I pulled out my tired, crumpled bag, then felt inside it. Stuffed in the corner, I felt the cracked framed photograph of my parents, tugged it out, and placed it on top of my table. Then I took out Rob's watch and traced the inscription with my finger. I longed for the comfort of his voice, then shook my head and placed the watch in one of the drawers. I put my weapon away and felt safe, hidden underground inside this impenetrable rock away from the enemy.

The nurses chatted with gaiety while they arranged their belongings. I further explored our quarters and saw indoor showers with hot water and real bars of soap, unlike the primitive hose showers we'd had in Baguio. The flush latrines were a marvel. I wandered around and saw electric lights that were kept on in the underground fortress.

The sergeant came by and walked us through the elaborate tunnels to get to chow. We got in line behind the many personnel. The hot food gave off comforting, enticing smells and we were told to take as much as we wanted. It was like we were in front of a pile of Christmas presents that came in the form of abundant food. We ate with a few of the nurses who had been there since last year. Our stomachs had shrunk from Baguio and most of us left a lot on our plates.

One of the nurses, who was about to leave, said, "Be sure to have a Coca-Cola and ice cream before you go!"

We had a little bit of soda with a spoonful of ice cream, and it was a delight. One nurse managed to drink an entire glass of the Coca-Cola float.

After chow, the sergeant gave us the rest of the tour. "Now…where was I? Oh yes, we covered the Topside. There are three levels on Corregidor—Topside, Middleside, and Bottomside. The Bottomside is the harbor area where there are 11 major gun batteries, anti-aircraft installations, and two concrete pits holding 12-inch mortars. Within the elaborate tunnel labyrinth is the Malinta Tunnel. The main corridor is 750 feet long, 25 feet wide and 15 feet high." He smiled. "Each lateral houses a special division of the fort."

We were shown the machine shops, refrigeration plants, and the doctors' quarters.

"Above you in each lateral archway are red lights that flash upon any attack on the island. The Japanese had been bombing the island since December, then stopped to take over Bataan. We have over 10,000 people on this island. The well-designed concrete tunnels are bomb-proof. As you can see, there are many ventilation shafts with blowers to bring in fresh air. This incredible underground fortress was built in secrecy years before the war. General Kilbourne negotiated with the Philippine government to ship hundreds of Filipino prisoners to build the facility. Corregidor has its own power and water supply. We also have an underground double-track electric car line to ferry supplies."

Molly burst out, "Wow—a train? In here?"

The sergeant continued, "The adjacent laterals are used to store food, medicine, and ordnance. The other laterals serve as barracks and administrative offices. What we have here is an incredible engineering feat. It was built after the Spanish-American War and became a U.S. military station. It was designed by American engineers and carved out with Philippine Scouts as the foremen, and Filipino convicts as workers, in 1922. It took 10 years to complete by blasting it with hand-rolled TNT cartridges." He ended the tour at the hospital. "I hope you'll all be comfortable here and will find our facility well equipped to care for our wounded soldiers. Ladies, I'd like you to meet Captain Ruth Burrows, who is in charge of the hospital. She will take over from here and give you the rest of the tour."

I introduced myself to an older, hunchbacked woman with stark white hair pulled back into a large bun under a small nursing cap. We followed the stoic captain, who must have been 50 years old—the mandatory age for retirement.

Captain Burrows said in a no-nonsense voice, "Our underground hospital is 100 yards long in the main section and includes eight smaller laterals that consist of convalescent and recovery wards. It is the largest hospital in the world and has a dental clinic, operating rooms, dining areas, and kitchen, plus a pharmacy. We are well equipped with refrigerators and cabinets." She opened the doors of a cabinet to display a huge assortment of surgical equipment.

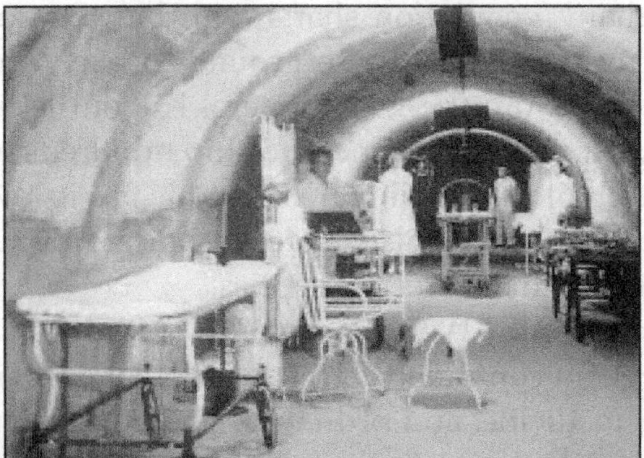

My mind drifted to Sternberg Hospital, then to Grace Hospital back home, and I was impressed. "How long have you been here?" I asked as we walked.

The captain said, "Since December."

"How many beds are here?"

"We have a 1,000-bed hospital." She gave a small, proud smile for the first time.

Our group of nurses followed Captain Burrows down the lateral into the convalescent wards.

"Chief Bea, Chief Bea!" I heard two patients exclaim.

I turned and saw Rosemary and Rita, who had been wounded by shrapnel at Baguio and were sent to Corregidor before we arrived.

"Oh girls, I'm very happy to see that you made it here! I've been worried about you. How are you both?"

Rita spoke up, "We're getting better. We can thank our lucky stars that the lieutenant general got us out of Bataan before the Japanese took over. We have received the best of care."

Rosemary added, "I think we'll be good enough to go to work tomorrow." She glanced at Captain Burrows.

The captain frowned. "Not yet, girls. You have to be fully recovered from your shrapnel wounds."

All the nurses gathered around Rosemary and Rita with happy smiles, glad to see they had made it to Corregidor.

I asked them if they had seen our medic, Davy. They hadn't.

Captain Burrows interrupted abruptly, "Chief Harrington, are your nurses ready to work?"

"Yes, of course, Captain," I said.

After our work shift, Captain Burrows informed me that we would be given new, clean nursing uniforms. Before I could say thank you, she left. It would take some getting used to, having a boss who was so impersonable.

We felt comforted by having 350 feet of solid rock above

us and three meals every day. None of us missed the creatures that roamed at night in the jungle and their scary noises. The nurses had regularly scheduled breaks, where they could go outside to smoke or catch some sun.

The next day, I saw Davy out of the corner of my eye. "Oh Davy, it's good to see you. You made it! I was worried about how you'd survive with the sharks in the water."

"Nice to see you, Chief Bea. I was happier to dodge sharks and end up here than in a Japanese prison camp."

"Davy, please don't mention that to Molly," I whispered. "She had to leave her husband behind."

"Don't you worry, I won't. Isn't it wonderful here?" He flashed his adorable grin.

"It is and I'm glad to work with you again."

Chapter Eighteen
Dottie
Tagap, Burma 1944

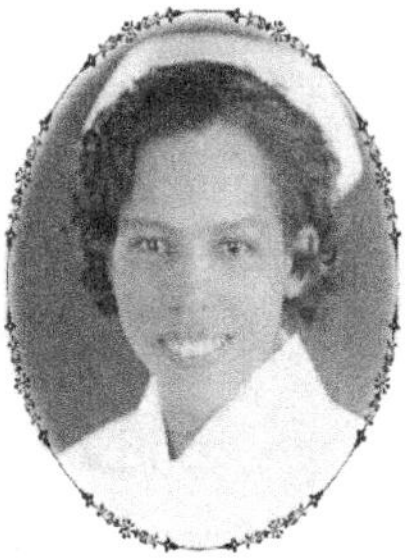

The next few weeks were filled with unexpected events. One night, while in a deep sleep in my tent after I had worked for over 12 hours, I woke to the sound of a shrill scream. I crawled out of my tent and yelled, "What's wrong? Who's screaming?"

Flashlight in hand, I shined it inside Mary and Hazel's tent. They held on to each other in fright.

Mary shouted and swatted her legs. "There's something in here that's jumping and climbing all over us—and it sure ain't mosquitoes!"

Hazel flung a creature at me. "Ewww, it's slimy! Get me outta here!" She ducked out of the tent and Mary crawled out behind her.

I caught the creature with one hand. "It's a lizard. I'm pretty sure they don't bite. But this one has weird, crossed eyes."

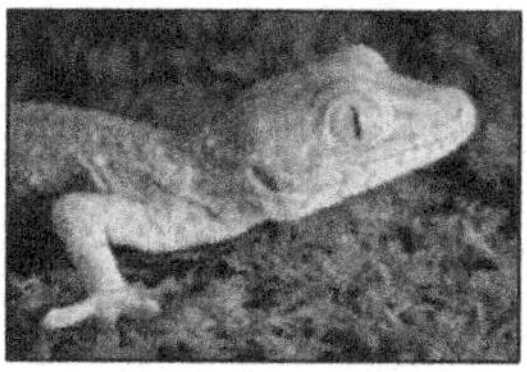

The "jumpers" in their tent were two frogs, the biggest I had ever seen—not like the cute little ones we had in Georgia. I tried to reassure the girls that they were harmless, even though I wasn't that certain. I captured the creatures and threw them out into the jungle. Handy Hazel found her flashlight. She shined it on her Red Cross kit and proceeded to safety pin the tent flaps together after I left.

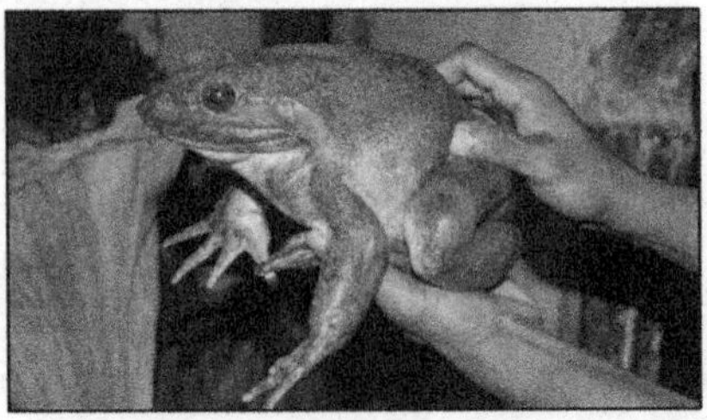

The next night, a different tent of girls screeched. This time there was a humongous, fat snake half in and half out of their tent. It must have been 20 feet long. I suppressed a gasp, then spun on my heels and ran to wake up Major John. He followed me back to the girls' tent, grabbed the snake by the tail, and flung it into the jungle. He told us it was a harmless python.

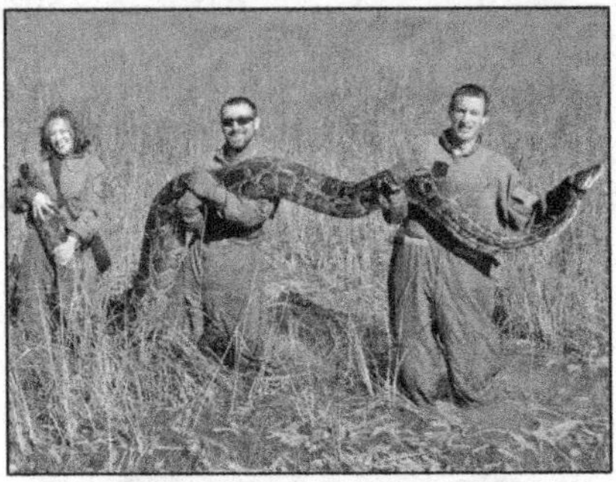

The next morning, the nurses shook out their clothes and looked for hitchhiker creatures in need of shelter. Many of the gals found some in their shoes. I ordered everyone to follow Hazel's example of safety pinning their tents closed at night so everyone could get a good night's sleep. We had to be able to do our jobs properly. I remembered from one of the Army's lectures that survival was the ability to adapt. How true this rang in this bizarre environment.

Later that day, Doc Samuel told me he'd read in one of his books that although pythons were not poisonous, they could kill a human by slowly squeezing them to death and were categorized as constrictors. He added that they didn't usually bite but if they did, it took very little time to recover from the wound. I kept my thoughts to myself, but that scary snake was taller than me and very fat. I hoped we wouldn't encounter another one.

The next night after work, sleep enveloped my tired body like a warm blanket. My legs ached from the hike up to chow and walking the length of the ward all day. Dreams did not come my way, which I preferred since when I did dream, they were usually disturbing.

I woke to an odd snorting noise and rolled over, thinking it was a nightmare. *How much more can I take?* I thought sleepily. From the tent next to me came a cry that pierced the jungle. I reached for my flashlight. After I heard another snort, I crawled outside and shined my light on the rear end of a massive creature with a cow-like tail that half poked out of the tent next to mine.

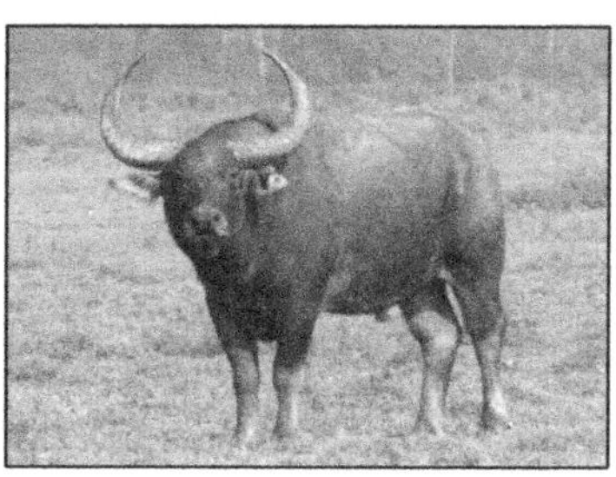

I screamed for help. The other nurses tumbled out of their tents, rubbing their eyes while Clara and Betty, trapped inside their tent by the creature, hollered for help as well.

I squinted. "I think it's a cow. No wait…it's what's called a water buffalo." I yelled to Betty and Clara, "Girls, stay calm. I don't think it will bite!" I then instructed, "Now, Clara, Betty, both of you are strong so push on its horns and face. The rest of us will pull on its tail and rear end, then steer it down the hill."

The nurses gingerly surrounded the buffalo's hind end and reached for its tail and hindquarters.

I shouted, "Push, push!" to Clara and Betty, then to the rest of the group, "Pull, pull!"

At last, the water buffalo backed out and lumbered back into the jungle.

I looked inside the tent. Near Betty's duffel bag was a package half full of chocolate chip cookies sent from home. I grabbed it. "Girls, this is why no food is allowed in our tents!" I said, waving it at the nurses. "There are too many hungry creatures here looking for a handout. For heaven's sake, we need our sleep. No food in the tents. Y'all got that?"

No one answered me. My patience was as thin as a scalpel blade. I shined my light on everyone until they nodded in agreement, then went back to my cot. I lay there, pleased that we had tackled that disaster without waking the doctors.

Chapter Nineteen
Bea
Corregidor, April 1942

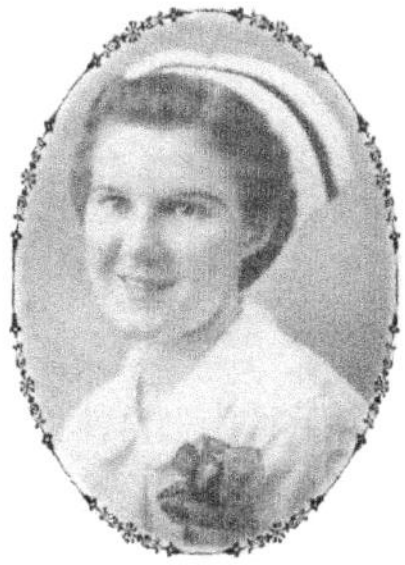

Josephina was our resident housekeeper. When there were enough nurses off-duty in our quarters, she pulled out boxes from under her bed and held an impromptu sale. One box contained dresses, another had skirts and blouses, and the third, various apparel items. She had obtained all these clothes from Corregidor nurses who had transferred before the war broke out.

When Josephina first saw our crew with our stained uniforms and raggedy coveralls, she became over-the-top excited to sell us everything. It had been a long time since we had seen civilian clothes and our group was thrilled about all the outfits.

She would show one dress and point to each nurse it would fit, then say in her broken English, "This good on you! Try on. How much you give me?"

Molly bought several dresses. She twirled around in her striped shirtwaist dress with a matching plaid jacket, and said, "My Charlie would love this one!"

We all clapped with gusto as her face lit up with excitement.

Veronica bought all the lipstick Josephina had and was

delighted because she had almost run out.

Josephina held up a taffeta ballgown. "Chief, this one look nice on you!"

I declined. There was nowhere to wear it. We weren't in Manila anymore, and besides, it was no longer peacetime.

Josephina insisted with a chuckle, "I give you scarf or belt free if you buy dress!"

Nurse Jane checked to see if I wanted it, then yelled out a number. This livened up all the nurses and a bidding war ensued.

Most of the nurses bought and assembled decent outfits even though we had no opportunity to wear them. It was a fun fantasy and did bring the gals a great deal of enjoyment. Sometimes at night, a few of the nurses would dress up in their new fancy clothes and have a fashion show as a form of relaxation.

Practical me bought nothing – not because of my large size but because I knew none of the outfits could be worn in the hospital. I was satisfied just to have a clean, new uniform.

The following day, one of the Corregidor nurses confided in me, "Stay friends with Josephina, she has set up her own personal business and gives manicures and shampoos, and can style finger waves!"

Mr. Wang was another asset on Corregidor. He was an older Chinese refugee and was a skilled tailor who resided in the tunnel behind ours. I loved to hear the echo of the sewing machine, which sounded like it went at top speed nonstop. His main job was to clean but when he had extra time, he sewed for everyone, including the resident quartermasters. He tailored many of the dresses that were purchased from Josephina and charged only a pittance for his services. This proved to be beneficial since most of us had lost a lot of weight. I heard Veronica whining, "I've lost my curves!"

Josephina established a smart business, giving shampoos and finger waves for two pesos, or $1, and manicures for 75 centavos, or 38 cents. It felt luxurious to indulge in these treats. We felt safe and secure with a ceiling over our heads and no monkeys, iguanas, ants, or snakes to bother the patients. Not only were we well fed with nutritious meals, but it was a relief to serve the patients as well. The last weeks of Baguio with only one meager meal a day were behind us. Everyone was happy to do their work without the fear of being bombed in the protective tunnel hospital. As a surgical nurse, it was a marvel to have unlimited supplies and sufficient lighting.

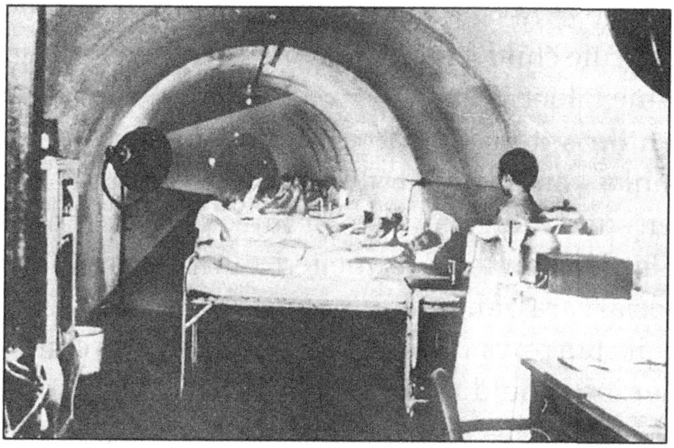

The state of the Bataan refugees that came in tugged at our hearts. They were hungry and their friends and families had often been killed. Captain Burrows found room in an empty tunnel where the refugees could live.

One day, a Filipino soldier brought in a cute little six-year-old he had found stowed away on a ship from Bataan. The soldier held him and spoke to the squirming boy in Tagalog to soothe him as I struggled to take his temperature.

"How did you get him to come here with you?" I asked.

The soldier blushed and showed me the candy he had in his pocket, then looked at me, his eyes filled with worry. "Will he live?"

I examined little Antonio. "He has a temperature of over 103 and has malaria."

"Please cure him. I got the story out of the boy that his entire family was killed and he wandered away and hid on a ship."

"Don't worry, we have medicine here for malaria. We'll take good care of him."

"Let me know when he's better and I'll take him with us back to the field camp." He smiled at the boy and gave him a piece of candy.

"There's no way I would allow that. It would be unsafe for the little tyke. After he's well, I'll see if he can stay here." I bathed the cute child's forehead with cool water and gave him an Atabrine tablet.

Poor little Antonio had a severe case of malaria. He would lie motionless and stare at all the nurses with his big brown eyes, then suddenly flash a small smile of affection, revealing his cute little dimples. He melted our hearts, and we took extra-special care of him.

Captain Burrows questioned me about the child. "When he's better, he should return to his family."

I told her he was an orphan and pleaded for him to stay. The nurses backed me up and the captain relented.

We ended up "adopting" him and as little Antonio got better, Carmelita gave him English lessons since he spoke only Tagalog. He was a wonderful diversion for all the nurses after they'd tended to the influx of sick and wounded soldiers from Bataan. When Antonio was cured, part of a lateral was cleared, and he was able to use an old bathtub with a mattress and blankets as a bed. Mr. Wang heard us talking about the little fellow and visited him, took out his measuring tape, then made several cute little outfits for our boy by piecing together used clothing.

One day, I had to supervise over 200 cases of food poisoning when an entire battery division arrived after eating contaminated meat. We didn't have enough emesis pans and in desperation, I found as many pails, bowls, and buckets as I could. The stuffy tunnel reeked with the smell of vomit. Thank God it lasted only two days. We quickly discovered that the tunnel's ventilation system did not work as well as Sergeant Hallahan claimed it did.

Captain Burrows was a tyrant and strict disciplinarian who demanded all the nurses follow the rules to the letter. It was hard on the nurses to have two bosses. I ended up obeying her orders and took the role of a nurse instead of chief when I was in her presence. She oversaw all breaks, and no one was allowed to ask for a bathroom break if it wasn't time. The captain scrutinized every shot given and every bandage applied.

I noticed that my nurses avoided eye contact with her and spoke behind her back about her meanness. Veronica called her the "old bag." I sympathized. Captain Burrows' bluntness was hard to bear. If only she would say please and thank you, it would have been a more pleasant atmosphere.

Each night before the captain went to bed, she drank half a bottle of whiskey, then fell asleep in a stupor and snored so loud it was difficult for the nurses to get a good night's sleep.

In the evenings, both soldiers and medical personnel ventured outside. If a bomber was sighted, the warning system of red lights would flash inside and we'd return to the safety of the tunnels. Break time was fun and I went outside with everyone when I could. I loved the sweet smell of the many flowers that bloomed on the island, and the lovely breezes of the tropical night, or sun-catching during the day. I noticed several gals flirting with the soldiers. I overheard them as they talked about spooning in the bushes—out of earshot of the captain, of course. I tried to remind them to be careful, that pregnancy would mean immediate dismissal from the Army, and they would nod in agreement, then ignore what I said.

One evening, three soldiers on their break hung out in the main portion of Malinta Tunnel, which looked like a large building with numerous corridors that fingered out from it. They played a harmonica, guitar, and trombone and the music uplifted everyone. Nurses and soldiers joined in, singing songs like "Home on the Range" and "The Yellow Rose of Texas." The song "You Are My Sunshine" was the most popular. It was a pleasure to watch many of the nurses dance with each other or with the men, and it was a much-needed escape since we were experiencing a brief reprieve from the war. Many of the nurses wore outfits they had bought from Josephina. We all had a great time since Captain Burrows was sound asleep, anesthetized by her liquor.

On April 26, only two weeks after the surrender of Bataan, two large 240 mm shells exploded near the main entrance, which slammed the tunnel's slatted iron gate shut. Screams were heard from the outside, where soldiers were taking a smoke break. Medical personnel ran toward the entrance and had to remove body parts from the gate to pry it open. Fourteen men lay dead and over 70 were wounded. A soldier's head rolled toward my feet. I didn't scream but jumped away, then threw up.

It was back to battlefield nursing again as we applied tourniquets and lanced off mangled fingers and toes, filling buckets with amputated flesh. All that night, the nurses and physicians worked endless, harrowing hours as we ripped off clothing to give injections, stitched gaping wounds, bandaged patients, and settled the treated patients in their beds. With sorrow, we covered those we could not save with sheets.

I still had not grown accustomed to seeing torn-up people—people who bled and died in great numbers with legs and arms wrenched off, jagged flesh wounds, and pieces of exploded shrapnel stuck in ugly wounds. A sense of numbness seemed to set in to keep us in the frantic pace of healing. When one patient died, it was agonizing, but when faced with such mass suffering and death, it left a crack inside of you and you wouldn't ever be quite the same again. Then, as a healer, you became robotic, somehow making the right decisions and automatically going through the motions. After that horrific night, no one went outside anymore, which made for a depressed atmosphere.

The heaviest artillery and air bombardment was two days later. The dust was horrendous and the entire island was on fire. The marvelous haven of The Rock became as hellish as Bataan with the incessant bombing. Medicine bottles fell out of cabinets and bunkbeds trembled from the concussive bombs. Every blast shook loose flakes of concrete and the dust spread through the ventilation system. Chronic coughs became prolific. Several times, the power plant that supplied the tunnel with electricity was hit and left us without electricity or lights. Sometimes the generators failed and we became moles in the dark.

It was ghastly in there. We felt the shock of each detonation and never knew when we would be in total darkness. When the electricity did fail, the corpsmen had to hold flashlights so the surgeons could operate. I felt like I was in an Egyptian tomb, and to cope, my mind drifted to the ride with Rob in the horse-drawn carriage in the open, fresh air with the smell of the ocean nearby.

The bombing and artillery attacks increased and the stale, muggy air mixed with the stench of disinfectants. Large amounts of people would gather at the tunnel's entrance to gulp the outdoor air in relief and to discover whether it was day or night.

The red lights that hung from the arched ceilings continued to flash warnings of impending attacks, but we worked through all the raids and only heard muffled thuds of bombs and shells from above. As bombs fell on Topside, a long parade of casualties came into the hospital. Our food supplies dwindled as the wounded soldiers poured in.

Veronica whined about the reduction in our meals to twice a day. "I liked the meals here and was just getting my weight back. Damn this war!" She puffed out her chest for all to see that her breast size was smaller.

On short breaks, we lost our sense of time and longed for the peaceful life we'd known in Manila before the war. I encouraged the nurses to talk about their families and hometowns and to avoid the subjects of food, love, or war.

The days crawled by as we worked at a frantic pace to try to help as many victims as possible. In surgery, a half-conscious boy's leg hung by shreds from his thigh. He said through gritted teeth, "Don't cut it off, don't cut it off..."

Nurse Annie stroked his arm. "We'll take good care of you, soldier, I promise."

I was proud of her reassuring manner but knew it was a hopeless case.

The litter-bearers brought in more and more soldiers every day. The tunnels were hot and cave-like. We were all cooped up with no natural light or air and felt disoriented, not knowing whether it was day or night. There was too much dirt and dust, and now large black flies swarmed in the tunnels and we started seeing rats. The odor of urine, sweat, and mildew combined with the fumes from the diesel generators was intolerable. The ventilation system became inadequate, and the walls dripped with moisture. Each shell or bomb that hit the area above the hospital loosened more dust and dirt and raised the dust level in the tunnels.

I went and spoke to our housekeepers about the flies and rats. The crowded tunnels were kept clean and as sanitary as possible by Josephina and Mr. Wang but as the number of patients increased, it was hard to keep up with. The Malinta Tunnel was a monumental feat of engineering, but it was not intended to have this many people in it. We were hidden away like tunnel rats in a claustrophobic maze.

Nurse Annie, our best complainer, would grumble to

anyone who would listen, "When the electricity goes out, I feel like I'm in a cave and this damp air makes me cough all the time. And I've got skin boils." She showed her bumpy arms to everyone.

Jane joined in. "Look at mine!" She rolled up her sleeve and several *ugh* noises could be heard from the nurses.

I nipped the gripes in the bud because complaints spread like molasses on a piece of bread. Almost all the personnel had impetigo, a contagious bacterial skin disease, with sores around the nose and mouth or other exposed areas of the body. These sores would break open, ooze, and then crust. We began to call it "tunnel disease" because it occurred in the underground, crowded spaces. It was hard to comfort Veronica, the former high school beauty queen, who cried over the impetigo on her face. And to top it all off, we couldn't shower due to the water shortage.

I said to the nurses, "Any of you with bad cases need to see Dr. Shibley and get your ailments taken care of. He'll lance the welts and apply mercurochrome and salicylic acid. Everyone get back to work or if you still have break time, there's a little library here. Go find a good escape book to read."

Captain Burrows came by to check on all the chatter. This made the nurses scatter and not another word was said.

A short time later, I was back in surgery, in the dark without a flashlight. I stooped down to give a morphine injection to a young man on a stretcher, and much to my horror, saw a body with no head. In shock, I yelled at the medical corpsman who had brought him in, "Why did you bring this body in?"

The young corpsman stammered, "It's dark out there, Chief, we can't use any flashlights and must feel for the wounded bodies, then roll them onto the stretchers. I didn't know he was dead."

"Next time feel for a head, for God's sake!" I was

exhausted and threw a sheet over the poor guy. "Get him out of here on the double." I found Agnes to replace me and left to get some rest to replenish my dwindling patience.

The nurses were given many of the cases that the doctors couldn't get to. The doctors would go down the long lines of bodies on stretchers, pointing and saying things like, "Take this one, nurse," and "You can handle that one."

Whenever the generators went out from the continuous bombing, the dark, damp tunnel felt claustrophobic, like a foxhole…or worse, a grave. The explosions reverberated throughout the tunnels and produced continual earaches and headaches. The walls and ceilings shook, and medicine fell out of cabinets that were not secured. I even thought I saw a bunk bed bounce.

This labyrinth became a suffocating, dark, malodorous environment with stale, muggy air mixed with the stench of disinfectants and anesthetics. An alarming number of staff continued to take desperate breaks at the tunnel's main entrance to catch some fresh air. I was too busy to do anything about it.

More beds were filled, and we could only serve the patients two meals a day, which meant we could now only have one. The food supply diminished, along with the medical supplies. The 500 patients turned into over 1,000 and we ran out of beds. As the shelling of Corregidor became heavier and more frequent, the population of casualties increased. The double-decked beds were welded into triple-decked beds. Civilian refugees slept packed in rows on the tunnel floors. It was a dreadful sign of the end drawing near. We had seen it all before, in Baguio.

The nurses continued to work endless hours, anesthetizing, helping with amputations, and sterilizing instruments. Our empty stomachs rumbled from near starvation. Days passed full of fatigue, lack of concentration, headaches, and lightheadedness. I couldn't prevent the nurses from continuous complaints since I wanted to join in myself. I was in a constant state of worry. How could we keep up the pace to heal all the wounded without proper nourishment?

The tunnel was full of gunpowder smoke and it was hard to breathe. The bombing hadn't ceased after the gate concussion, but for now, we were safely hidden in the underground rock hideout. Rumor had it that there was 350 feet of rock over us but in one place there was only 50. All the nurses wanted to know where that one place was, and would we be buried alive? No one seemed to know.

On a short break, Molly and I reminisced about fresh air, tropical breezes, and greenery, then dream-talked about the dances at the officers' club with our tropical cocktails. We agreed that even the sticky, humid outside air would be a welcome relief from the air inside the tunnels.

After a short night of sleep, I got back at it again. As I dressed, I overheard Angelica say in a loud, panic-stricken voice, "Those Japs are bombing my people out there and murdering them. When will this endless war stop?"

We all wondered the same thing. I touched her shoulder to reassure her. "We'll get through this." That was all the time I had to comfort her before I rushed back to work.

Water was scarce since it was brought in by barges from Bataan, which was now impossible. I took a quick inventory and saw that we had enough dressings and sulfa drugs, but would they last?

The narrow hospital corridors were crammed with the wounded, sick, and dying. And the raids continued. The basics of water, food, air, light, and supplies were essential for a hospital to run properly. And we had none of them.

The end of April was worse. Casualties were prolific. We had 14 air raids in one day, which started at 7:30 in the morning. There were three entrances to the hospital and the wounded were brought in from all of them. The entire island was under attack and was pounded relentlessly. I looked out the entrance and saw total devastation. Trees were down, roads were buried by debris, and the air was heavy with dust.

The Japanese blasted the field units, refrigerator plants, and warehouses on the outside. An entire unit of soldiers would likely die as they couldn't escape the shelling outside except for a few in some well-dug foxholes. Severely shell-shocked soldiers began stumbling into our hospital.

The water supply got lower and lower. We rationed water and washed our clothes in our helmets, then took wash-rag baths from them as well.

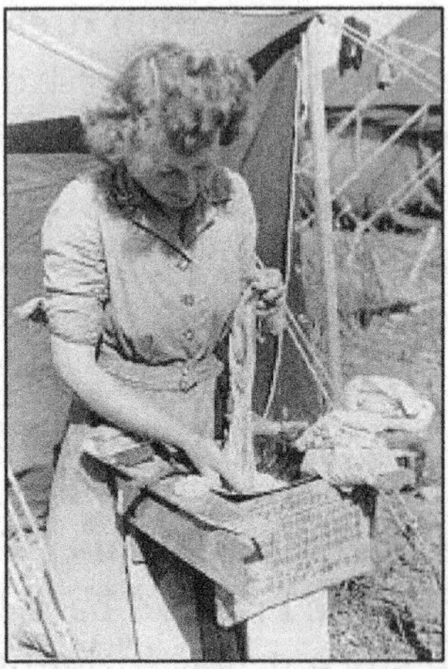

Washing clothes in a helmet.

Terrible rumors surfaced that our enemy could put poison gas in the air ducts or throw incendiary devices down the laterals. This did not help our already weakened morale at all. To say that everyone was on edge was an understatement. The only food left was several cans of meat and tomatoes, but we still had sacks of rice.

Lt. General Wainwright, commander of the Allied forces in the Philippines, made frequent visits to the hospital to cheer up the soldiers, thank them for their service, and praise all the nurses for their dedicated work. He always added, "We will win this war!"

I personally did not buy his optimism and thought our rock fortress was a bullseye just waiting to collapse.

The "Voice of Freedom" radio programs were broadcast three times a day. Every transmission ended with the statement, "Corregidor still stands! We encourage all the staff and soldiers to hold their ground."

On April 28, Lt. General Wainwright came into the hospital and took Captain Burrows and me aside. "Surrender to the Japanese is imminent. I received orders from General MacArthur to send 20 of our nurses to escape by Navy Catalina PBY seaplanes. They are to pack up and be prepared to fly to Melbourne, Australia where MacArthur is based. Do not tell anyone."

We both answered, "Yes, sir."

Captain Burrows and I were left in a quandary. We were unprepared for this, especially since Lt. General Wainwright said there was only room for 20. We decided to select the American nurses instead of the Filipina nurses because the Filipina nurses didn't want to leave their country. Then we narrowed it down to the older nurses in their 40s or 50s who wilted under the duress of war or nurses who were the sickest.

I chose my words carefully and said to Captain Burrows, "Captain, you deserve to leave and have served the Army well. Are you close to retirement age?"

The tired old nurse answered in a most quiet voice. "I suppose you're right, Chief, and I think I will leave."

Much to my relief, she went to pack. I could have picked myself to leave but as chief, I would not abandon my patients or the nurses that remained. I naturally chose Rosemary and Rita, who still convalesced from their shrapnel wounds. They were both grateful as well as relieved.

Caroline, one of the nurses I selected, took me aside. "Chief Bea, I want to go but I don't want to go because I'm sure I'll never see any of the nurses again. I'd rather face whatever is to happen here because we've been through a lot together. Plus, I don't want to leave my patients."

I answered, "I understand how you feel and am honored by your patriotism; however, you've been sick and this is why you were chosen. I wish you the best of luck and we will all miss you." I marched away to hide my tearful face.

Jane and Molly came into the dorm on a break.

Jane asked the nurses who were packing, "What are you doing and where are you going? You're leaving us, aren't you?"

Molly broke down in tears. "I want to go. I've had enough of war and I want to stay alive to be with my husband."

I interrupted and lied, "I'm sorry, girls, these are strict Army orders from Lt. General Wainwright, who made up the list. I had no choice."

Susie, who had a fever, tried to pack up but could barely open her eyes. "I don't want to leave my wounded soldiers."

"The Army commander has ordered you to leave," I lied once again to move her into action. She was of no use here and would get proper medical care in Australia.

Those who were ordered to leave had survivor's guilt and wanted to stay, and those who stayed wanted to leave. It was a problematic situation.

"Why can't I go?" Nurse Agnes asked. "I don't want to be here when the Japanese come. I heard they maim and rape nurses."

This remark caused a great deal of hysteria. I tried to be sympathetic but to no avail.

A sergeant came in and whispered in my ear that Colonel William Carter, an older department surgeon, had decided to leave. It was a dreadful job for me to have to "unpick" one nurse. But when all was said and done, the nurses who remained sadly agreed with the plan and frantically wrote letters home so they could be mailed from Australia. Letters were pressed into the hands of the group before they left, with pleas of, "Mail this to my Johnny, I want him to know I'm still alive," and "Send this to my family, I'm sure they're sick with worry."

The 19 nurses, with sad and tired faces, waved goodbye to those who stayed behind, and followed the colonel out of the tunnel. As I watched them go, I knew the odds of flying to Australia were slim and I prayed that it would not be a suicide mission. They left under cover of darkness.

On May 2, the Japanese attacked for 12 straight hours with 500-pound shells and over a million pounds of explosives. The bombs pounded us from outside and never let up. I tended to a wounded soldier brought in that day who told me there was total devastation outside, with downed trees and a gaping crater deep in the rock of Corregidor.

The explosions from outside flung bottles, dishes, and any loose objects off of shelves and onto the floor. Several people were knocked to the ground from the concussions. A few officers and privates came into the smoke-filled tunnel and told us they had been relieved of duty and knew that surrender was to occur. They lay on any available bed and either dropped into exhausted sleep or stared blankly from severe shellshock with weary, bloodshot eyes.

General MacArthur requested that the submarine *USS Spearfish* transport more nurses to Australia. He told me to pick 12 nurses to escape on the secret submarine. I hoped that the submarine would be safer than the two planes that had left a few days ago.

Annie came into the barracks after her shift and stormed right up to my face. "I heard about the submarine and I want to leave on it. I didn't ask to go on the planes because they'd most likely be shot down anyway."

"I'm sorry, Annie, the general gave me a specific list of the nurses who are to leave."

"Chief Bea, my fiancé died in this outrageous war, and I

deserve to leave. I want to see my family."

I sighed. "I have no choice in this matter. Army orders."

I left her as she cried. I no longer had the strength to comfort her.

After the next group of nurses left, the ones who remained behind languished in despair. A thick hopelessness hung in the stale air.

Chapter Twenty
Dottie
Tagap, Burma 1944

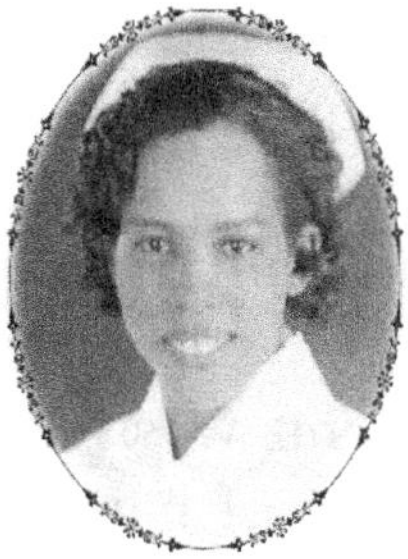

When on duty, I wore my Army cap, shirt, tie, and skirt, and pinned my Grady name tag on my shirt. I wanted all the patients to identify that I was in charge. We kept our hair rolled up as it was sticky hot all the time. Some of us fashioned rolls on the top and back of our heads, others just bunched their hair up and wrapped it in a white snood. I had one roll of hair in the back and my cap kept the rest out of my face at work.

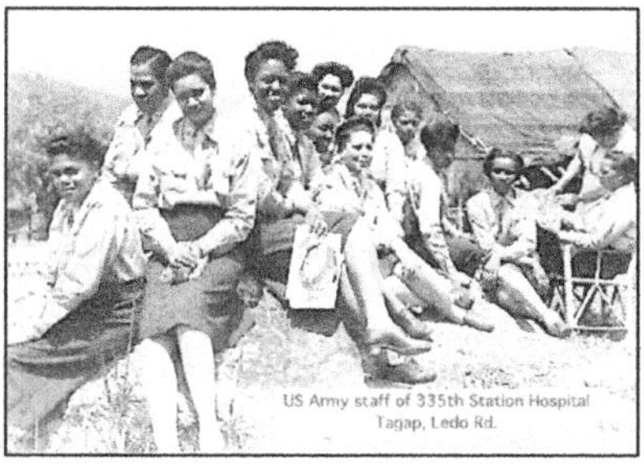
US Army staff of 335th Station Hospital
Tagap, Ledo Rd.

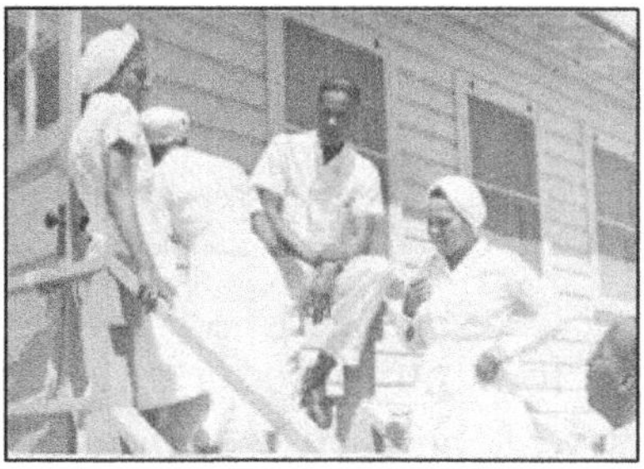

The primitive showers consisted of a hose connected to a #10 can with nail holes punched in the bottom to make a shower spray. The makeshift shower was enclosed in a shed.

We were smart pioneers and used our large metal helmets to wash our clothes in. The climate was so hot it took only 30 minutes for our clothes to dry hanging from a tree branch. We grew accustomed to living this way.

The ward was not the sterile environment we were used to. All the nurses protested the dirt floors and open sides.

I brushed off their comments and reminded them, "After all, we work in a jungle."

I tried not to be upset about the horrific conditions but the first night I was on duty I saw giant rats running up and down the rows between beds. This was worse than Liberia! Before me stretched endless rows of bamboo beds. Bamboo poles held up a palm-frond roof. There were no sides, no dividers or privacy for the sick or injured patients. Of course, I had to keep any negative, worrisome thoughts to myself. The most important thing was to be alert and ready for construction accidents or war wounds as well as a variety of mysterious diseases.

As the days went by, I divided up patient care by snake bites, construction accidents, war injuries, disease, and of course, leeches.

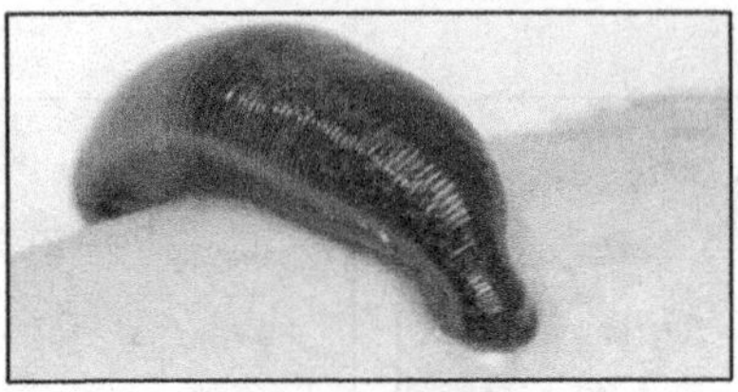

It took all my energy to deal with the nasty leech critters. Many of the battle soldiers had gotten them in the rainforests as they fought in Burma. Stevie, with his sweet laugh, called them the Draculas of the jungle because they were so skilled at sucking blood. He knew all about leeches and told me he had learned from Major John to never just yank them off.

"Come, I'll explain to all the nurses how to pull them off," he told me, happy to show off his skills.

The nurses gathered around a Chinese soldier on a cot with about 20 leeches all over his legs. The bloodsuckers pumped up and down as they sucked the soldier's blood. Stevie enjoyed the spotlight and shared his knowledge with us in his cute, animated way, and waved his arms about as he talked.

"Leeches are sneaky and sometimes you can't even feel them sucking your blood. It takes about 10 minutes of attachment, then you feel a twinge, scratch it, and discover the engorged bloodsucker hanging from your flesh."

Lorna said, "Yuck," after she heard the words "engorged bloodsucker" and put a hand over her eyes.

Stevie continued, "On my first day here, I explored deep into the jungle. When I felt a twinge on my arm, I tore off the slimy worm and ground the bloody mess onto a rock. This was a mistake, because the suction site left a ragged circle that bled for the rest of the day, and I itched for over a week!"

After that explanation, Lorna left for the bathroom and reluctantly came back a short time later.

The nurses observed the leeches on the Chinese soldier and either whined in disgust or closed their eyes.

"Stevie, tell us the proper method to get the dang things off," I said. I loved the guy but he was such a slow talker and lapped up the attention. The subject in general, plus the sight of the pulsating leeches, nauseated me. I gagged like I had done in nursing school and tried to slow my breathing to control it.

Throughout Stevie's dissertation, we watched the dark-green, spotted worm creatures with suction cups on each end of their bodies wiggle, pump, and suck.

I glanced over at Lorna as she held her stomach. She exclaimed, "This is too disgusting." She looked at me with a desperate grimace, as if to say, *I can't do this!*

Stevie continued and reveled in the female attention. "Do not tear them off. Just find its sucker mouth, which is the smaller, thinner end of its body." He pointed to the correct end. "Nurse Polly, get me a pan and put salt in it."

Polly was glad to leave.

When she returned, Stevie said, "Now, put a finger on the patient's skin next to the leech's thin end, which is its mouth. Slowly slide your fingernail under it, push it sideways, like so..." He demonstrated. "...then do the other larger end. This cleanly breaks the seal."

He adeptly flipped the leech into the pan and it met its demise in the salt. Polly's hands shook after it plopped into the container and she averted her eyes. At least she didn't groan or gag like everyone else did.

"Leeches have a permeable skin and salt causes their cells to lose moisture. That's why it has shriveled up like a raisin!" Stevie's face registered accomplishment as he watched the leech wither in the salt.

The nurses did not have the same reaction and remained squeamish.

He continued his lecture. "After you remove them all from a patient's body, place adhesive bandages on the wounds. Remember, always flick it off so it cannot reattach itself." Stevie beamed at his female audience, then scanned our sour faces and continued detaching more leeches.

The Chinese soldier sat up the entire time and watched what was happening on his legs with total fascination. Stevie seemed to calm him with a few Chinese words he had learned.

I stepped out into the jungle and found thin bamboo branches. I broke them all equally except for one, then returned to the ward. "Gals, I need you all to pick a stick. Whoever gets the shortest one needs to push leeches off the soldiers with Stevie."

The nurses all stood there, terrified. But we had many

cases of leeches to attend to and I had to pick someone to help Stevie.

"I'd rather throw a snake out of my tent," Clara mumbled.

"I'd rather have a gecko crawl on my body than deal with those revolting worms," Hilary added.

All the nurses displayed pitiful faces but obeyed my orders and drew sticks. Hazel picked the short stick.

When I saw a little tremble on her eyelid, I said, "Just assist him for today, then we'll all take turns the rest of the week."

Hazel seemed relieved. She gave a heavy sigh but pitched in without complaining and helped Stevie.

"On to the snake bites!" I announced, glad to get away from the nasty bloodsuckers.

I sang a cheerful song on the way to the snake ward and Betty's melodic voice joined in.

There's nothing worse than a bad nurse

There's nothing better than a good nurse

It takes a good nurse to keep 'em fighting.

We walked down the expansive ward and found all the snake bite victims, and I assigned Alma to take care of those.

After evening chow, we returned to our tents and found bars hammered to all our cots and a roll of mosquito netting. Progress! Maybe we'd be bitten less now. I praised the two nurses who had supervised the installation of the cot bars, and they beamed back at me with pride.

That night not only did the mosquitoes stay off us, but none of the night creatures nosed in since everyone remembered to pin their tent flaps.

Chapter Twenty-One
Bea
Corregidor, 1942

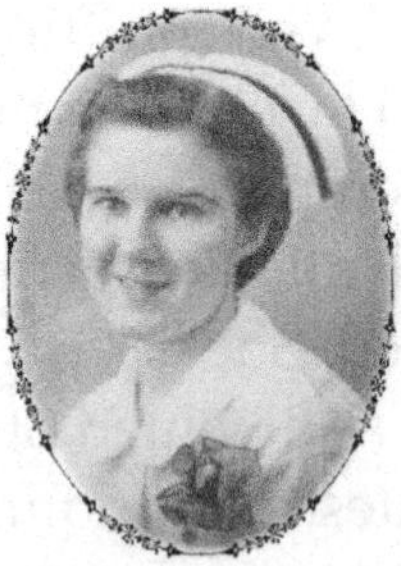

On May 6, 1942, Lieutenant General Jonathan M. Wainwright, Commander of Allied Forces in the Philippines, surrendered the island of Corregidor to General Homa Masaharu, chief of the Imperial Japanese Forces, in Luzon, Philippines. He surrendered 11,500 troops. When he returned to Corregidor, he ordered two of our soldiers to take down our precious American flag and replace it with a white bedsheet that signified surrender. Upon the lowering of the flag, a bugler played "Taps."

The surrender produced high anxiety because we did not know what would happen next. If the Japanese threw gas bombs into the tunnels, it would mean a slow death for us all. I ordered all the nurses to keep their gas masks at hand. We had heard rumors that the Japanese soldiers had raped and murdered British nurses in Hong Kong last December, and tried to push those thoughts from our minds.

Lieutenant General Wainwright informed me that on April 9, after Bataan was surrendered, all the American and Filipino soldiers were forced to walk over 60 miles to the Camp O'Donnell internment camp. He told me it was known as the Bataan Death March because no rest was allowed in the heat of the day. With no food or water, scores of troops perished. The march lasted from 5 - 10 days, depending on where a soldier was forced to join in. The Japanese subjected the troops to unspeakable torture and brutality during the march. The captives were beaten, shot, bayoneted, and beheaded. Many American and Filipino soldiers died or were left to die in the sun. Those who made it to the camp died of starvation and disease.

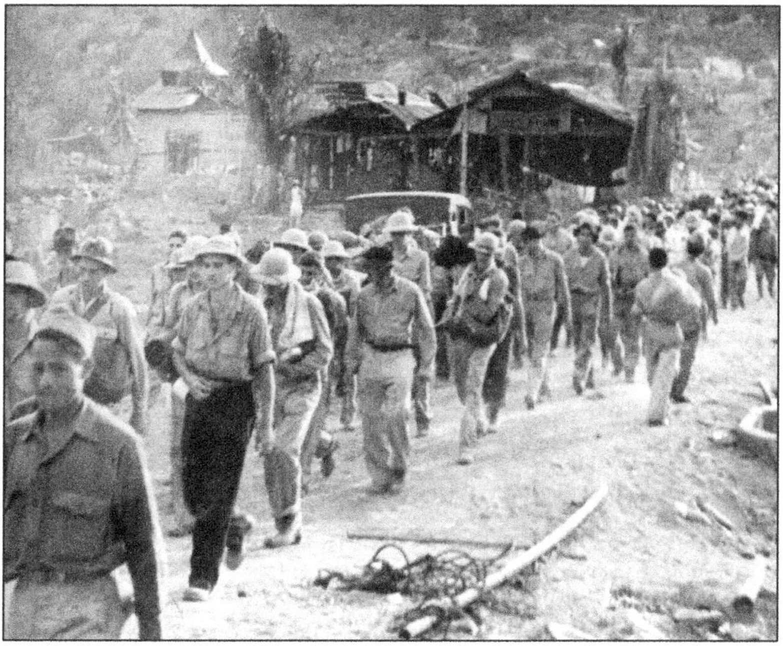

The Bataan Death March

After he told me about this torturous event, he said, "I'm telling you so you will make sure all the nurses remain on high alert when the Japanese enter the tunnels."

This piece of news I kept to myself, but I was overcome with severe anxiety.

The nurses asked me all sorts of questions.

"Where are the Japanese?"

"Will they come inside?"

"What will they do to us?"

I had no answers for them. We had to keep doing our jobs to prevent the intense butterflies from beating in our hearts as well as our stomachs. The nurses were jittery and deathly afraid of the enemy coming into the tunnels the Japanese now owned.

What kind of people bomb hospitals? ran through my mind.

The bombing had stopped, and more questions were thrown at me by my nurses. Would the Japanese shoot their way into the tunnel? Would they point their flamethrowers down the laterals and turn the tunnels into infernos? Or would they put poison gas in the air ducts, then march everyone outside and shoot us?

I finally stopped the worry fest. I ordered everyone to wear their Red Cross armbands, hoping the Japanese might respect the universal symbol that we were non-combatants. We were informed that, according to the Geneva Convention, as non-combatants we would be put on a Red Cross ship and sent home if we were captured. The last thing I said was that we should never be caught alone if the Japanese came inside.

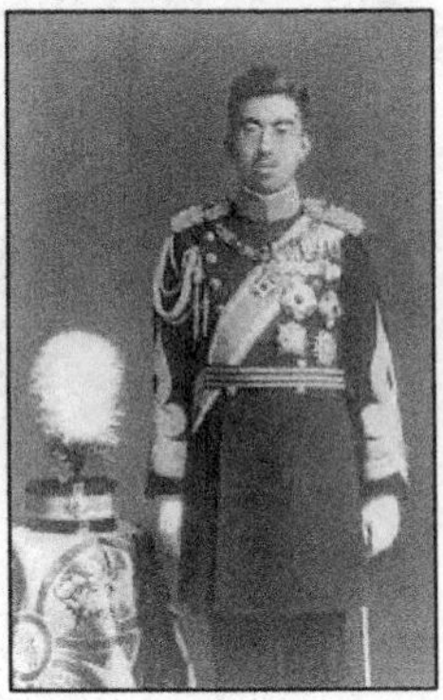

We now had over 900 patients in the tunnel and supplies were very low.

On May 9, Japanese officers and their enlisted soldiers marched into the tunnel in full regalia with bayonets.

We were not harmed but were shaken to the core with fear. They told us to fall into formation. The nurses left their patients and stood mute.

The Japanese walked by us and inspected us like cattle. One officer felt the hem of my nurse's uniform. They told the nurses, doctors, and corpsmen to continue to treat the patients while they inspected the fortress.

In every area, they posted signs that read: THIS IS THE PROPERTY OF THE IMPERIAL JAPANESE GOVERNMENT.

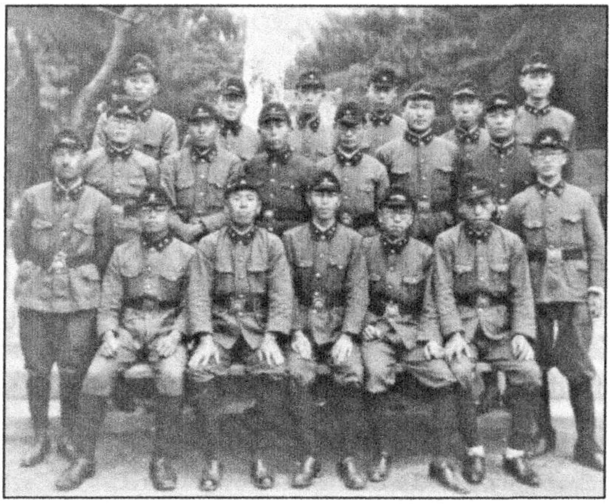

Whenever a Japanese officer came in, the nurses stiffened in fright from the uncertainty of what they would do to us. We were only allowed outside for air under supervision.

The next day, our captors ordered all Americans to bow to them to show our obeisance. Most of us bowed fast to get it over with. A Japanese sign was placed on the lateral where we all slept—NURSES OF THE U.S. ARMY.

On Tuesday, the Japanese Imperial Army took 10 nurses and me outside. Most of us thought it was the end and that we would be shot. We were told to line up outside in front of the entrance to Malinta Tunnel and smile. It was a shock to see all the splintered trees among the scores of bloated corpses of our soldiers, which were covered by swarms of black and green flies.

A Japanese officer said in excellent English, "We will take your picture and we're going to send it to MacArthur to show that you are alive and that we take good care of you. Don't be afraid, I graduated from one of your universities."

Of course, this did nothing to alleviate our fear. We stood there with forced smiles and frightened faces.

For the first few weeks, we continued to do our jobs and stayed busy and alert. Then the looting began. The Japanese soldiers would pilfer anything of value, day or night. Annie slipped her engagement ring onto a safety pin and secured it inside her blouse. Veronica fashioned a fancy curl on her head and placed a watch inside her hair.

The Japanese stole radios, wristwatches, binoculars, jewelry, pens, cigarette lighters—even the silver picture frame around the photo of my parents. One soldier removed a ring from a nurse's finger while she slept and woke her up. I left my glasses out and they were stolen. Now I wouldn't be able to read the charts.

I ordered the nurses to sleep in their uniforms because of possible rape. Two Japanese soldiers would frequently enter our quarters in the middle of the night, point their bayonet rifles at us, and count and watch us. One Japanese soldier looked at Molly's photo of her husband in his medical U.S. Army uniform. He laughed. "Ah, an American officer. Killed on Bataan! Ha, ha, ha."

Molly controlled herself but as soon as he left, she wept into her pillow. I comforted her and told her that he'd said that just to scare her.

I whispered to everyone, "Remember, keep all your valuables hidden and never be caught alone. We need to stick together at all times." I stuffed my lucky charm gun and sock full of bullets plus my two watches inside my pillowcase and slept on top of it at night.

The nurses took turns keeping watch at night. They rang a bell the minute a Japanese soldier appeared. We sat up every time we heard that bell ring and didn't get much sleep.

As the weeks went by, the Japanese Imperial Army inspected all 900 patients in the wards and forced many to leave the hospital. If a corpsman or doctor tried to intervene, they were knocked to the ground as the guard forced the patient out of the tunnel. Only 400 American men were left in the hospital—those who were extremely sick or wounded.

What are they doing to our patients? I fumed to myself.

The nurses were slapped with the side of a bayonet if they did not follow orders immediately. Thank God none of us had been raped. We were fed only twice a day with cracked-wheat cereal and cracked-wheat "coffee" for breakfast. Lunch was always corned beef hash and dirty rice, and our weight continued to drop.

In June, all we had for breakfast was cooked cracked wheat full of weevils. We tried to get the weevils out when they floated to the top but then the nurses agreed that the weevils were protein and ate them.

We made a remembrance sheet from a muslin bedsheet to mark our existence. It had the heading "Members of the Army Nurse Corps and civilian nurses who were in the Malinta Tunnel when Corregidor fell." In columns, 69 women embroidered their names. It was a solemn occasion, but we wanted to leave a record in case we were killed.

The Remembrance Sheet

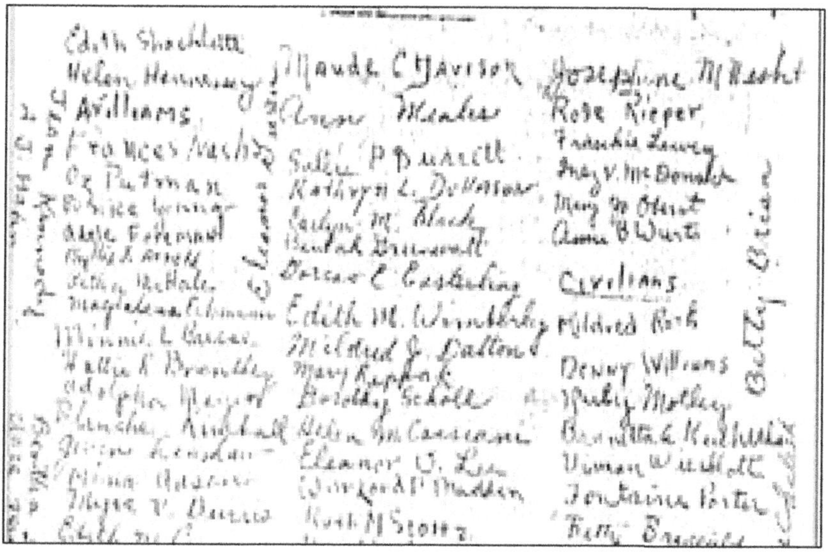

After Annie signed her name, she cried out, "You Jap bastards!"

The outburst startled Carmelita. She crossed herself and prayed in Spanish. When all 69 women had finished the remembrance, she took the sheet and hid it in an empty lateral.

It was a dismal existence in our captured tunnel. We were fearful that we would be shot at any time. With most of our patients sent outside, we had very little work to do.

On June 25, Lt. General Wainwright came into the barracks to talk to the droopy-faced nurses. "I have good news. I have convinced the Japanese commander to allow the entire hospital to be moved to Topside to the former Fort Mills Hospital. I'm convinced we will be happier outside as captives than in this dreary place."

This announcement produced applause from everyone. We packed our musette bags among cheerful chatter and followed Wainwright and the Japanese commander outside into the tropical sun and fresh air. The few remaining gardenia trees were in full bloom and exuded a perfumed smell all around us. We were sick of the stinky hot tunnels with no air circulation.

Fort Mills Hospital, much to our dismay, was just a shell of a building that was no longer a hospital, and our previous patients were nowhere to be found. The corpsmen carried up beds and the 400 remaining patients were put in their new quarters with the blue sky as a ceiling and the delicious smell of the sea air. We used mosquito netting to protect our patients from unwanted insects in the roofless facility. Carmelita and Angelica picked a gardenia for every patient so they could enjoy the smell of the flowers.

But, although we were out of the suffocating tunnels, we were still captives. The fear and tension of what would become of us remained.

Chapter Twenty-Two
Dottie
Tagap, Burma 1944

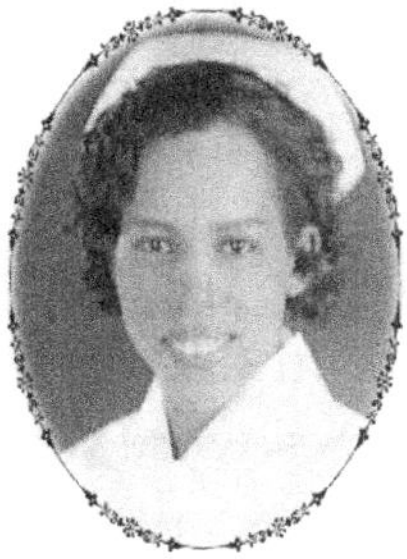

We were able to put together a Christmas party in one of the original buildings that still needed to be renovated. Medic Stevie brought a native tree inside, and Handy Hazel cut stars out of empty plasma cans to decorate it. Soldiers from the nearby ordnance and engineering units came to celebrate with us.

A buffet table was filled with rations from the PX and special treats came from anyone who received a package from home. I shared decorated sugar cookies made by my family and Polly's family had sent a fruit cake. The soldiers also contributed quite a few goodies they had received.

One soldier brought in an old wind-up phonograph and records from the 1930s. It was fun to have that much male company. The men far outnumbered the nurses so we danced every dance and the soldiers had to wait their turn.

Major John asked Clara to dance, and Doc Samuel asked me. I was quite surprised by how well he danced because I'd always thought of him as such a studious guy. Even Lorna danced despite having a boyfriend back home.

The record "It Don't Mean a Thing (If It Ain't Got That Swing)" by Duke Ellington was an absolute delight to dance to. Bing Crosby's song "Silent Night, Holy Night" ended the festivities and brought tears to our eyes. Everyone left quietly to go to sleep in their tents.

Many of the patients on the ward were not American Negroes but our duty was to fix them up and send them out to make room for more wounded. I asked Major John at chow the next morning what races were represented there.

He told me, "We care for all workers employed by the American and British armies, which includes the American Negroes, Chinese, British, Indians, and Africans. Plus, the local Burmese tribesmen—Nagas, Karens, Shans, and Kachins."

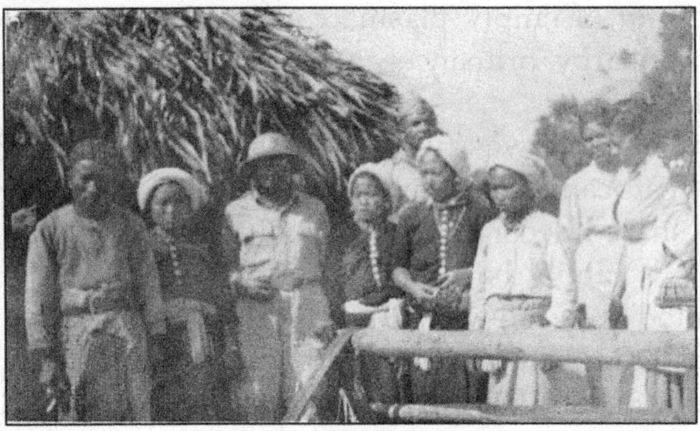

"What a cultural heterogeneity!" I blushed after I showed off my vocabulary.

"Indeed," the doctor replied. "It makes it complicated at times, what with the differences in dietary habits, customs, castes, and taboos of religion, to provide proper care for such a variety of people. You'll see." He smiled and stood.

"Oh my, you must have been a basketball player with that height." I blushed as I felt blood rush to my cheeks.

"I was in college but had to drop out even though my team won. I chose medicine over sports."

"Lucky us…I mean, it's good you did since you seem like such a competent physician." I stood up with my metal plate in my hand as the doctor looked down at me. Goose bumps spread up and down my body as I rushed off, embarrassed.

When the first basha was built, we had quite a celebration. We took turns and climbed the bamboo ladder, poked our heads out of the uncovered open windows, then waved to everyone down below.

"It's so cute, hope mine will be built soon," Lorna raved.

My roommate, Clara, said, "I wonder why it's built up so high?" Then she added, "I wish we had a table and chairs."

I too was curious about why the basha was high up and not on the ground, but was glad about it and thought, *Good, no more roaming creatures can get in!*

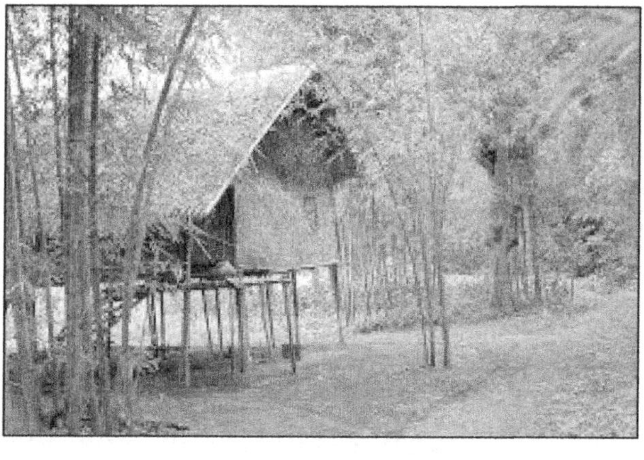

Back at work, I strolled through the multicultural ward and nodded and smiled at the variety of faces that greeted my gaze. I counted over 36 Chinese and a handful of native workers, but the majority of the patients were Negroes.

Our 16 American nurses and the Chinese patients experienced a clash of cultures, which made our jobs difficult. Stevie, who had picked up some of the Chinese language, told me that they did not like the nurses and wondered why a "high type" kind of woman would perform the menial tasks of bedside care.

The nurses found it hard to maintain proper discipline among the wards because the Chinese did not feel it necessary to follow a woman's orders. To top it off, very few of them understood English.

Hilary was with me on the ward one day. I always enjoyed her company as she was a true practicing nurse with experience and learned new nursing skills with ease.

She complained to me in a nasty whisper, "These Chinese soldiers are the worst. I think they are an intolerable race and I don't like dealing with them. Believe you me, Chief Dottie, I've tried my best."

"Tell me the problems you have with the Chinese." I tried to listen but was concerned when she said, "intolerable race."

"Just to keep them in the so-called isolated malaria ward for rest is a hopeless task. I caught one of them with a high malarial fever playing cards with another patient who had wounds. They are a race of obsessive gamblers and no matter how many times I separate them, they are sneaky bastards and always join back together again."

"Hmm, that is disturbing..." I used a sympathetic tone but when she said "sneaky bastards" another alarm went off for me.

"And these people! As soon as your back is turned, they unwrap their dressings to scrutinize the condition of their wounds. I yelled at a few of them about this, but they pretended they didn't understand English."

"What else have you tried to do to alleviate this situation?" I asked.

Hilary answered candidly, "I put a bandage on myself, then peeled it up and yelled 'NO!' while I shook my finger at them to show them it's wrong."

"Did that work?"

"Not at all. They just snickered and talked in their weird sing-song voices. One Chinese yelled back at me, 'NO, NO, NO!' and shook his finger while all his friends burst out in laughter." She threw up her hands.

"I'll have to think about this problem, Hilary. Thanks for letting me know." I felt nervous, which was unusual for me, but I did not know how to deal with Hilary's prejudice—or the unruly Chinese patients, for that matter.

Fueled by my attention, Hilary continued to complain. "I think they're a stupid group of people and only know how to use a gun because they're paid. Also, what's wrong with their eyes? Why are they slanted like that?"

After that comment, I knew this was a problematic situation and would further escalate if I didn't do something about it. *Now.*

I walked the length of the ward with Lorna, Hilary, and Betty. Most of the Chinese chattered away like it was a party. I realized then that I hadn't watched the patients and had just supervised the nurses at their jobs to make sure they gave proper care.

Hilary declared loudly, "Look at how they carry on when they should be resting." She walked up to one bed and looked under it. "Chief Bea, look at all the food garbage under their beds!"

I bent over and saw piles of orange peels, eggshells, and vegetables under each patient's bed. I was about to suggest a solution when Lorna pointed.

"There are even chicken feathers!" She scooped up a

bunch of feathers and threw them into the air.

Exasperated, I yelled, "Pick those up!" Then asked, "I wonder where the chickens are?"

Lorna picked up the feathers. "They keep chickens, ducks, and other live animals hidden in the jungle, then cook them and sneak back to the ward to eat them. All their hidden food supplies have made the rats overrun the wards."

"Those Chinese tame the rats and keep them as pets or eat them," Hilary joined in.

Betty kept quiet, which was a relief.

That night, alone in my new basha while Clara worked the night shift, I did some soul-searching. This was a new experience for most of us. We usually received the brunt of people's prejudice, not the other way around.

The next morning, Hilary came in and went to work on dressing a Negro soldier's wounds. I observed her as she applied new bandages with compassion and touched his shoulder. "You're healing well, Johnny, just one more day to go. I know how much you want to leave and help get that road rebuilt."

It warmed my heart to hear Hilary's compassion after her verbal bashing of the Chinese soldiers.

At supper chow, I was happy to see Major John cooking a can of beans on the fire.

He greeted me, "Hello there, Chief Dottie, how's everything going on the ward?" He gave me that special smile of his.

"Pretty good, just a few minor problems."

"Like what? Anything I can help you with? Let's sit over there, I'll share some of my hot food with you and we can talk alone."

We sat at a bamboo table away from everyone else amid the glorious mountain range and with the colors of the night sky about to descend upon us. I told him about the messy food problems and the need for a sufficient isolation ward. I wasn't sure I wanted to discuss the prejudice problem yet.

Major John was glad to help. "First, I'll talk with the soldiers. I have picked up some Chinese and can speak a little of their language. We do have a rat problem and I will tell them that. The issue of an isolation ward for very sick patients is a great idea. Pretty soon we'll have a ward that has concrete floors and closed sides, which will also help keep the rats out. I have some building ideas and I'll get back to you."

I gazed into his eyes gratefully. "That's terrific. We sure would appreciate it."

I had an easier time that night while I slept and dreamed of slow dancing in Major John's arms. When I awoke, I was surprised at how infatuated I had become with him.

In the ward the next day, a mother and father from the Naga tribe brought us a screaming little boy, perhaps two years old, who was bitten from head to toe by chiggers. The bites were severe and infected. While the child howled in pain, Hilary cleaned the wounds with iodine. Stevie helped and found a convalescing Naga patient who could tell the parents that a drug called penicillin would be given as a shot to heal the child. Hilary gave the boy the shot and the parents left and displayed much gratitude.

We did have many malaria cases to deal with, just like in Liberia. The Army sprayed DDT on all mosquito-infested areas. The personnel were ordered to wear long sleeves and pants. The nurses gave up wearing skirts and stockings, and reluctantly put on fatigues. All the troops were issued daily Atabrine. The nurses were diligent about protective clothing and took the preventive medicine because none of us wanted a repeat of Liberia, when we lost half of our nurses to the disease and were all sent home. Thank the Lord that malaria was not spread from human to human.

On Tuesday, Major John came to find me and asked the nurses which patients had malaria. Then he looked under a few beds and saw the piles of food garbage. I heard him speak in broken Chinese as he pointed to the garbage under the beds. He laughed with one of the patients and I thought he was such a helpful, jovial man.

The next morning, I looked under one of the Chinese soldier's beds to see if Major John's talk had helped any. I jumped back and suppressed a scream after I saw a fist-sized, monster spider with pointed legs and enormous fangs on top of a pile of garbage.

Stevie was nearby and was able to stomp it dead. I inspected the soldier's body, and he had patches of bites on his legs, arms, and back, all from that dreadful creature. It was hard enough to fix up the men after battle and road accidents, but the harmful critters from the jungle attacked them as well. With a sigh, I accepted it as yet another thing we had to contend with.

Chapter Twenty-Three
Bea
Corregidor – Santo Tomas
1942

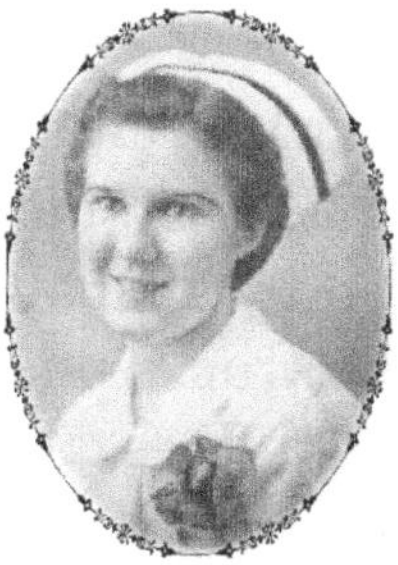

Our happiness was short-lived. On July 2, 1942, the Japanese commander informed our colonel that the nurses would be loaded on a freighter that afternoon for Manila.

I balled my fists. "What will happen to everyone else?"

Lt. General Wainwright said, "Chief Bea, we have lost the war and are captives, as you are well aware." He gave me a stern look. "I can only tell you what the Japanese commander has ordered. Now, go pack up." He turned away and left.

We were driven to the dock and waited in the hot, sticky weather for the boats to arrive. An hour went by before the small boats finally appeared and took us to an old steamer with *Lima Maru* painted on the side.

We were as skinny as reeds and suffered from many ailments. It was a hard climb up a long rope ladder to get on board the steamer. My body swayed as I climbed, and I felt dizzy and weak. My musette bag hung around my neck and I gripped the rope with all my might so I wouldn't drop into the shark-infested sea. Once aboard, we shook out our nurses' capes and laid them out on the wet deck, then sat on them in silence.

When the boat docked in Manila, our 64 nurses were transported in the backs of three trucks. The devastation we saw was hard to bear. The once beautiful harbor was now a filthy cove littered with the steel hulls of partially submerged ships. I hid my reaction but thought, *This can't be our Pearl of the Orient!*

Once we passed the harbor, all three trucks stopped. The 25 Filipina nurses, who had been placed together in the first truck, were told to get out by a Japanese guard. We watched as they piled out, then our trucks pulled away and they were left behind with bewildered faces.

In the back of our truck, the nurses threw questions at me.

"Chief, why aren't they going with us?"

"Will the nurses go home?"

I answered in a solemn voice, "I don't know."

Our trucks drove on and we approached Sternberg Hospital.

Molly yelled out, "There's our hospital! Now we can work and wait out the end of the war, then go home!"

But as we passed the hospital and drove on, Veronica cried out, "Oh no…where are they taking us?"

The once-bustling city of Manila now had only sparse traffic, and grass grew in the middle and along the sides of the streets. Much to my surprise, we were driven through the gates of Santo Tomas University, where I'd had my first date with Rob. But now this once-vibrant college campus was littered with strange wooden huts and many Japanese guards stood around holding bayonets. I saw a few thin Americans who went in and out of the huts, and had a small flash of hope that maybe Rob had been captured and sent there. Then we would be reunited at last.

The trucks stopped in front of the Japanese commandant's office. It was late afternoon when we were herded into a cramped room. We stood there in our wrinkled nurses' uniforms, still wearing our Red Cross armbands. I was sick with worry that we would be tortured right there by the vicious Japanese.

Our meager musette bags were searched and our names were put on a large roster. Then a Japanese officer, in a heavy foreign accent, grilled us like spies. He asked each one of us, "What were you doing on Corregidor?" and "Who do you work for?"

All of us were tired, hot, thirsty, and many were sick. Three hours went by before I finally mustered up the confidence to say, "Sir, we need to go to the bathroom."

"Only one at a time," a Japanese guard answered in a fierce voice, then grabbed my arm and dragged me outside.

As I looked around, I was overcome by the fact that I had been there before with Rob, and memories of our date flooded my mind.

On the way to the bathroom, I searched for an American uniform but there were only ragtag civilians milling about. The guard and I passed the odd-looking handmade shacks with open sides. They were adorned with silly signs displaying names like "Glamorville" and "Hollywood."

The soldier led me into one of the campus buildings and up several flights of stairs to join a long line of women who waited to use one toilet. I got in line behind a tiny, wafer-thin woman with scraggly white hair and dressed in tattered clothes.

She whispered in a British accent, "Do you know if the war's over?"

I shook my head discreetly when the guard glanced my way. The woman asked if I'd seen her husband, Richard. I shook my head again.

"What is this place?" I whispered to her.

"Don't you know? It's the Santo Tomas Internment Camp."

Her answer was what I had feared. "How long have you all been here?"

"Since January."

"What's it like?"

"They keep us crowded together and supervised at all times."

The guard yelled out, "Quiet over there—and keep moving!"

When the Japanese guard wasn't paying attention, I whispered, "How's everyone treated here? Is there any... torture?" I choked on the last word.

"We are treated all right given the fact that we were all civilians who lived in Manila and just got caught in the war. The Japanese have even allowed us to form an executive and advisory committee."

My eyebrows rose in surprise. "How does that work?"

"The committee was elected by us and is made up of 15 Americans and six other nationalities who were businessmen on the island before they were captured and interned here. The Japanese army gives them a pittance of 35 cents per person per day to run the camp, and to purchase food and medical supplies."

"How many people live here?" I asked.

"Over 3,000, I think."

"That amount of money doesn't seem feasible."

"No, it isn't, but we did receive supplies and food from the Red Cross. We're luckier than the military men who were captured in Bataan. I heard they've faced a lot of starvation and brutality."

I thought about all the doctors and medics from Baguio and my mind swam with worry. Were they safe? I glanced at the guard. When he wasn't looking my way, I asked, "How do you know all this?"

"My husband is on the committee and when I meet with him, he keeps me informed."

"Meet with him? Don't you stay with your husband?"

"No, the Japanese keep the sexes separated."

"How awful for you!"

"Unfortunately, nothing can be done about that. The Japanese have their own sense of rules and order. The committee is trying to solve that problem."

The guard yelled our way, "Silence over there!"

I whispered to her when the guard looked away, "Thank you."

"It was nice to meet you. Please let me know if your nurses need anything and when I see my husband, I'll put in a good word for you."

When my turn came to use the toilet, I was given four squares of toilet paper. I found out later that the one bathroom was shared by 300 women.

The guard took me back. Because I was caught talking, the commandant did not allow anyone else to go to the bathroom. After everyone was checked in, we were told to get back into the trucks.

Oh my God. Where are we going? I worried.

We were driven a block away to a building that had a cross on a steeple and a sign in front that read *Santa Catalina Convent*. There we were housed on the second floor in two rooms jammed with cots. Thank goodness there was a bathroom. When the guard left the convent, it was locked. The nurses fell asleep after an arduous, emotion-filled day. But I couldn't sleep. I lay awake and wondered if there would be food brought to us.

In the morning, two guards brought us a small but sufficient meal of noodles, vegetable soup, hot chocolate, and pineapple. We felt refreshed to have food, but there was not enough protein and it would not sustain us for long.

The nurses were happy to heal themselves and stayed on the cots. Most of us suffered from malaria, dysentery, arthritis, hepatitis, stomach cramps, leg ulcers, or dengue fever—and sometimes a combination of those. As the weeks went by, we asked for books, playing cards, and yarn to pass the time. Molly and Jane were clever enough to knit needed socks and underpants for everyone. I was glad to see Molly keeping busy, which kept her from fretting about Dr. Charlie.

As we began to recover and felt better, we wanted to work. We missed caring for patients. Every day a guard came by and allowed us to go outside behind the convent for two hours of exercise. Cheerleader Veronica conducted a few sing-a-longs, and she got Annie to help her organize skits and talent shows.

In late August, after over a month of confinement in the convent, we were moved to the old hospital on the college campus. We packed up our musette bags and were walked over by a guard to the Santo Tomas Internment Camp. On the way, we saw volunteer internees who carried over beds and other equipment from the convent. We were led into spacious quarters, and much to our surprise, found 10 of our nurses from Corregidor there making beds.

I gasped, "What are you doing here? You're supposed to be in Australia!"

Nurse Caroline, who had a few more wrinkles on her face, answered in a subdued voice, "We left on the seaplane for a stopover in Lake Lanao, then hid until sunset. When the pilot took off under the cover of darkness to avoid the enemy, our plane hit a stiff wind and turbulence blew it back to shore. It hit a rock that ripped a hole in the fuselage and the cabin filled with water. All of us plus the pilot tried to evade the Japanese for two weeks, and went from one farm to another to stay and eat with the families. We were caught by the Japanese and brought here…except for the pilot."

"Did the other seaplane make it?" I asked.

Thelma answered, "We have no idea whether they made it to Australia or not."

Molly interrupted, "Do you know where my husband was taken to in Bataan?"

Caroline said, "Most likely to one of the many prison camps. We're lucky to have been brought here. The military prisons can be barbaric places."

Molly burst out, "Oh no…"

I took Molly aside. "They don't know that for sure. Let's continue to work and do our jobs. I'm sure we'll find our men after the war is over. Go help Susie put away the medicine in the cabinets."

As we got set up, Caroline asked, "What happened in Corregidor after we left?"

"After Lt. General Wainwright surrendered, the Japanese took over the island and we were brought here."

Eleanor asked, "Where are the Filipina nurses?"

"They were brought on the boat to Manila, and I think they went home." I changed the subject. "Do you know what the wooden huts are all over the grounds?"

Thelma explained, "Our executive committee, through negotiations, got the Japanese commandant to allow internees to build structures made of scrap lumber and tin where families could spend the day together and have a secluded sanctuary away from the crowded rooms. At first, the commandant would not agree, but then he allowed the shanties to be built with the restriction of open sides so the guards could inspect them. They are permitted for daytime use only."

Caroline added, "Susie and I built one with a small flower garden around it to make it look more attractive."

Veronica chimed in, "I love the cute, creative signs people put on them, like Garden Court, Broadway, and Jungle Town."

"We call our shack MacArthur Drive!" Caroline laughed.

Susie said, "The silliest names I've seen are Hollywood Boulevard and Papaya Street."

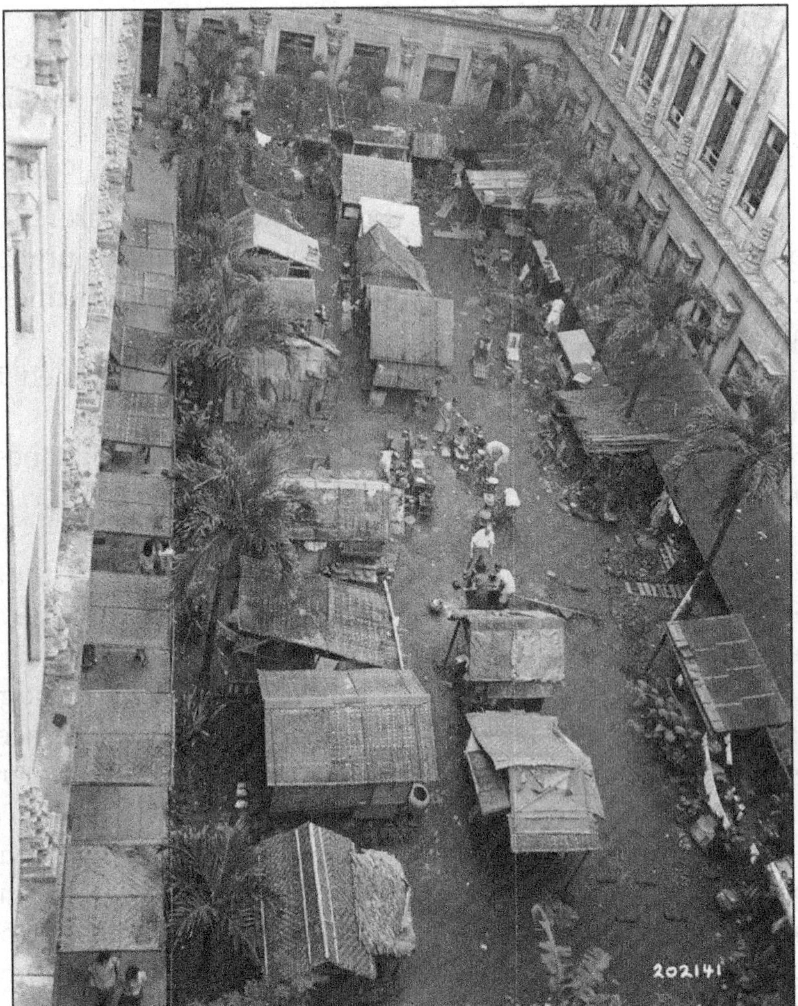

The nurses took up their duties in the internment camp hospital and most of us were happy to do what we did best—heal people. Before the nurses arrived, the hospital was run by one civilian nurse who had been sent from Stotsenburg Hospital and oversaw 700 sick internees by herself.

When the war broke out, many of the businessmen's wives with children remained in their houses in Manila. The Japanese brought more of the families to stay in the convent, which was why our group had been moved. Our staff consisted of an optometrist and dentist with very few surgeons. A Filipina nurse who was married to an American internee also worked with us.

We found our new quarters in the old hospital more spacious than being locked up in the convent, and it was a nice sense of freedom for the nurses to mingle with the civilian internees during their breaks. With the constant increase of new internees brought in by the Imperial Army, I requested that the executive committee ask the commandant for more surgeons. My request was granted and I was told that two physicians would be sent in from Camp O'Donnell, one of the military prisons.

A few weeks later, while the nurses tended to the patients, in walked a Japanese guard with Dr. Bloom and Dr. Charlie! Molly saw her husband and dropped in a dead faint. Dr. Charlie scooped her up and when she came to in his arms, her face beamed with joy. The Japanese guard immediately told him to put her down. But after the guard left, Molly and the doc resumed their embrace.

Molly exclaimed, "I missed you terribly, Charlie. I'm so relieved to see you. I was worried that you were tortured there."

"No, darling, nothing like that."

"What was Camp O'Donnell like? You look very thin."

"The food was worse than at Santo Tomas. It was a sanitation disaster with lice, bed bugs, and rats. There were no brooms or mops to clean with, so we had to use rags. We organized an emergency crew from our prisoners to build latrines because there were none. The Japanese guards were strict but not too abusive."

"Oh, good," Molly said.

Dr. Charlie continued and we all listened with rapt attention. "It was overcrowded and many of us got bacillary or amoebic dysentery from contaminated water. At first, there wasn't enough to eat and no soap or blankets. Thanks to Colonel Duckworth's leadership, he got the Japanese to sanction the building of a hospital since there were over 4,000 Filipino and 150 sick Americans. The colonel, with help from the medics, salvaged pipes for a water system and an assortment of medical equipment plus unearthed emergency food rations from bombed-out Baguio. Before I left, a hospital was in the process of being built. We also received parcels from the British and American Red Cross. The worst for me was not having any news about the war and…" He looked at Molly. "…missing you, my dear." He kissed his wife deeply.

"Oh, Charlie, it sounds dreadful." Molly kissed him up and down his cheeks.

"Molly, honey, let's put that behind us. We are together now."

Molly and Dr. Charlie were over the moon to be reunited but they were not allowed to sleep together according to the Japanese rules at the camp. They did build an open shanty, but this did not allow them to have the intimacy they strongly desired and needed.

The monsoons of late summer and early fall brought torrential rains. We had 27 inches, which caused many of the shanties to fall apart. That included Doc and Molly's, which they called "Love Nest." Once the monsoon season subsided, everyone rebuilt their hideouts.

One morning, the new Japanese commandant announced over the camp loudspeaker, "We will enforce a bowing procedure. All prisoners, including children, must bow to the officers in uniform. You are wards of the Imperial Japanese

Army and have received our protection, and must bow deeply from the waist to show respect. Anyone who does not follow this law will be punished."

There were a lot of grumbles after hearing this. Most of the internees, due to the lack of a proper diet, were ill and no one felt like they could perform this deep bowing to the many Japanese personnel who passed by us frequently.

The next day, about 30 internees decided to play a prank on the Japanese soldiers. A few at a time would pass the guards at short intervals and bow, which required the guards to return the gesture. Then the next group passed by, which made the guards bow again. After a few dozen rounds of bowing, the guards left and walked away. When they saw more internees approach, they got wise to it and turned their backs to avoid the bowing escapade. Our internees got a good laugh after tormenting our captors.

A camp announcement from Commandant Kuroda came over the loudspeaker a few weeks before Thanksgiving: "The interiors of the shanties must remain open to view on two sides and at no time be closed when in use. All prisoners must obey the camp rule that the shanties are permitted only for daytime use, and this will be enforced. The Imperial military is not in the business of making babies. No sexual relations are allowed. If this rule is disobeyed, jail time will occur. All room monitors will report any pregnancies."

Pregnant women, married or not, were sent to hospitals outside the camp until they gave birth. A young internee came to our hospital pregnant and had been engaged before the internment. She begged me to help her get married or the Japanese would send her away permanently. There was only one priest there and he refused to perform the ceremony. He had to obey the rules. The internee room monitors reported six pregnancies that month.

Twenty-three Navy nurses were brought in from an emergency hospital in Manila to join the ANC nurses. This was a godsend as we needed more help at the hospital because the patient load was increasing. I was happy to have the extra support for my already exhausted nurses.

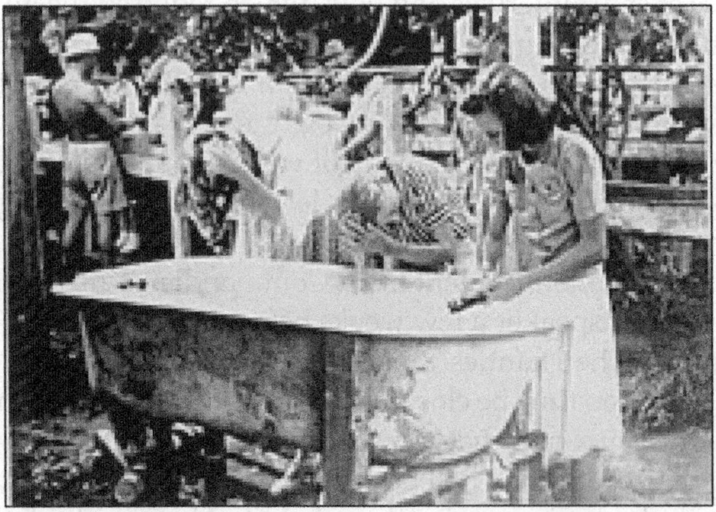

Washing hair at the internment camp.

Chapter Twenty-Four
Dottie
Tagap, Burma, January 1945

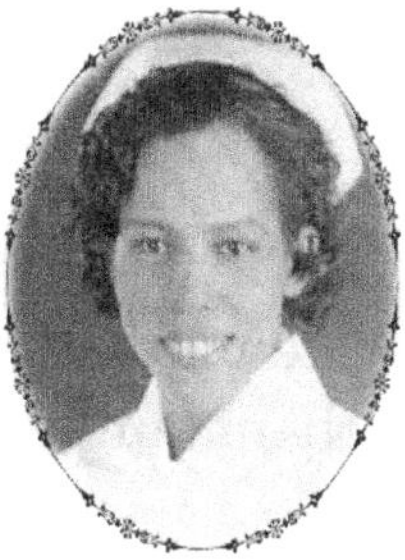

In the New Year of January 1945, at the end of the month, our entire compound at the 335th Station Hospital was complete. The location in the middle of the jungle required several months of hard work to build, and much time was spent clearing the land and repairing or replacing the dilapidated buildings. The good news was, we had a medical laboratory, dental clinic, pharmacy, operating rooms, patient rooms, a finished mess hall, and new medic living quarters. The surgical buildings and wards no longer had dirt floors but concrete foundations, and were powered by generators.

Major John obtained salvaged pipes and the nearby pipeline engineers instructed the natives on how to install a complete water system that ran from the watersheds in the upper mountains to the hospital, plus a drainage system to help manage the flooding during the monsoons. The medics and a few physicians also improvised a hot-water electrical power source.

The nurses were thrilled that the hospital was finished and up and running, complete with 150 beds. In other sections, we had a library that doubled as a game and reading room. We were isolated there in the mountains, but many activities were instituted like volleyball, tennis, ping-pong, horseshoes, basketball, and baseball.

Twice a month, we had Saturday-evening dances in an old makeshift building that was redesigned into a new officers' club with a fresh coat of paint and a bar added. Sam and I attended all the dances and adored each other's company, especially the intimate, slow dances. The recreation committee events and the shows from the USO and GI programs helped keep morale high for the entire staff. I spied Major John and Hilary playing tennis together on their breaks. It was a pleasure to watch them laugh and enjoy one another's company.

The incredible feat of Ledo Road, constructed by Allied soldiers, began in December 1942. The road started in Assam, India and went to the Burma Road, then connected to Kunming, China. The entire length of 1,072 miles was finished in January 1945 and was renamed Stilwell Road after U.S. Army General Joseph Stilwell, commander of the China-Burma-India Theater.

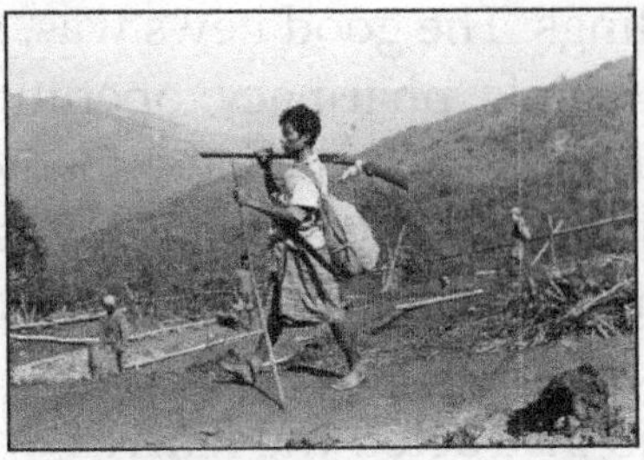

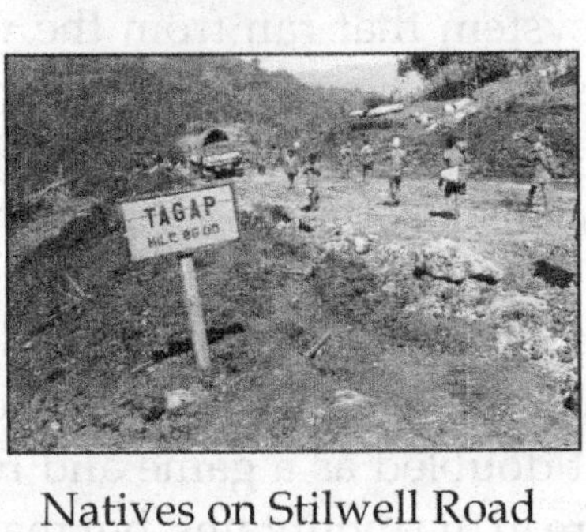

Natives on Stilwell Road

Thanks to Major John, the native workers brought in tall bamboo room dividers and the major set them up to separate the farthest part of the ward. He had all the malaria patients, plus a few cases of scrub typhus, move to the isolation ward to get proper rest and to heal. The patients who had contagious illnesses like tuberculosis or measles were kept isolated behind the room dividers as well. I labeled the dividers with signs that stated the patients' various ailments to help the nurses care for and keep track of them better.

Next, the native workers gave every patient a handmade palm-frond garbage bin. Major John asked Li Jie, who spoke English and Chinese, to interpret for him. He instructed all the patients to use the bins and stay in their assigned wards, and added that if anyone disobeyed the rules, they would be discharged early to go back and fight while still sick or recovering.

Major John threatened, "We'll also get rid of your animals and gardens that you are hiding in the jungle if you don't use the bins and empty them every day in the outside garbage pits." He had the interpreter add, "Does everyone understand the rules?" He scanned the entire ward. There was complete silence.

I thanked the good doctor.

He grinned. "I could tell they didn't like the idea of being discharged early!"

"Yes, that was a fine way to get them to cooperate. Thanks, Major John."

The next day, the major visited the ward and took me aside. "Are the garbage baskets being used for the food scraps?"

"Pretty well. As long as the medics keep them emptied and the nurses remind the soldiers to use them every day."

Major John looked at me directly. "Since you're the chief, you must prepare your nurses for the monsoons—and believe you me, it's nothing like you ever experienced in Georgia. It's a devastating yearly event in this part of the world. Imagine an exaggerated form of a storm with drenching rain that goes on for months, nonstop. The good news is that the Chinese patients will lose interest in their outside food sources, which will alleviate that problem."

"Our nurses experienced the monsoon season in Liberia, and it was horrific weather, but we'll persevere, don't you worry," I assured him.

"Glad to hear that. I didn't know you were stationed in Liberia. What was that like?" Major John leaned toward me.

"We were overstaffed with medics and there was no war activity there. Our nurses didn't feel needed. When half of our nurses ended up with god-awful malaria, we were recalled back to the States."

"One of the main problems we have here is the monsoons cause our trucks to get stuck in the mud, and we've had bulldozers roll over the banks of the roads. You'll have to tell your staff to get ready for an influx of accident victims this time of the year—some with gruesome injuries. Our Negroes drive the trucks hard, day and night, and use heavy equipment to build the Ledo Road to China. They end up with broken bones and sprained backs. The push is on to finish the road while our Allied Chinese soldiers beat back the Japanese in this terrible climate. We'll get 140 inches during the monsoon season, which will start this month, May, and end in November." Major John explained.

"Don't you worry about us. Liberia has the worst monsoons in the world." I put my hand on my hip.

"I want you to know that Burma can be a horrible place. When the monsoons descend, it brings out all the pests—mosquitoes, scorpions, leeches, snakes..."

"I'm glad we'll have the bashas to live in. It doesn't sound like tents would hold up well."

"No, they wouldn't. I'd better make sure the last of the bashas are done." He turned to leave.

"Thank you, Major."

Major John faced me with a big, flirtatious smile. Now I knew he was interested in me! I hummed a little ditty and continued with my work.

After the doctor left, I pondered what I would tell the staff about the rainy season. But we were in the Army, and we would have to adapt. We'd done it before.

Stevie came and told me, "Mong's missing."

A Chinese soldier said, "He left for the bazaar to get a good deal. He'll be back."

"There's a bazaar here?" I marveled.

"On the other side of Tagap." Stevie pointed west.

My nurses had settled into a good routine, so I borrowed a jeep and took Lorna with me to visit the local bazaar. I thought the excursion might get her mind off her boyfriend back home. When we arrived, I was unable to speak the language but found a native who knew a little English and paid him to help us bargain and shop.

"Look, high rubber boots!" I pointed. "These are perfect for us. Help me pick out the right sizes for all the nurses."

"What would we need those ugly things for in this hot climate?" Lorna said, wrinkling her nose.

"Remember the monsoons in Liberia? Well, they have them here too. And they're coming."

"I hated all that rain in Liberia."

"Major John told me that buckets of rain will pour down and cause accidents for the soldiers building the road."

Lorna found canned butter and Lipton Chicken Noodle Soup. I added fresh fruit to the basket—papayas, mangoes, bananas, coconuts, guavas, limes, lemons, grapes, musk melons, jack fruit, pineapple, and a giant watermelon.

When we returned to camp, we parked the jeep and began unpacking our market items.

Hilary greeted us. "Chief, all the bashas are done. We can say goodbye to the tents!"

I was so busy unpacking that I didn't notice all the huts sitting neatly in a row, finished at last. "That's wonderful news! I'd like to see everyone's new houses. But first, everyone, please take the supplies over to the table and we'll have a celebration."

Polly sang out, "No more tents, no more tents!"

Hilary inspected the box of boots. "Those are ugly-looking things."

I sighed. "The monsoon season will come this month and you'll all be glad to have the rubber boots then." I looked at all the new bashas. "At least we have decent shelter now. I saw some items at the bazaar we can furnish them with and I'll go to the market again next week. Look—we have fruit that's not in a can! Everyone, please eat. I'll get a knife from my basha." I hurried to retrieve the knife and returned to the excited girls.

Betty leaned into the jeep and lifted the watermelon over her head. "Let's have watermelon first."

Clara, full of cheer, said, "I've never had a watermelon."

"I suppose you wouldn't since you're from New York City," I said. "My family grew watermelons in our backyard in Georgia. I love 'em." I cut a slice for everyone, then took a juicy bite from the bright-red fruit, which brought memories of meals with my brothers and sisters in our backyard.

The next day on the ward, in walked Major John. I was busy bandaging a patient and heard him start up a conversation with Clara. Out of the corner of my eye, I saw that he had his boyish flirt going on. After I watched him touch Clara's arm, I was prickled with jealousy but continued with my nursing tasks. I waited for the major to ask me how I liked all his improvements, but much to my disappointment, he left without giving me the time of day. I was ready to talk to him about the issue of Chinese prejudice among the nurses, but that would have to wait.

Doc Samuel came into the ward with a patient of his who

had been in a road accident and had just had his arm amputated. He gave me instructions for the care of this poor man. While he spoke, I was once again riveted by his lovely, multicolored eyes.

"I'll personally make sure he heals well. How've you been, Doctor? I don't get to talk to you very often." I moved closer to him.

"I've been in surgery nonstop since the monsoons arrived. Many of the truck drivers swerve off the road and careen into the jungle—lots of accidents. I do feel very needed here." He smiled at me. "How've you been, Chief Dottie? I've been meaning to come and see you."

"As busy as you. We've established a good routine here. I just have a few problems that I'm trying to figure out." I gave him my best smile and experienced that same delicious, warm sensation I felt when we had traveled together.

"Do you have time to take a break? I miss our conversations." Doc Samuel grinned.

"I could." My entire body quivered as I straightened my army cap.

"If you have enough staff here, why don't we go for a walk? It's one of those rare days that it's not too wet out."

"I'd like that. Let me go talk to Clara and put her in charge."

A short time later, we took the jungle path up to chow. I slipped on the uneven ground and the doc caught me before I landed on my bottom. His grip on my arm was strong but gentle.

"Careful, Dottie, you're sorely needed here. I wouldn't want you to end up becoming one of the patients!" He gave a little chuckle and held my hand the rest of the way up.

"Thanks for catching me," I said, batting my eyelashes.

As I held Doc Samuel's hand, it brought up the only memory I had of being close to a boy. At home, I never had the time to go out on dates what with chores, family time, and work. When I was 13, Elijah, the boy next door, came over while I was outside and said hello. Much to my surprise, he helped me hang the wash. When we were almost done, his mother called for him to come home. He looked straight into my eyes, grabbed me, kissed me firmly on the lips, then ran off. At first, I was startled, but then I touched my lips with my finger and felt my cheeks flush. It was just like the feeling I had now.

We were all alone, high above the hospital, and since it was between mealtimes, we sat next to each other on a makeshift bamboo bench with a view of the mountains.

"Those snow-capped mountains are breathtaking," I marveled. "Real snow!"

"Yes, I'm amazed to see snow on the mountains in this humid jungle. I like sitting here with you away from our hectic jobs. I always admired how sensitive and positive you were when you trained your nurses back at Fort Huachuca."

"I've missed the conversations we had when we traveled together." I tilted my head and smiled.

"You helped pass the time. I loved sharing all my book knowledge with you about Burma." He sighed. "I've been frustrated having to perform so many amputations. I wish I could do more for the soldiers…save their limbs. Poor guys will be sent home now as invalids. Tell me…you mentioned you had a problem. I'd be glad to help."

I told Doc Samuel every detail of the conversations I'd had with Hilary, happy to have a confidant while we sat on the bench and observed the surreal, seemingly endless panoramic landscape. "For the most part, the nurses do their jobs well and have had to overcome the squeamish parts of nursing care in a jungle environment, like removing leeches. But I can't seem to figure out how to change a few of the nurses' outright prejudice against the Chinese soldiers."

"Tell me more so I can help." He touched my hand and looked at me intently.

"The Chinese soldiers are from an unusual culture. They don't like to be told what to do, especially by women. They obey the physicians and medics more than us. One of my nurses has no patience for the Chinese and even asked me what was wrong with their eyes!"

"Always remind your nurses that the Chinese soldiers do risk their lives to help us win this war. As soon as they are healed, they go right back into fierce warfare in the jungle with the knowledge that they could be shot or killed."

"How true, Doc. And I'll tell my nurses that. Hilary seems to be the main problem and I feel that if I can change her opinion, then the other nurses will follow." I surprised myself and leaned closer to him.

"Prejudice causes discrimination along with preformed negative judgments and attitudes. I've found it's all a matter of education to get a person to see a different side and step into someone else's shoes, so to speak. It's unfortunate that most races tend to think they are the superior ones."

I nodded. "Yes, it's odd to hear coloreds acting so prejudiced when we've always been on the receiving end of that kind of behavior, don't you think?"

Doc Samuel agreed. "It's important to not stereotype an entire group because of one person's actions. When nurses choose this profession, a good nurse must check her negative opinions and look for the positive traits of an individual as much as possible. And remember, a little bit of praise for good behavior goes a long way."

"Well said. You've given me a lot to think about. Now I can pass your fine ideas along to the nurses. Thanks, Doc, for helping me with this difficult problem."

"And thank you for being such an understanding chief. Your nurses are very fortunate to have you." He paused. "This is off the subject, but I can't keep from admiring your brown eyes. I feel like I could sink in them!"

He took off his glasses and put them in his pocket, then

held my gaze. I turned away to hide my awkwardness.

"Sorry," he said softly. "I didn't mean to be that forward."

"I'm not used to receiving compliments," I admitted with a weak smile.

"Your big, brown, beautiful eyes have incredible yellow sparkles in them and shine when you smile. I thought my mother's brown eyes were big but yours are sensationally larger." He latched his eyes to mine.

I said, "Your eyes are quite a captivating color as well—such an unusual mix of colors."

He chuckled. "My father's White and my mother's colored, and I must've received a mix of their eye color."

"When I first met you, I was so distracted by them! I observed you during your lectures at the base and tried to figure out whether you were White or Negro. Your skin color has quite a light-brown tone. I wasn't sure which race you were."

Doc Samuel grinned. "I'm sure you know that if you have one drop of Negro blood, you are labeled a Negro. My Mom used to say, 'One drop of Negro blood means one hate from the White folks.'"

"Yes, I do know about the one-sixteenth or one-drop rule because I worked in Georgia."

I wanted to ask him if his parents were married, since racial mixing was illegal. But instead, I brashly asked, "I'm curious, and please don't feel you have to answer this question, but have you ever tried to pass for White?"

He displayed a noticeable blush. "Yes, I have, but I've never told anyone because when a colored passes for good and gets away with it, they lose all their relatives and friends. What's so sad about that is they would lose their family stories, memories, and traditions. I passed for a while to actually help Negro patients since White doctors were allowed and Negro doctors were not."

"I imagine that it helps you see both Negro and White

worlds. Do you mind telling me when you did this?"

"Well, that's how I got into the library in Huachuca to research Burma."

"Oh. When you told me you went to the library, I thought it was unusual because that town was not a place that would have had a library just for Negroes."

"How was your day leave in Huachuca?" Doc Samuel adeptly changed the subject.

"I ended up in jail there on a day pass."

Doc Samuel gave me an astonished look and I explained what had happened that day.

"Dottie," he said, then hesitated. "May I call you that?"

"Yes," I said in an eager but quiet tone.

"Please call me Sam. I'm sorry you were treated like that in a nurse's uniform—and especially because you have the high rank of chief." He rubbed my shoulders with affection and put his arm around me.

We sat for a little while longer and I felt like I was floating over those white mountains in the distance.

"Well," the doctor finally said, "guess we'd better get back to work."

We hiked back down the trail.

Outside the ward, Sam gave me a sweet little kiss on my cheek and said, "Let's get together again next week."

That night, I dreamed I was White-skinned, and the doctor was my color. It always amazed me how dreams mixed up elements of your real life, but in the dream it all seemed believable.

Chapter Twenty-Five
Bea
Santo Tomas, 1942-1943

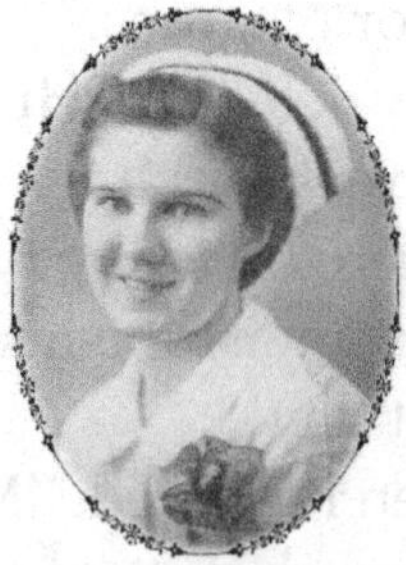

For Thanksgiving, we were lucky to receive truckloads of food labeled PRISONER PARCEL, thanks to the South African Red Cross. Each package contained cans of bacon, meat spread, margarine, condensed milk, tomatoes, marmalade, cheese pudding, soda, tea, crackers, a chocolate cake, and a piece of soap.

The executive committee approved the purchase of turkeys. The camp cook roasted them all but there wasn't enough for our burgeoning population. At the athletic field, a football game was played by our men and hundreds of internees cheered the teams on. After the game, we ate dinner and everyone had a small taste of turkey.

Hopeful whispers were heard during the meal.

"I sure hope our troops are coming…"

"They'll make it by Christmas, for sure..."

Before Christmas arrived, a wood whittler carved wooden crosses for the children. One of the nurses organized sewing rag dolls for all the little girls. The Navy nurses made jelly from native limes for presents. Caroline embroidered images of shanties and flowers on scrap linen. It brought me great pleasure to see everyone trying to keep the faith. I was surprised at how much I missed my mother as the nurses talked about what their Christmases were like back home. I reflected on mine and realized how spoiled I had been.

In the New Year of 1943, a New Year's Eve play of Cinderella was staged with handmade costumes. The production gave all the internees a positive attitude.

One day, I saw Mary with her husband outside. He was a member of the executive committee, and I told him that our nurses did not have any money to buy items we needed from the camp store.

Mary's husband, Oscar, said, "Your nurses can borrow money from the committee that can be paid back after the war is over. I'm sure your pay is held in an American bank."

"That's reassuring," I replied.

"Have you seen the camp store yet?"

"No."

"It's run by internees, and you can buy used clothing, soap, housewares, ice cream, sugar, flour, and so on. The goods are only cost plus 10 percent."

"I can't wait to tell the nurses!"

At the camp hospital, our nurses were required to put in four-hour shifts. We were grateful for the work, and it gave the nurses stability and purpose while we waited to be liberated, which we hoped would occur any time now. It was a relief that we no longer had to do intensive battlefield nursing with its endless emotional trauma and weary hours.

We were fast running out of medical supplies due to so many ill camp internees. We treated dysentery, jaundice, dengue fever, and the seemingly ever-present malaria. Many of the nurses were sick but we carried on and kept calm, like the stoic British said.

Molly continued to complain to me about not being able to sleep with her husband. I finally lost patience with her and said, "Be thankful your husband's alive!"

Her complaints stopped after that outburst.

On my shifts at the hospital, I saw intestinal maladies, heart problems due to anxiety, and chronic depression with emotional distress. In my opinion, this was all due to forced crowding. The internees looked gaunt and those in stained clothes looked like hobos. With the increase in population and food shortages, the executive and advisory committee drafted a letter to the Rockefeller Foundation and asked for money to buy supplies. The commandant accepted it because the committee also asked for money for all the small hospitals in the city of Manila.

The Rockefeller Foundation approved the request and sent the money to the executive committee. The committee agreed to give the nurses money each month, but we were required to pay it back as soon as the war was over. The money allowed the nurses to build shanties and buy extra food from Filipino vendors or the camp canteen.

Every day, the Filipino people came to the gate to give us free fruit or to sell us cooked items. On my day off, I went to the gate to buy food and there was Carmelita with her family. I was delighted to learn from her that our Filipina nurses from Corregidor did return to their homes after we had left them. I bought all the adobo Carmelita had made, and she told me it was the national dish of her people. I shared it with the nurses at the hospital, who ate it with gusto and were happy to hear the news that our Filipina colleagues were safe and well.

More and more civilian prisoners were brought into the camp. Commandant Kuroda ordered the nurses to move into the main women's building. They were loath to move again because everyone liked how spacious our area was compared to the two rooms we'd had at the convent. I protested to the executive committee, who said we had no choice because more women, children, and elderly had been "found" and needed to be relocated there.

We were packed in rooms with cots less than six inches apart, with barely any room to dress. We slept head to toe. There were still empty classrooms available, but the Japanese wanted everyone close together so they could be monitored. The chaos inside of babies crying and youngsters arguing left most of the nurses begging to work longer shifts at the hospital just to escape the chaos.

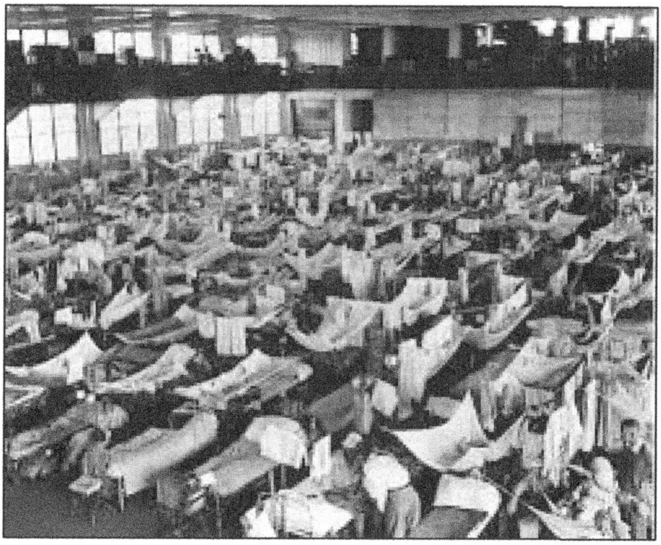

Over 200 more people were brought into Santo Tomas plus the Japanese commandant transferred in the sickest patients from Philippine General Hospital. There were continuous shortages of food and our innovative nurses planted gardens to help feed the patients. For the first time in my life, I was at the perfect weight, and now worried about becoming too thin.

The Japanese Imperial Army changed the commandant of the internment camp every six months. The new commandant arrived and announced on the camp loudspeaker: "No outside Filipino doctors and nurses will be allowed into the camp. No internees may get care at the eight outside hospitals for special services. Any internees at these hospitals must return. Married couples with or without children are permitted to live in their shanties."

There was an outburst of claps from the internees and Molly yelled, "Yippee! At last, I can sleep with my husband!"

I wasn't too surprised by this announcement since we had over 500 children without any vacant classrooms to live in.

The executive committee suggested that classes be formed to ease the prolonged tension of the internment. Many of the captives had been imprisoned there for almost two years, since January 1942. Spanish classes were taught. Father O'Leary had a class on the Catholic view of art. Two golf pros had been captured and a golf class was formed. Camp baseball games were held. Singing lessons were offered, and a choral group performed for the camp.

All these leisure activities helped pass the time but we were always still under the watchful eyes of the armed Japanese guards. And we were all still prisoners of war.

Chapter Twenty-Six
Dottie
Tagap, Burma 1945

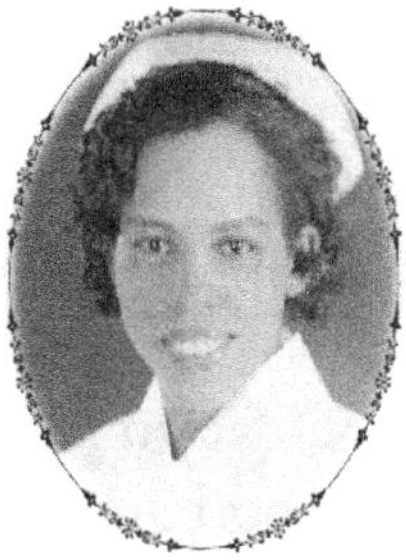

I took Hilary with me to the bazaar to have some alone time and to get closer to her before I broached the serious subject of prejudice.

I asked her how she was, and Hilary replied, "Good. That dreamboat Major John was smart to supply isolation partitions and garbage bins, and we've formed a great relationship." She giggled.

That remark floated through my mind. *I'd better not waste my time on a polygamous flirter.* Not only did he flirt with me and Clara, but now Hilary too. Mama always called men like those philanderers and womanizers.

We wandered around the exotic native bazaar and bought inexpensive bamboo chairs, tables, and colorful camel-hair rugs for our new abodes. I bought more fresh fruit and vegetables. Hilary had a grand time and helped me pick out colorful pieces of material to make into curtains and tablecloths. She called me over to a table where a small native woman was selling precious British sanitary napkins.

"Great find, Hilary. The girls will love those." I bought the entire supply.

When we finished shopping, we got back into the jeep and

had a native help pile in the supplies for the nurses. When we arrived back in camp, the nurses were ecstatic to see all the packages.

Polly stared at our loaded vehicle. "Everyone's gonna get birthday presents!"

Lorna added, "Those cute tables and chairs can replace the crappy crates and boxes we have."

I saved the best gift for last. "Look what we found." I brought out the sanitary napkins.

Oohs and ahhs sounded out as Clara bounced up and down in glee and shouted, "No more rags!"

After everyone took a good supply of the napkins, I told the gals I would store the rest in the hospital.

The next day, two nurses came in to replace us for lunch and I invited Hilary to hike up to chow with me. On the way up the hill, in a soft voice, I said, "Tell me, Hilary, where are you from?"

"Biloxi, Mississippi. Southern, just like you." She smiled.

"Have you ever experienced anyone of a different race that was nasty to you?"

"Of course! White people. All the time. That's a silly question."

This was my opportunity to explain to her the advice that Sam had given me. I told her how our country relied on the Chinese to help end the war and added what a skilled nurse she was. "Hilary, I would like you to try harder with the Chinese and keep in mind what their lives must be like on the battlefield. And…" I reiterated, "…how to appreciate their help in this war."

She stopped on the trail. "I'll try."

That evening, with most of the nurses present at chow, I stood up and said, "I know it is hard for all of you to understand the unusual behavior of the Chinese soldiers, but these men are risking their lives to win this war. When they gamble or eat their own kind of food, it is their relief from fighting and a way to feel better. As soon as they are healed, they must go right back into fierce combat knowing they can easily be shot or killed."

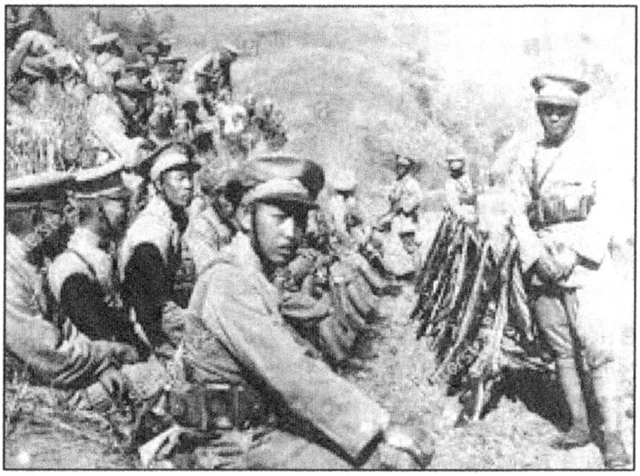

I saw a few expressions of agreement.

I continued, "As nurses, we must check our negative judgment and look for the positive traits of cultures different than ours. As colored people, we know what it's like to be negatively judged but that doesn't give us the right to do the same to another race."

I sat down and ate some beans and rice, and listened to the nurses, who discussed the circumstances when they had experienced discrimination.

I showed my gratitude and said, "Thank you, everyone, for choosing nursing as a career. I know it is not an easy job, but not one day goes by that one of the doctors doesn't tell me how skilled and competent you all are, and that you are all a pleasure to work with."

Sam came into the ward the next week and whispered in my ear, "Can you take a break now?"

Heat rushed onto my face as I beamed, "Sure can, give me five minutes."

My heart beat a little quicker as I hurried to find Betty and put her in charge.

She said with a mischievous smile, "Everyone thinks you two must be an item!"

I looked behind me to see if the doc had overheard but he was waiting outside the ward.

On our way up the mountain, a smile spread on my face as I thought, *Oh my goodness. I think we're going on a date – as much as dates can exist in this primitive environment!*

On the path, he talked about the lovely flowers of the jungle, like the lush purple butterfly orchids that hung from the trees and cascaded down from the branches. The vines were three feet long with many deep-purple flowers up and down them, plus bright-red, tongue-like petals on each flower. Sam told me he had read about jungle flowers in the Huachuca library.

I felt one of the soft purple petals. "I love that it's called a butterfly orchid because of its two wings."

Sam picked one of the profusions of yellow blossoms called hibiscus, and put it gently behind my ear, then placed a butterfly-wing flower behind the other ear.

I whispered, "Thank you. The flowers smell heavenly."

"And you look beautiful with them in your hair." He touched my cheek, then kissed me as we stood at the top of the hill and took in the breathtaking view. His mustache tickled my nose.

Sam and I sat close together on the bench and stared out at the magnificent sight of the mountain range. He cuddled toward me, and I rested my head on his chest and listened to the patter of his heartbeat.

"I sure like you, Dottie." Sam took off his glasses.

We looked into each other's eyes, then fell into a long, sensual kiss. I shut my eyes tight and saw tiny stars twinkling.

When our break time was over, we left with our arms around each other and headed back to our duties.

When I returned to the hospital, I saw several of the Chinese soldiers cleaning their guns, which wasn't unusual. But…they were using our Kotex! I was furious that they had wasted our precious napkins to clean their weapons. In a huff, I grabbed up the extras to store inside my basha for safety. After I calmed down, I realized that the soldiers probably had no clue why we needed them so badly.

Later that night, Clara whispered to me in private, "I'm happy for you, Chief. I think you and Doc make a good match."

I was a bit shy but felt a sense of pride to have someone I cared for in this awful place.

My nurses grew close to each other. We were in small, confined areas day and night, which resulted in close bonds and friendships. And whenever someone received a package from home, it was shared, no matter how small. Even a jar of mustard!

Chapter Twenty-Seven
Bea
Santo Tomas, 1944

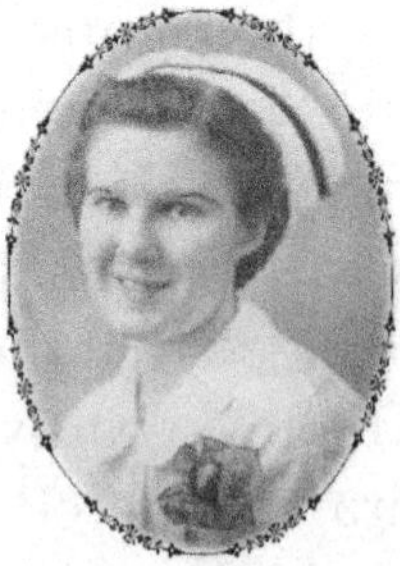

As we faced the year 1944 in the POW camp, our hopes of rescue were dashed. Many of us looked up at the sky for our shiny silver planes with stars on them. Occasionally, one was spotted but that was the problem—only one! I waved my arms at the vast blue sky and yelled, "Where are you, Uncle Sam?"

This was our second year in captivity and Nurse Susie announced to anyone who would listen, "The Japs are systematically starving us to death."

I gave her a stern stare but noticed how everyone agreed with her.

More and more gardens were planted in February and seven acres were cleared. Swiss chard, beans, tomatoes, and native camotes—a root similar to a sweet potato—were planted. The nurses who had the energy to work in the gardens helped but many were unable.

The rice reserves were exhausted. Many of the internees sat around and did nothing. The new commandant suggested that anyone who stayed in bed all day should be given less food to eat. He announced: "All able men, women, and children need to garden in every available space on the campus. Manila has only a small amount of food available to buy. In the dry season, expect fewer vegetables."

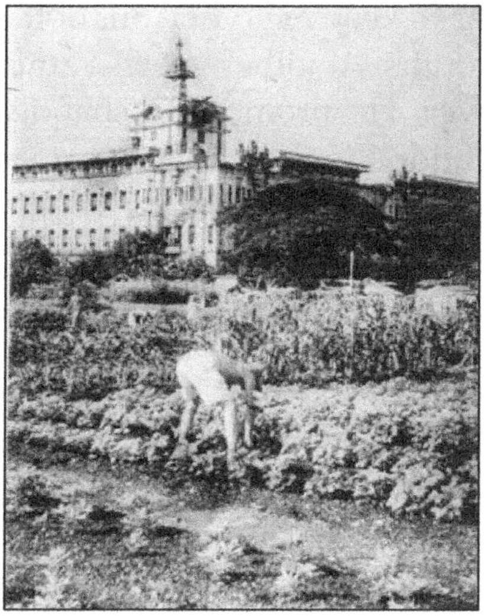

Dr. Bloom suggested that the dogs and cats in the camp be collected and killed, then eaten, and that the children should be fed first. His suggestion was taken and within the week, there were no dogs and cats seen roaming about.

The commandant allowed every corner of Santo Tomas to be used for garden space. Shifts of men worked hard in the gardens—even the commandant himself worked in one of them. The older, weaker men could not do as much. Soon depression and starvation were the main illnesses in the hospital.

In February of 1944, from the window of the highest floor of the dorms, we saw American planes bombing and strafing the city of Manila. We endured constant bombing and air raids. The next week brought the longest air raid. In the morning, American planes were seen diving and bombing in the area of Manila Bay. The question on our minds was...were we winning?

A Japanese general's Cadillac had been brought into the camp to store. One day, the children were caught playing in it so the commandant, outraged, ordered that a special shelter be built for the car to keep everyone out of it.

After six months, another new camp commandant, Onozaki, took over. He promptly disbanded the executive committee and added more Japanese guards with guns. Charcoal and wood supplies used for cooking were cut off. All the stores and shops were closed. We had to line up to get meal tickets stamped, and meat was only used as a flavoring. Noontime meals were stopped for the adults and were only available for the children. Some people believed this radical change meant we must be winning the war.

In the sweltering summer, many of us were weak and dizzy. Someone built a bench we could sit on between the flights of stairs leading to where we slept. That way, we could rest halfway up. One super-positive Navy nurse, Sue, made a large rag doll dressed in scrap khaki fabric and put a large sign on it that said, "Any Day Now, Doll!"

On June 6, we heard on the "secret radio" the wonderful news that the Allies had invaded France and liberated it from the Nazis. This hidden radio set was bolted inside a five-gallon oil can with a tight cover, and there was a replacement set inside a pressure cooker. Our camp electrician, Jim, oversaw both. It was turned on infrequently, and only in safe times away from the guards.

A week later, eight Allied Marine Corps bombers buzzed low in formation over the campus and dropped a flurry of notes and a pair of aviator's goggles, which a nurse found with a note attached that read "Roll out the barrel, Santa Claus is coming!"

The Japanese guards ordered everyone to stay inside after close gunfire was heard outside the Santo Tomas walls. All night long we heard sounds of shelling and detonations across the city, and through our windows on the top floors, we saw fires that burned in the distance.

As the summer got hotter, we saw many Japanese Zeros fly by. We spotted an American plane, which "waved" at us with its wings, and many of the internees cheered. I thought, *I dare you to come down here and take me home!*

Molly recorded 75 cases of beriberi for the month, a nutritional deficiency disease caused by low levels of vitamin B-1 and thiamine. There were also cases of wet beriberi that made the extremities swell and patients immobile. I tallied four cases of scurvy, which was a deficiency of vitamins B and C, and 12 cases of pellagra, a niacin deficiency affecting the gastrointestinal tract. As chief, I was required to record, but since my eyeglasses had been stolen on Corregidor, I was unable to read and write.

Our diet was slowly killing us. There were falling accidents from not having enough food. Everyone I saw had thin jawlines and sunken cheeks. My positive attitude took a nosedive. Susie was right—the Japanese were systematically starving us to death and being malnourished taxed our metabolism, muscles, and cardiovascular systems. I was tired, weak, and irritable with joint and leg pain and swollen and bleeding gums. Bruises appeared all over my skin and my hair turned prematurely gray. I became a tall, spindle of a gal. Most of the women weighed under a hundred pounds and the average male internee lost a staggering 51 pounds. One of the Japanese guards told me they were given the same amount of food as the internees. I saw the lie on his face and his healthy body, and knew that wasn't true.

The patients in our camp hospital who were expected to die were usually sent away to the city hospitals. The Japanese wouldn't permit that now because of a lack of fuel available to transport them. If anyone was near death, the nurses would put up a white sheet around their bed and let them die right there in the hospital. The tropical weather made the dead bodies decay fast and large rats preyed upon them. This had a profound, depressing effect on all the patients until a nurse would go out and beg one of the guards to carry the dead out to be buried.

A friend of an elderly patient asked if he could be given a little more food. Dr. Bloom answered, "I'd rather give it to the children."

The Imperial Army cut further amounts of food from the internees. The number of deaths for the month of October, 1944 was nine, all older men.

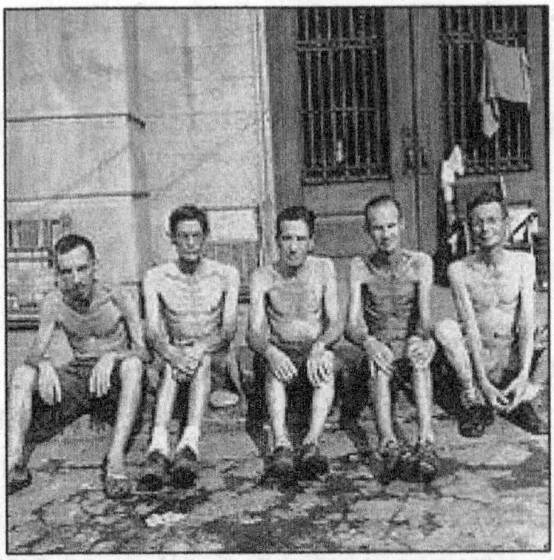

I confided to Molly, "I can feel my intestines and stomach bounce with every pathetic step I take. Plus I have a limp that I'm sure I got from having beriberi."

At the end of October, we heard over the secret radio that American troops were at the Leyte Gulf to liberate the Philippines. We held any piece of good news close to our skinny bodies and repeated it to everyone with faith that we would be rescued soon.

Thanksgiving came and the International YMCA sent over 200 ducks. Unfortunately, they were scrawny and did not feed enough people. I turned a blind eye when I caught one of the nurses eating cold cream out of her Red Cross kit.

My dedicated nurses continued to work their shifts, although we had to sit down and rest between tending to the patients. With only one cup of gruel a day, the act of changing a simple bandage exhausted us. The gruel was made from soybean meal that was customarily used to feed cattle, and had little nutritional value.

Dr. Charlie made a camp announcement. "Parents, you must watch your children. Do not allow them to eat any poisonous plants like hibiscus leaves or canna lily bulbs. Your children scoop up spilled mush from the ground and are eating garbage. I repeat—everyone watch your children. There have been many cases of food poisoning."

The longer the war continued, the more restrictions the Imperial Army enforced. Everyone was ordered into their buildings by 7 p.m. with lights off by 8 p.m. Our sources of entertainment, like bridge or chess, were not possible in the unlit interiors of the buildings. Only small lights were allowed in the toilets and hallways because of the blackouts. The Japanese were on the hunt and confiscated electric razors, several electric light bulbs, and over 50 library books were censored. Hot water was discontinued because of the fuel shortage for the boiler.

Everyone was frustrated and arguments broke out among the internees.

"They're doing this because we're losing the war!" Arthur yelled as he paced outside.

"That's not true. The Japs are punishing us because we're winning the war!" Jim screamed back.

Unfortunately, this did not improve morale and plunged many internees further into despair.

Chapter Twenty-Eight
Dottie
Tagap, Burma 1945

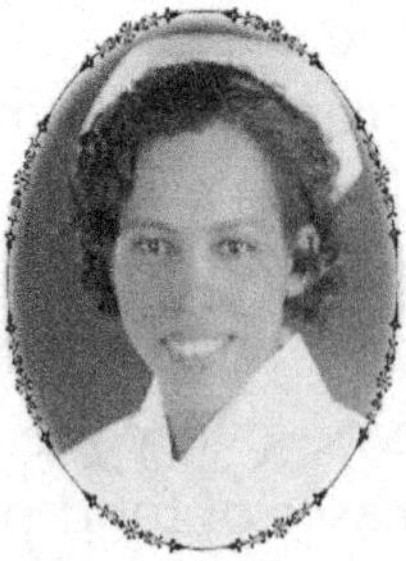

Doc Sam came by the ward and picked me up for another date. After hiking the trail to the chow area, we sat on "our" bench, looked out at the distant Tibetan snow-capped mountains, and shared our week. It was a good feeling for both of us to have a confidant. He held my face in his hands and we shared a long, deep, dreamy kiss. Then we sat in silence, observed the unending landscape, and enjoyed each other's company.

"How's it going with your nurse…Hilary, I believe was her name?" Sam put his arm around me.

"I used all your helpful suggestions, and she was quiet during most of the conversation, which I think meant she was listening. I know Hilary is capable of compassion and change. I asked if she had ever experienced prejudice herself and what it felt like. The next day, I saw her trying to talk to one of the Chinese soldiers to tell him to keep his bandages on, and I could tell by the kind tone of her voice that she had listened to me."

"That was very astute of you to ask her if she had ever experienced prejudice. This helps a person reflect on what it's like to be on the receiving end. In wartime, we all share the same goal—to bring peace to the world and end the war. It's important to focus on this essential, long-term goal and not get distracted by small problems that can be fixed with a proper attitude." Sam paused. "Sorry, I didn't mean to lecture..."

"Not at all. I agree with every word. Well put."

"Dottie, continue to praise her when she is compassionate, as well as all the other nurses. Which I'm sure you do."

I nodded. "Sometimes when she says mean things about the Chinese—especially to the other nurses—I give her my *don't talk like that* look and she stops. Do you think that's all right to do?"

"Definitely," Sam said and kissed me once again.

This might be the day I lose my virginity... I thought. Caught up in the rush of the moment, I whispered, "I think I'm falling—"

He pulled away and raised his eyebrows.

"I think...I think I'm falling for you." I had almost blurted out, *I think I'm falling in love.*

"Yes, I understand." He took my hand and led me into the bamboo dining hall. His gaze pierced into mine as he unbuttoned my shirt and I unbuttoned his.

I stopped and said, "Do you have..."

He answered in a joking voice, "What do you think? Don't you remember the lecture I gave on venereal disease?"

"Of course," I blushed.

The doc reached into his pocket and pulled out protection, then we stripped off the rest of our clothes and lay on the dining table. Sam climaxed and I didn't, but I did feel a satisfied contentment afterward—especially since he was such a careful, gentle man.

Sam lightly tickled my arm, then kissed my cheek. "I adore the color of your skin. It reminds me of my mama's."

"What's she like?"

"My memory of her is hazy. She died from influenza when

I was a young boy. Your skin color matches hers and reminds me of a delicious chocolate bar."

"How sad for you that she passed away when you were just a kid. My daddy died of influenza too, when I was a teenager." I gingerly tickled him "When I feel your chest, its pale color makes me feel like I'm touching forbidden fruit."

As we lay there, naked and exposed, a breeze blew through the back of the dining basha.

"I think I hear someone." I jumped up and quickly put my clothes back on.

Sam did the same and looked outside the hut. "I think it was just one of the jungle animals."

We strolled back to the bench and sat close together.

"Tell me, Sam, have you ever been with a White girl?"

He hesitated. "I'd rather not say." He glanced at his watch. "We'd better get back to work."

That night, I lay in bed and wondered if Sam knew I didn't climax. Or maybe he didn't care. I decided it didn't really matter and savored the intimate moment between us.

I was deep in thought the next day as I worked on charts. My mind drifted and I relived my rendezvous with Sam. I felt certain that he had been with a White girl in the past since he wouldn't talk about it when I asked.

"Chief Dottie, should I take his temperature or not?" Clara said for the second time.

Embarrassment washed over my face. "Sorry, I've been deep in thought…" I answered her question, then contemplated, *So, this is love. Love at last! I mustn't let it take over my work or a disaster could occur.*

On the ward that day, I overheard two Negro patients who were recovering from accidents talking about their work. The soldier with a broken arm asked the boy next to him, "Have you ever had trouble with Sgt. Michaels?"

"Yeah, I was kicked by him while I was building the road because I wasn't moving fast enough as far as he was concerned."

"I had the same thing happen."

"I'm tired of these White officers who act like they're hot shit and think they're better than us."

"The major said to me that Negroes do not make strong leaders and your group will be successful only if White men lead them."

"What burns me is we rarely get promoted in rank even though we've put in the time and work."

"That's for sure!"

"I do like Chief Road Engineer Colonel Pick. He once caught a White officer who shoved one of my buddies and Pick told him in front of everyone that if he ever did that again, he'd get demoted."

"Yeah, he's an outstanding chief. I always feel that he respects Negroes anytime he's around."

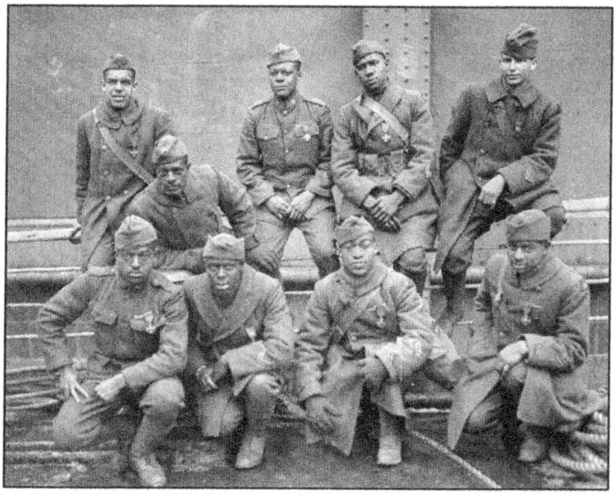

93rd Division soldiers who worked on Ledo Road

A short time later, Stevie and another medic brought in a White soldier on a stretcher. I gasped as they transferred him to an empty bed.

I took Stevie aside. "What are you doing in here with a

White soldier? You know it's not allowed."

Stevie held his ground. "He's hemorrhaging and demanded to be taken to our hospital since he would've died by the time we got him to the 20th General White Hospital."

"Go get Doc John. We must get permission to treat him," I ordered.

A short time later, Major John stormed into the ward. He looked at the man, who had soaked bandage after bandage from his bleeding wounds. Alarmed, he said, "What's happened to this man?"

Stevie answered, "He was attacked by a tiger."

"Give him blood before he bleeds to death!"

"But Doctor," I said, "we only have Negro blood—no White blood." I squeezed my hands nervously.

The patient pleaded, "Don't let me die. I don't give a damn if it's Negro blood!"

Major John yelled, "What are you waiting for, Stevie? Go get the 'N' blood!"

Stevie came back with a glass bottle of blood labeled "N" and handed it to Clara, who began the transfusion.

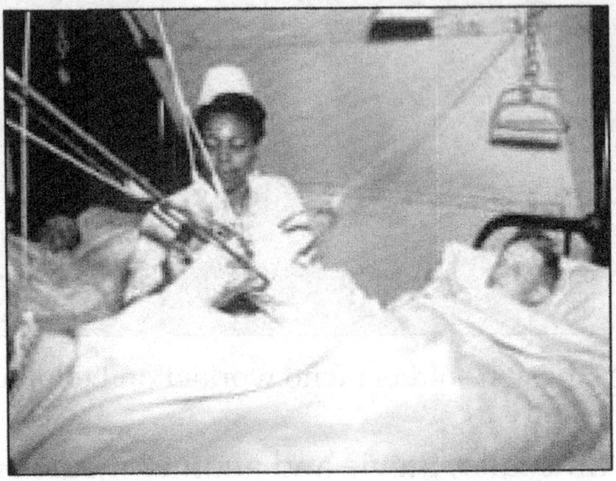

Hazel spoke up, "Will it make his skin black?"

"No!" I snapped. "When I was at Grady Hospital, we had a similar situation, and the 'N' blood did not turn the patient black. As far as I'm concerned, all the races are the same color inside. RED!"

After the White man was sewn up in the operating room, he was brought back into the ward to recover and told us about his attack. "I was deep in the jungle getting the natives to clear it so I could put in better drainage pipes. I passed by a tiger hidden in a large cluster of bushes with her family of cubs. Before I knew it, she attacked me from behind. Her big canine teeth pierced the muscles of my neck, and she clamped down with the full force of her jaws. There was no sound from the animal—no hiss or growl. Then she shook me like I was a captured deer. I remembered that someone once told me if I ever was attacked by a savage dog, to put my hand behind its lower teeth and pull down. I managed to do that, and it tore up my hand, but it worked. A few Naga workers hit the tiger with giant bamboo poles and chased her away. But I was bleeding profusely and covered with blood."

The nurses on the ward were dumbstruck by this event. I shook my head as I listened to the story with the other patients and nurses. *There's never a dull moment caring for patients in a jungle,* I thought.

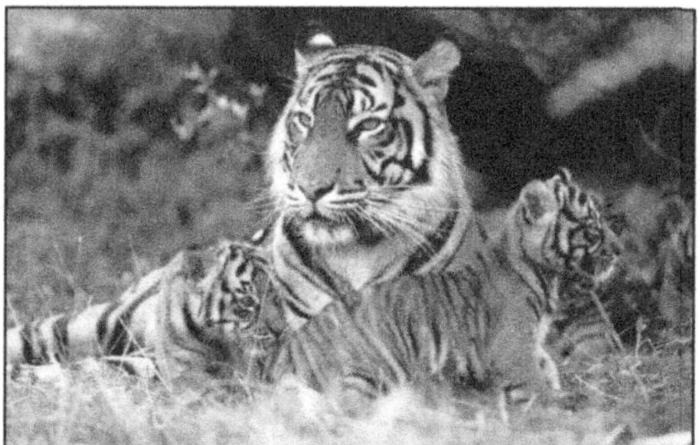

Chapter Twenty-Nine

Bea

Santo Tomas 1944-1945

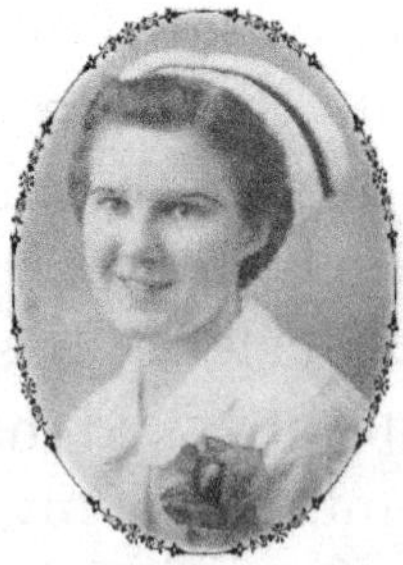

The month of December brought flights of Japanese Zeros that swarmed the airspace above our camp. Shortly thereafter, we spotted 19 Flying Fortresses and 40 P-38s. My heart beat faster when I saw the American planes.

Maybe Rob will come and rescue me…

Our Allies dropped bombs north of the camp. We all applauded and heaved sighs of relief. It was the first time we had seen more than one of our Allied planes nearby.

Our Japanese captives delivered over a thousand letters dated from months ago, and dumped the pile outside in front of the dorms. I was on duty at the hospital doing my rounds when Arthur came in.

"Chief Bea, here are all the letters addressed to the medical personnel."

"Thank you," I said. "It was kind of you to sort them."

On my break, I asked Molly to read the only letter I had received from my mother since my internment.

Dear Beatrice,

I will keep this letter short since you have not answered any of my previous letters.

France has been liberated and all the ladies in the bridge group consider this to mean we will win the war. Please write me as soon as possible. Did you get the hat I mailed to you? I don't even know where you are. I wish you were home with me safe and sound. I truly feel it was a big mistake that you joined the Army.

Love, Mom

I thanked Molly, then stuffed the letter into my pocket. I did not have the energy or the right attitude to respond. And I was still angry about my glasses. It was doubtful that my mother had received any of my letters since Corregidor.

There was good news and bad news. First the good news. On December 7, the Japanese brought in three truckloads of food, which included 10 kilos of rice, 400 kilos of sweet potato-like camotes, 100 coconuts, and salt. The commandant announced that any men who performed labor, like building a boardwalk, should receive extra rations. Most of the men did not feel well enough to work—especially on unnecessary projects that the commandant insisted were necessary.

The bad news occurred when the Japanese military police marched into camp and arrested all the members of the former executive committee. Their shanties and sleeping quarters were searched. We all wondered what they were looking for. Papers? The hidden radio? They found nothing, but took the members to the tiny jail room behind the commandant's office. Mary, the wife of one of the men, became a nervous wreck and worried that her husband would be shot.

On December 24, the air raid alarm sounded. A solemn, Christmas Eve Mass was conducted by Father O'Leary in the hospital chapel but not at midnight. Music was postponed because of the bombing. And so, another Christmas season in Japanese captivity was celebrated in despair. The Red Cross had nothing to give because of the black market. Sugar and margarine cost an extreme amount per pound.

Members of the Neutral Welfare Committee of the International YMCA were permitted into the camp and brought in a small amount of food items, tobacco, clothing, phonograph records, and medicines. But there was never enough food for our bulging population.

Very early on Christmas morning, under cover of darkness, leaflets were dropped from an American plane. As others scrambled about picking them up, I grabbed one off the ground and managed to read it with squinted eyes.

> *The Commander in Chief, the officers, and the men of the American Forces of Liberation in the Pacific wish their gallant allies, the People of the Philippines, all the blessings of Christmas and the realization of their fervent hopes for the New Year.*
>
> *— Christmas 1944*

We held the leaflets tight in our hands and mumbled prayers that we would be rescued soon.

Molly, full of glee, said, "Our troops are coming! Maybe we'll make it home for a New Year's celebration!"

On Christmas Day, the children were given two teaspoons of jam, one small disk of native chocolate, and two pieces each of bocayo candy, which was made from coconut and sugar. This was possible because the parents had chipped in money and the Japanese brought the items into camp. Some of the fortunate children received homemade toys and dolls from their parents. Only the elderly and children received three meals that day. Breakfast was mush and coconut milk with a small amount of chocolate, and a cup of so-called coffee. Lunch was thick soybean soup. Dinner was a double serving of fried rice, camotes, and canned meat. It was a meager

Christmas for the rest of us.

The day after Christmas, an air raid sounded at 10 a.m. Five American Pursuit planes flew over the city. Our faith was like a seesaw; up when we spotted our planes and down when a few days later, the sky was filled with Zeros.

It was now January 1945. We'd been imprisoned since July 1942—almost two-and-a-half years. Other internees had been there since January 1942, a full three years. It was a strange reality to grasp. Dr. Bloom reported 23 deaths for the month of December.

Are we all going to die here? I worried to myself.

Deaths continued to rise at an alarming rate. The hospital saw tuberculosis, measles, whooping cough, bacillary dysentery, edema, and anemia. The nurses witnessed mental breakdowns and suicide attempts from many of the patients. On one particularly gloomy day, all of it hit me. I went into the small bathroom in the hospital, locked the door, and sat on the toilet. I wanted to cry— I needed the release...but didn't have the strength to do it.

After a knock sounded on the door, I threw cold water on my face, then forced a false smile. When I opened the door, Dr. Stevenson stood there. I averted my eyes and left to immerse myself in my work.

Our captives pretended that we were treated well and did not want to be indicted for war crimes. The commandant ordered the physicians to remove the words "starvation" and "malnutrition" from all internee death certificates. When Dr. Stevenson refused, an armed guard came into the hospital and put him in the one-room camp jail for 10 days. When he returned, he reported that he was only given water, no food, the entire time.

Since the executive committee had been abolished, the guards began implementing punishments. For minor offenses, an internee was slapped several times in a public display. For major offenses, a person was taken outside of the camp, beaten, then brought back and hospitalized.

Four members of the executive committee continued to be jailed. I tried to find out from one of the wives why they were being held. She told me between sobs that they had no reason whatsoever to hold them in jail and that she could not find out from the Japanese commandant what the charges were.

At the end of January, 32 deaths were reported, most from heart failure due to starvation. Of course, Dr. Stevenson was ordered to leave the word "starvation" off the death certificates.

In February, the entire horizon was ringed with fire and smoke. The sound of demolition explosions was heard all night long. One day at noon, there was heavy bombing of the Manila waterfront. The Japanese commandant ordered the strongest internees to slaughter the last camp carabao. It was psychological torture when the meat was devoured by the Japanese in front of us and we were given only two sacks of inedible, fermented rice. The duck farm sheds were torn down for fuel. And the four members of the executive committee were still not released from jail.

On February 4, 1945, a hundred Allied men climbed over the wall and attacked the Japanese guards from behind. When we heard a loud metallic clap and banging, we knew the iron gates to the camp had been crashed down by American Army tanks. Everyone rushed to their windows to look outside. The flying column of the 8th Regiment 1st Brigade and Cavalry Division Rolled right up to the front door of our dorms—200 American Army men with five tanks.

The unmistakable sound of an American accent brought joy to our ears as a soldier called up to us in English, "Hello, folks! We're here!"

Several people sang out, "They're here! Our boys are here!"

Joyful cheers erupted throughout the dorms and tears rolled down our haggard faces. It was a happy, crazy scene as hundreds of internees raced down the stairs and jammed the lobby of the main building. But the Japanese guards, who stood inside with bayonets, would not let us out. The sentries fired their rifles out of the windows at the tanks. They put out the lights on one tank, killed one American soldier, and wounded three more.

Many of the internees leaned out of the second- and third-story windows and shouted repeatedly, "Let us out!"

The commandant refused to surrender and held both the men's and women's buildings hostage. The Japanese soldiers broke up furniture to barricade the doors, and guards with machine guns were posted at each end of the buildings.

The campus was crowded with tanks, guns, trucks, and jeeps. Tents went up and fires were made for cooking. At 1 p.m., kettles of stew made from corned beef, mung beans, and cornmeal were left outside the entrance to the building by our Allied soldiers. The Japanese took some, then left the rest for the internees upstairs. Later that day, six American soldiers were killed on campus and several internees who had climbed out of a window on a sheet were shot to death.

The Japanese continued to shell the campus. Someone said Dr. Bloom had been killed when he came out of the hospital. The priest was a patient in the hospital and a Japanese shell killed him in bed. Our Allied soldiers killed several Japanese.

The Santo Tomas Internment Camp became an active war zone with foxholes dug and shots fired from both sides. Shells crashed down on us, and concrete fragments and mortar dust blew in the air. We were in an excited state of bewilderment. What would happen? Would we win?

Many internees slept on the floors away from the windows. Throughout the night, large-caliber artillery boomed. We were caught in the war, and it was not over yet.

Within a few days, Santo Tomas was liberated and Colonel Brady negotiated to escort all the Japanese outside the camp to the city limits. The four members of the executive committee were executed by the Japanese and their bodies were found by our soldiers.

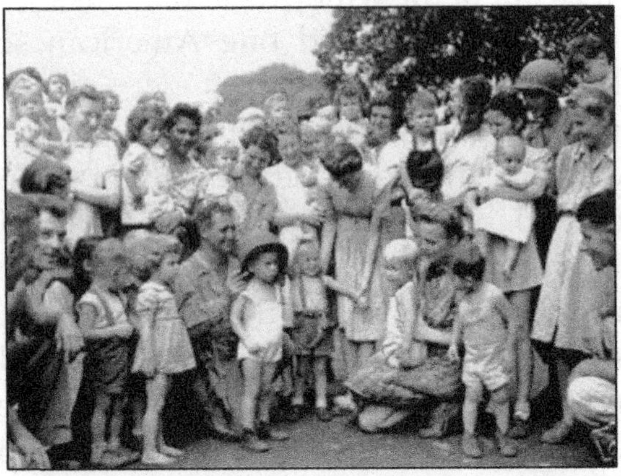

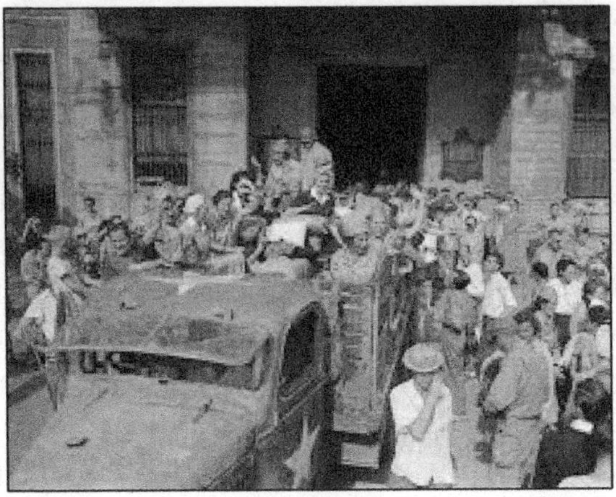

On February 5, 1945, our entire group of internees was released from both buildings. We stood in ceremony as the Japanese flag was taken down, followed by the hoisting of our beautiful Stars and Stripes. Our entire group of over 4,000 internees sang as loud as possible "God Bless America" followed by "The Star-Spangled Banner." Tears flowed in a mix of pride and relief.

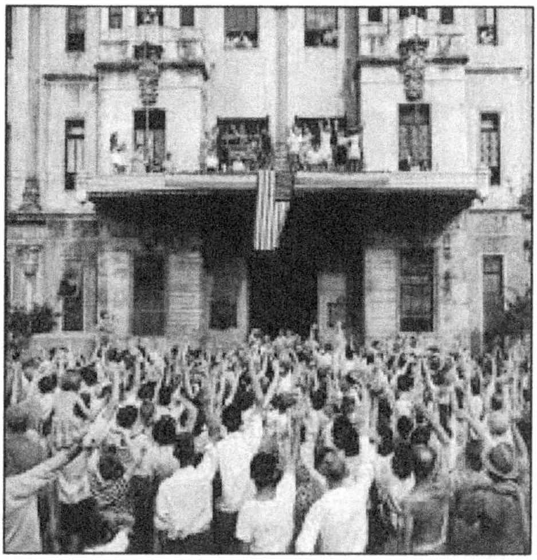

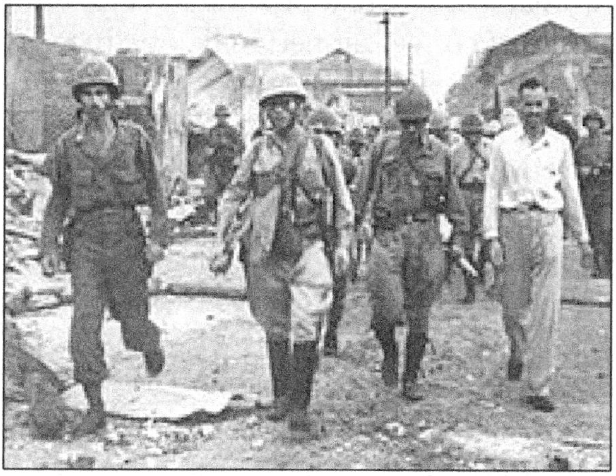

Liberation

Our Allied soldiers looked like giants compared to our emaciated camp men. Veronica felt the cuff of a soldier's uniform to make sure he was real and that she wasn't hallucinating from hunger. I asked as many U.S. Army soldiers as I could if they knew my Rob, but nobody did.

After the Japanese were gone, we were given what was called military K-rations. They consisted of three complete, compact, balanced meals that totaled 3,000 calories a day. Each meal was in a box the size of a Cracker Jacks box, wrapped in a waterproof carton impregnated with a synthetic wax paste. They were labeled, "breakfast," "dinner," and "supper." We found it incredible that an entire meal could be packed into one small box.

The supper and dinner meals contained one four-ounce tin of meat or fish. The meat was either ham, veal, Spam, or sausage. Vegetables came in a tin as well, either tomatoes or peas. There were two types of Nabisco hard biscuits, and a confection that included either chewing gum, caramels, or a chocolate bar. Drinks were either powdered beef bouillon, lemon powder, or a sugary drink. All could be mixed with hot or cold water. Waxed-wrapped Domino sugar cubes were included. A breakfast box had powdered eggs, butter, cheese spread, a packet of coffee, canned milk, one bar of fruit paste or compressed cereal, and salt tablets to ward off dehydration. In addition, there was wooden cutlery and a packet of toilet paper, plus a pack of four Old Gold, Chelsea, or Chesterfield cigarettes.

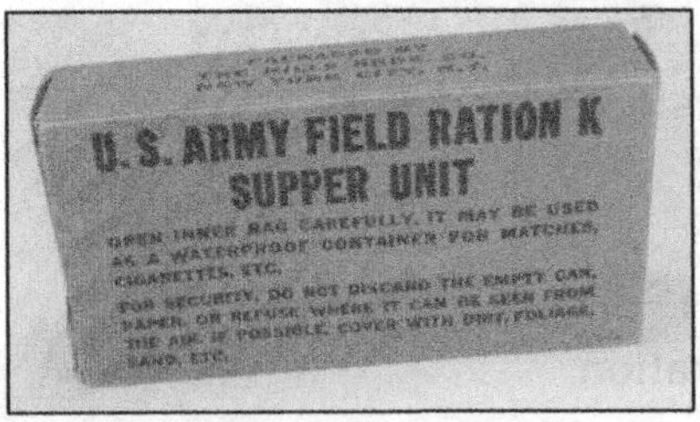

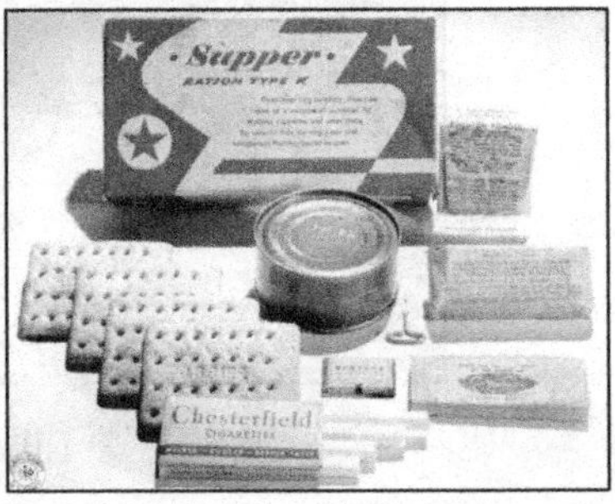

Our mess kit consisted of a small metal tray with compartments, a metal cup that doubled as a measuring cup, a foldable small metal stand to put a cup on, and fuel tablets to light and produce a fire.

Veronica exclaimed, "It's adorable!"

We were thrilled that we no longer had to bow or stand in line for roll call or meals. The taste of real coffee and chocolate was quite a treat.

Later that day, a large, cheerful soldier came into the hospital. "Chief, would your nurses like to send a message home?"

"That would be wonderful!" I replied. "How many words are allowed?"

He looked at me with a quizzical expression. "As many as you'd like."

I said, "The Japanese only allowed 25 words and the letter was censored."

"That's all over, Chief. Write whatever you'd like."

"Thank you, Lieutenant."

I squinted my eyes and wrote a simple note to Mom, as I didn't want to frighten her. I wrote that I was well and would be home soon.

Chapter Thirty
Dottie
Tagap, Burma 1945

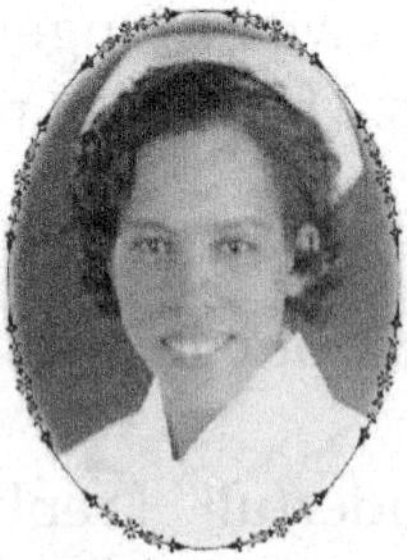

After a few days, our White patient was close to recovery and was driven down the mountain to the 20th General White Hospital to convalesce. Major John came into the ward after the patient was gone to talk to the nurses and medics.

"The wounded come in many colors in Burma, and our hospitals may be segregated but anyone brought into *my* hospital—particularly in an emergency—will receive equal treatment. Everyone in the human race shares pain and suffering and deserves our equal care and medical attention, regardless of skin color. I joined the Army to help our country win this war. Most Negroes in the service work above and beyond to prove their ability, and we expect to return home and be treated as equals to the Whites."

After Major John finished his speech, all the Negro patients, medics, and nurses clapped.

With pride, I shouted out, "Amen!"

Major John gave a slight grin. "Nurses, we will continue to serve every person who needs our services. We are all well-trained American citizens who happen to be colored, but we are proud to have been chosen to serve our country."

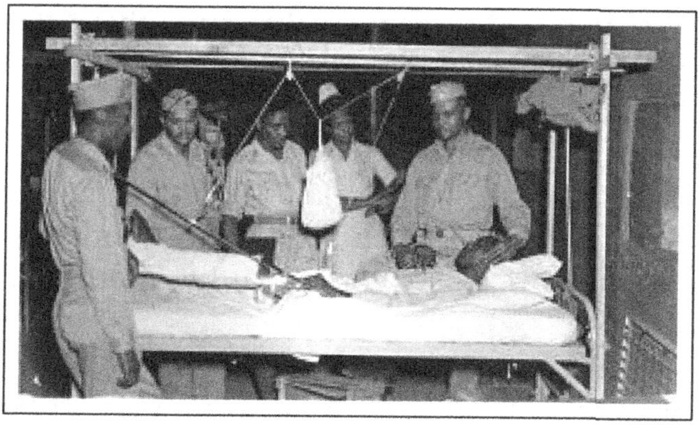

With that, the doc left abruptly and returned to surgery.

The next day, Major John came to find me on the ward. "Chief, I need you to go to the Chinese troop camp near the battlefield. We're almost out of blood needed for transfusions for the White, Chinese, and native patients. Take another nurse with you and try to collect 300 ccs from each soldier, and try to get about 75 donors before you come back."

"But sir, I don't understand why Negro blood is the only one labeled and segregated, and not the blood from other races."

He answered, "We are required by the U.S. Army to segregate our blood and in our hospital, we will follow that rule unless we have no other choice and need to save a patient's life. As a Negro general told me when I enlisted, 'Negroes fight two wars; the one overseas against fascism for our country and the one at home for equal rights to end segregation.' The general called it fighting for the double victory."

"How very true this is, Doc, and I want you to know all of our nurses share your beliefs. We have been fortunate to serve under your command."

"Why thanks, Chief Dottie. And I appreciate everyone's service in our exceptional hospital here."

I decided to take Hilary with me to expose her to the

Chinese soldiers who generously gave their blood for transfusions. We packed the jeep with boxes of tourniquets, solutions, and bandages, then headed off early in the morning on the rough, winding Ledo Road. Our jeep bumped and slid on the road in the frightful blackness of the early morning. I breathed a sigh of relief when the magical sunrise appeared over the mountains. The colorful sky lifted our spirits and guided our way.

We found the camp and were greeted by two Chinese soldiers who recognized our U.S. Army uniforms. I explained why we were there, and they helped us with our equipment and provided us with a large tent to set up in. Hilary and I were alarmed to hear artillery close by.

The first volunteer blood donor came into the tent and Hilary took his temperature to rule out any sickness. I took 300 ccs of blood. There was a long line of volunteers, and we tried to block out the noise of battle while we worked.

A soldier came in and brought us lunch rations. We ate under a tree with an audience of monkeys above us, and after a quick meal, thanked the soldier on our way back to the tent.

He answered, "We soldiers thank *you!*"

We continued to receive donations of blood and almost reached our quota of 75 soldiers but had to quit to allow time to arrive back home before nightfall.

There were many bridges to go over and I drove with concentrated care. We passed convoys of truck drivers carrying men who were working to build the road. A few honked with big grins, happy to see two women in uniform. Hilary waved back, thrilled by the attention.

A short time later, she said, "Chief Dottie, all the Chinese soldiers were remarkable and eager to donate blood. I was very impressed with the turnout."

"Yes, it was a rewarding day. It would be helpful if you could share our experience with our nurses since I will have to go back twice a month with someone. For now, we have enough blood for combat wounds from artillery, landmines, road construction accidents, and of course, the usual snake bites and animal attacks."

"I'd be glad to tell them and wouldn't even mind returning myself. The Chinese sure have rough jobs to perform and I can see why the patients need to relax while they recover at the hospital."

I gave Hilary a warm smile and was glad that my goal to dispel her prejudice had worked by taking her along with me. I couldn't wait to get back to tell Sam about Hilary's progress.

Chapter Thirty-One
Bea
Santo Tomas – Leyte, Philippines
1945

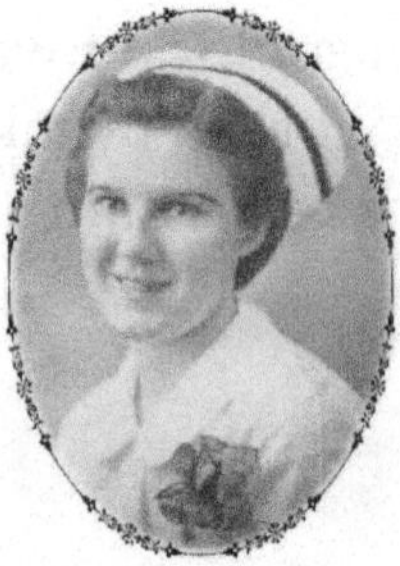

Colonel Howard F. Smith, head of the U.S. Army Medical Corps, came to the hospital with good news. "Chief, I'm here to inform you that all the imprisoned Army nurses will be the first to leave Manila and go home. All the nurses have been a tremendous asset to the Army. Your group will leave on February 16 and be flown to Leyte, Philippines in twin-engine C-47s, with a stopover in Honolulu, then on to San Francisco."

Before we left, the lower floors of the main building were made into a new hospital to serve the Army and a steady stream of wounded Filipino civilians and soldiers. Filipino Red Cross physicians and nurses came from various Manila hospitals, and over a hundred U.S. Army nurses were sent to replace us. When the new nurses arrived on campus, we heard catcalls and piercing whistles from the soldiers, along with assorted comments.

"Get a look at that blonde bombshell!"

"I like the brunette babe with the waves!"

All our faces dropped. We were gaunt and haggard. These

sharp-looking women had luscious new lipstick and new uniforms. Their skin had a healthy pink hue, unlike our pasty gray skin. Their hair was soft with rich-colored curls. We felt like weathered grandmothers.

My nurses perked up a bit when the American nurses gave us their spare khaki blouses and skirts. Several of them asked what it had been like for us to be captives there for almost two-and-a-half years. We told our stories about Limay and Baguio in the jungles, then the underground hospital in Corregidor. The women were not only astonished but made us feel like heroines. They expressed their profuse gratitude and admiration for our service. I watched the glow of pride on my nurses' faces and felt thankful that only two of us had been wounded and none of us had died.

Colonel Smith informed us that more than half of the medical personnel we had worked with on Bataan and Corregidor were dead. This was difficult for us to hear. We choked back our tears in silence. We had given our service to our country, even when our energy ran out. We almost starved to death and were grateful to leave, even though the war still raged on in Iwo Jima, Japan. But the Allies were winning. Molly mentioned how grateful she was that her husband had been transferred to Santo Tomas, and that she could spend time with him there. It was hard for her to leave Charlie behind but knew she would see him soon in the States.

Our nurses were transported by truck to cargo planes that flew south to Leyte, and we were taken to the 126th General Hospital.

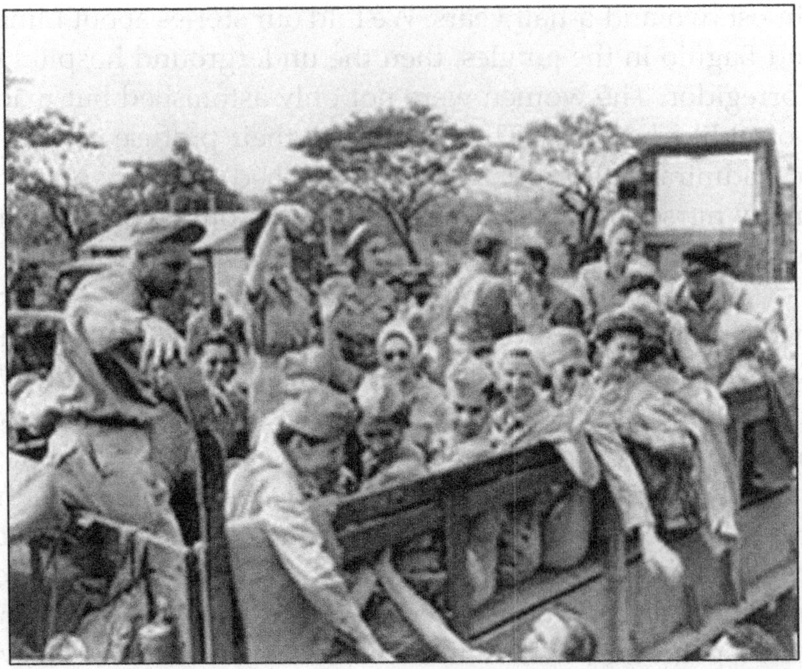

Chapter Thirty-Two
Dottie
Tagap, Burma 1945

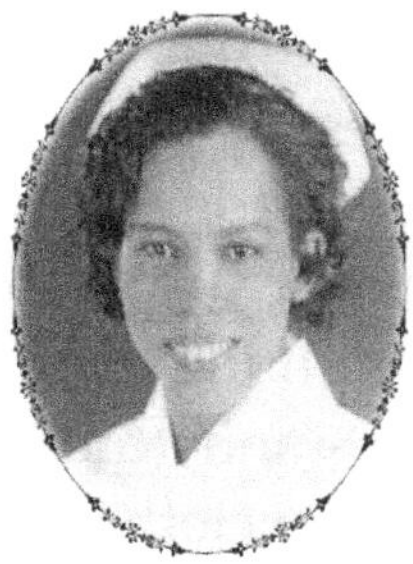

In April, Doc Samuel spotted a helicopter high in the sky above the hospital. Most of the nurses had no idea what it was. It didn't sound like an airplane, more like an intense, thrumming, eggbeater sound. It was sent to rescue a crashed C-46 transport plane that carried a pilot, four airmen, and eight soldiers. Three of the soldiers were wounded along with the pilot. The plane had lost an engine and had crash landed behind enemy lines in the dense jungle. The Sikorsky R-4 helicopter, nicknamed the "hover fly," was taxed to its limits and it took a few trips to rescue the crew. The wounded were brought into our hospital for care, and we were told it was the first aerial rescue using a helicopter under combat conditions.

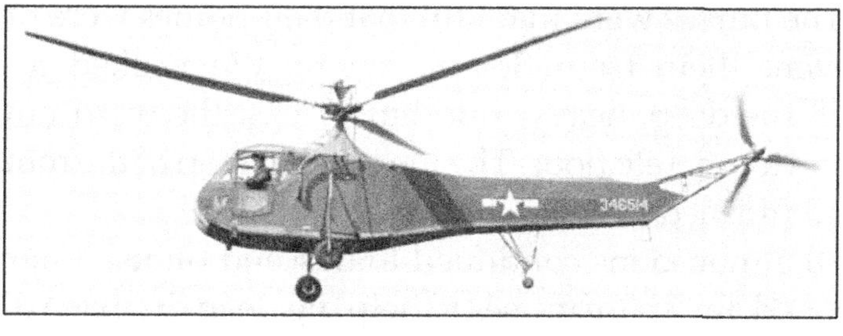

The monsoon season began in May as predicted, and I had hoped that the rain would make it cooler but it didn't. Instead, it brought oppressive, monstrous humidity. As Mama used to say, "It's hotter than Hades."

The torrential rains made doing laundry an almost impossible task. We used our surplus World War One helmets to wash our clothes in and hung them up in our bashas. They never completely dried and the nurses soon resigned themselves to wearing damp clothes.

As the months wore on, the complaints about the monsoons became unbearable and finally, I'd had enough of it. I announced to my nurses, "The monsoon season will last all the way into fall, and we are commissioned here to work. And work you will – with vigor, enthusiasm, courage, and devotion to duty." My face burned after that lecture but at least it kept everyone silent for a while. After further complaints the next week, I gave another similar lecture again, but this time with extra sentiments like, "Count your blessings that at least all the buildings are finished."

Yes, conditions in Burma were harsh as we slogged from our bashas to the ward in our high rubber boots, which were no longer called "ugly." We wore raincoats that had been issued in the New York hospital and used umbrellas as walking sticks. It was a sorry plight if anyone slipped in the mud. The nurses were thankful that their homes were on stilts to prevent them from floating away. We walked to work through the deep, heavy mud but at least the ward now had sides and a concrete floor. The mess hall on top of the mountain also had finished walls and a concrete floor.

As the monsoons continued to descend on us, Major John summoned any spare nurses to help dig deep drainage ditches, or at least supervise natives in carrying off the tons of water that rushed down the precipitous mountainsides. Our entire area was reworked to provide better drainage. He knew the monsoons were a hardship and praised all the nurses as much as possible for their help.

Stevie, our favorite medical corpsman, had developed big muscles from all the hard labor and the good doctor complimented his work every chance he got.

One day, Stevie came into the ward and announced, "At least the tea and rice crops are happy!"

I answered for all the nurses to hear, "How right you are! And thank goodness for the necessary rainfall."

Just as Major John predicted, the jungle creatures found their way into the cozy, dry ward to escape the deluge. Lorna let out a scream as a one-foot-long cobra slithered past her while she tended to a patient. Medic Donny threw it out the door into the jungle.

He asked, "How did it get in here? The ward's sealed up now." He walked up and down the spacious building, inspecting every corner, then announced, "I found a hole! I'll patch it up before some other creature seeks a comfortable home away from the downpour."

The next week, another shriek was heard from a nurse in the kitchen within the hospital. Donny ran to investigate and found that a young tiger had ventured inside through an open door. Donny rushed off to find Stevie, who got some meat and threw it out into the jungle. The tiger lumbered out after it and we were grateful that no one was attacked.

Inside, the mildew took over our books and nursing charts. Outside, the jungle trees and their leaves shook as the rain poured down. Every stream and river bulged with water. The steady drone of machines on the Stilman/Ledo Road no longer penetrated the overgrown jungle. Instead, the sound of rainfall and wild birds reigned. Even the pack mules that carried supplies to China sank into the mud and the natives had to pull them out.

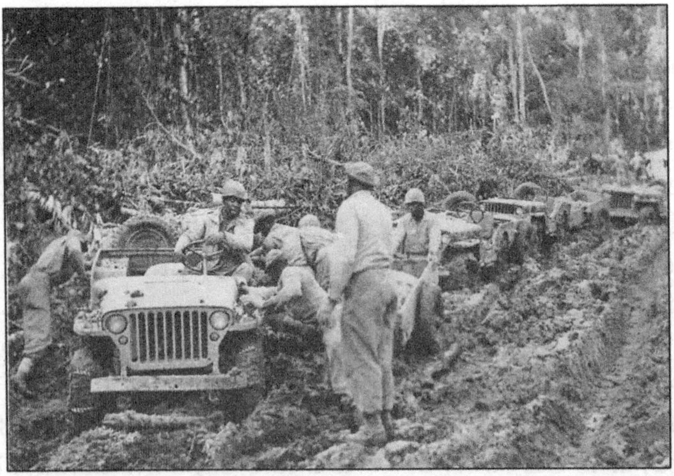

In the first two months of the monsoon season, approximately 400 patients were admitted to our hospital. Of those, over a hundred were operative cases. During the next three-and-a-half months, our station hospital treated over 500 accident victims. The terrain and monsoons in Burma caused frequent plane crashes and truck accidents.

The rainy season continued and brought in the most serious accidents from the road. Pfc. Robinson drove a huge cargo vehicle fully loaded with supplies. As the rain poured down from low-hanging clouds, he inched his way around a sharp, dangerous curve. Suddenly, he couldn't see where he was and his truck had skidded and flew into the air. The soldier was pinned under his truck, which landed way down the mountainside. Two truck drivers saw him go over and called our ambulance service on a nearby camp telephone and told them the mile marker of where the accident had occurred. The strong men climbed down the mountain and were able to pull out Robinson. The ambulance was only five miles away and drove him to our hospital.

I gave him a shot of morphine after the medics told me the details of the horrific event. Major John was summoned, and diagnosed that the soldier had a broken pelvis and fractured legs, and the recovery period would most likely take two months.

I said to Major John later, "It is fortunate that our hospital established a 24-hour ambulance station and was able to rescue him in time."

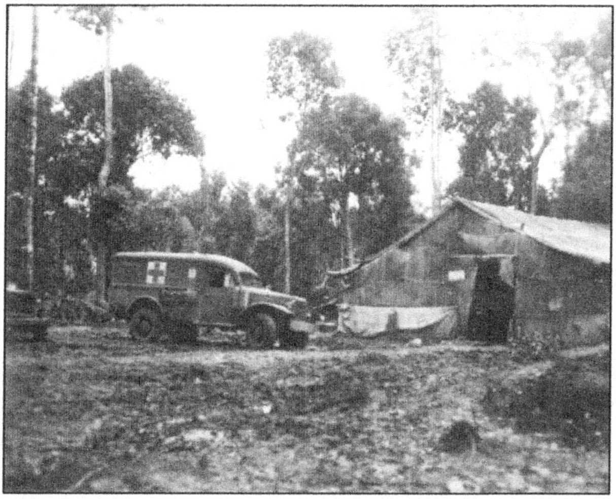

The monsoons raged on along with the war and the patient census increased. Our neighbor, the 20th General White Hospital, reported the admission of 12,000 malaria patients.

Soon the nurses were required to work three eight-hour shifts each week, which was difficult in the afternoons because of the heat. When corpsmen were available, they assisted us and treated routine cases, which freed the rest of us to treat patients with more serious issues. The Chinese soldiers had so many wounds—most from artillery, tanks, and landmines. But Major John was right. With the heavy rainfall, the Chinese lost interest in going out into the jungle for their hidden food supplies.

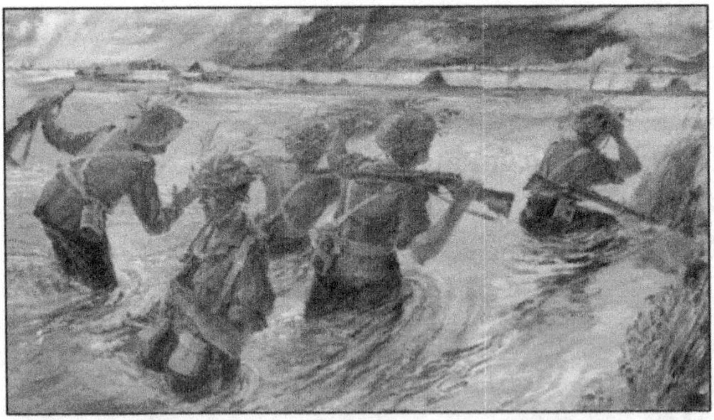

My only complaint was not being able to have a date with Sam because we were both so overworked. With only 16 nurses to treat patients, it was clear that we'd have to step up to assume greater responsibility. We learned how to identify the signs and symptoms of all the different tropical diseases. The surgical nurses dressed wounds without the presence of the doctors and the medical nurses instituted intravenous fluids plus routine courses of medication without a physician's help. Penicillin, the precious new drug we were using for the first time, was a very effective treatment for rapid venereal disease and was lifesaving for serious wounds. It was a well-known fact that disease had killed more soldiers there than the enemy.

Many of our Negro soldiers lost their lives on the road either by building it or through accidents, malaria, sniper bullets, insects, or wild animals. A prolific number of gravesite markers were posted alongside the road instead of mile markers. On the Stilwell/Ledo Road, one marker read, "Here lies Sgt. Morgan, dead from a sniper bullet. Mile 97." It was commonly said that Stilwell/Ledo Road lost a man a mile.

The airplane drops of food became few and far between. At first, food supplies were adequate but monotonous. Our hospital was at the end of a long supply route, and we were usually short-changed. We supplemented our food supplies with wild turkeys that a few of the medics or natives hunted. Fish was purchased from the native Naga tribe as they caught it by dynamiting the local streams, then carried the food in by elephant. It was frightening how much weight we lost, and I prayed that the monsoon season would end soon.

Chapter Thirty-Three
Bea
Leyte, Philippines 1945

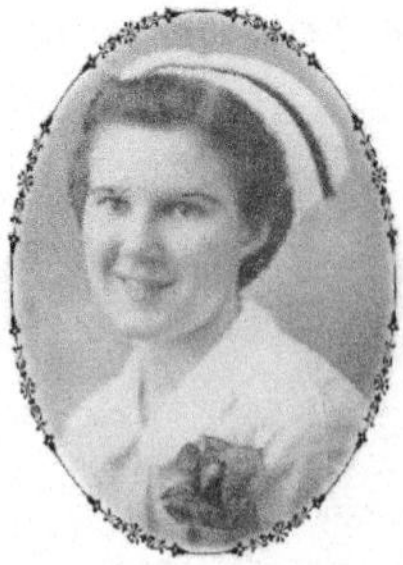

We were fed steak dinners and the smell was divine. We cut the juicy meat into small pieces because our jaws were not used to chewing that much. We were fed as much as we could eat, which was not a lot since our stomachs had shrunk.

The next day, we were interviewed by the media. The nurses at the hospital gave us cosmetics and nail polish. We felt like Hollywood stars when a dozen newspaper reporters arrived and flashed cameras at us, and there was one newsreel cameraman.

The reporters asked us difficult questions like, "Were any of you raped?" "Were you beaten?"

"We were never molested by the Japanese," I answered for everyone.

"I got slapped in the face for not bowing, but it wasn't too bad," Susie volunteered.

"No, but we were fed evil-smelling fish!" Molly said.

"And rice with weevils," Veronica added.

"I never thought I'd make it out alive," Annie exclaimed.

A convalescent hospital was set up for us in the middle of pineapple palm groves. We strolled on a lovely beach that stretched for miles, listening to the rhythmic waves that soothed our minds. The Leyte Hospital nurses loaned us swimsuits, but it frightened us to look at our skin-and-bones bodies without our usual curves. We sunbathed and swam in the surf. That night, we were shown a private viewing of a movie starring Fred Astaire and Ginger Rogers while we snacked on cookies and ice cream.

Our official Class A olive-green ANC uniforms were flown in from Australia for a ceremony. The first official uniform had been distributed in late 1943, but we were locked away at Santo Tomas by then, so had to wear our old nurses' uniforms for years.

I opened the first box, which contained the Army Nurse Corps formal olive, wool garrison wide-brim peak caps. Displayed in the center of the cap was the great seal of the United States, which was gold and several inches high. We loved the eagle with a scroll in its beak that read *E Pluribus Unum* —out of many, one. In one claw it held an olive branch, a symbol of peace; and in the other it held 13 arrows, a symbol of war.

We paraded around in our brand-new underclothes and our Army Nurse Corps caps. We whooped it up and practiced saluting. Next, we traded around the sharp, stylish service jackets, skirts, and khaki shirts to get the best fit.

I opened the box of neckties and asked amid the laughter, "Who knows how to tie these?"

Molly shouted, "I do! I had to help my younger brothers tie them. My father made the boys wear ties to church." She grabbed a tie and demonstrated on me how it was done. "I love the tie. It really spruces up the uniform and makes it look formal as well as official."

After everyone was in uniform, I opened the white box of jewelry, which came with instructions for how the items were to be pinned on the uniforms. I handed out two small gold block U.S. pieces for everyone to place on each side of the top lapel of their jacket. The best piece was the grand one-inch caduceus. The stunning gold piece had a short staff entwined by two serpents, with glorious wings of Greek gods on top that represented healing. We each put two on our bottom lapels. Boy, did we look sensational.

After we were dressed, the Leyte nurses painted our nails, put their makeup on us, then fussed with our scraggly hair. Brigadier General Guy Denit, chief surgeon in the Southwest Pacific, was to arrive and perform a ceremony. We looked like heroines in our brand-spanking-new uniforms and felt proud. But we were still a bit dismayed by how skinny we were.

Under the palm trees, we stood at attention when the Army officials arrived.

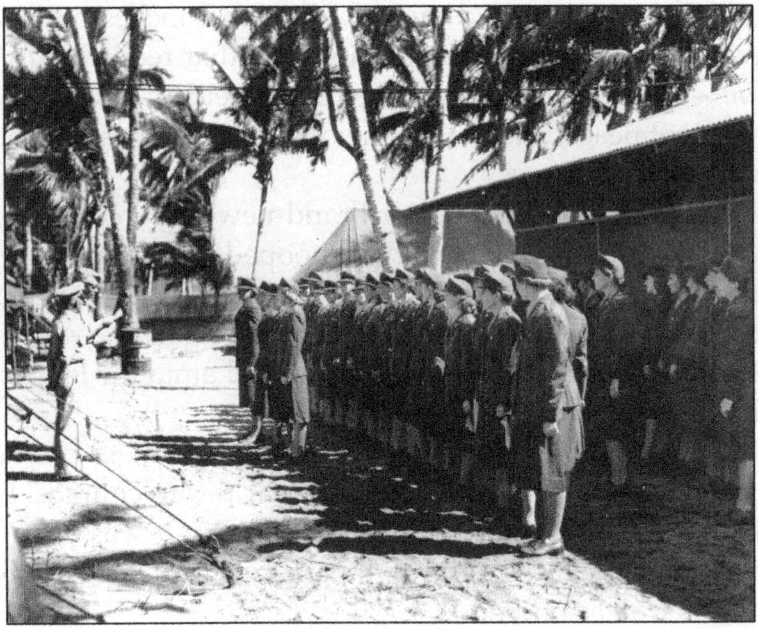

After a few speeches of gratitude for our service, the nurses were promoted to one higher grade in rank as first lieutenants, and I was promoted to major. We were each given a battle ribbon with the Bronze Star for valor.

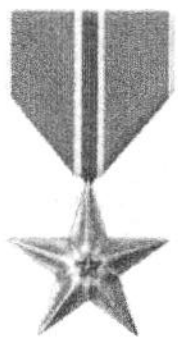

After the ceremony, we were interrogated individually about the war crimes of the Japanese Imperial Army. A form was filled out titled "Testimony in the Matter of Imprisonment of Civilian Internees and American Prisoners of War Under Improper Conditions at Santo Tomas Interment Camp in Manila, Philippines 1942-1945."

I stated my rank, and dates and places where I had served. Then I pledged in an oath that all my answers were true to the best of my knowledge and belief. The interrogation was certified by an agent from the Security Intelligence Corps.

The general told all the nurses that telegrams had been sent home to our families, informing them that we had been rescued by our Army Forces and were enjoying a brief rest, then would return to the United States by the first available air transport. We were all relieved and couldn't wait to see our loved ones.

Chapter Thirty-Four
Dottie
Tagap, Burma
August – September 1945

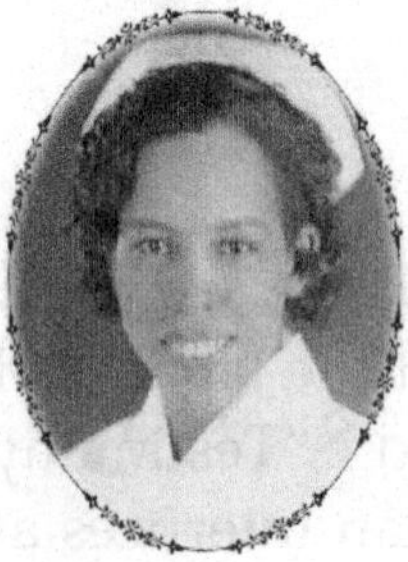

After heavy fighting, the British troops, along with our Chinese Allies, ended the Burmese Campaign and defeated the Japanese by August 1945. The 335th Station Hospital was notified that two atomic bombs had fallen on Japan and World War II was coming to an end at last.

On September 2, 1945, the Japanese surrendered and we were honored by a visit from the China-Burma-India Theater surgeon general. All the physicians, medics, and nurses assembled to hear his speech. The nurses wore their full uniforms for the first time since our arrival in the jungle.

The surgeon general spoke with enthusiasm. "The War Department is pleased with the work of the 335th Station Hospital, which you have all done under primitive conditions in an extremely trying climate. Because the war against the Nazis in the European and African continents took precedence over the war against the Japanese, those who were stationed in the China-Burma-India Theater were faced with a longer war with fewer resources. Everyone's rank will be raised one level higher. Thank you all for your patriotism in helping to win this war."

We had a party in the officers' club and celebrated the end of the war. The nurses were thrilled to have risen to the rank of first lieutenant, and I was given the rank of major, as was Sam. The jungle that surrounded our hospital was lush and green with the end of the monsoon season. Major John asked Clara to dance twice. Sam and I delighted in a sensual, slow dance to a song called "I'm in The Mood for Love." At the end of the dance, he gave me a long kiss in front of everyone. I was star-struck and stunned and when our audience clapped for us, I blushed.

The day after the party, Major John came into the ward and announced, "Nurses, I want to thank you for your services in Burma. With your help, our hospital was transformed into a fine facility and in doing so, you contributed significantly to the low mortality rate of all the patients. Thank you for your outstanding service to our country."

After the nurses were done applauding, the major continued with a grim face, "The surgeon general has informed me that the 335th Station Hospital is no longer needed and I have been instructed to disassemble it completely."

I protested, "What about the patients here?"

Clara added, "What do you mean *disassemble* – the hospital was only recently finished!"

Lorna said, "It's a perfectly good hospital. We shouldn't tear it down!"

The major said in a quiet voice, "Our Negro patients will be sent home and the Chinese returned to their country. Ladies, the war is over. The hospital is no longer needed. The U.S. Army has ordered the station hospital to be removed. I'll send over boxes, and I need everyone to help pack up all the equipment before you are shipped back to the United States on October 1. You will board the ship *USS General C.G. Morton* and arrive in the New York Port of Embarkation by October 23."

After Major John left, we were in a state of shock over this dismal event. Our nurses had arrived in October and by January 1945, the 335th had been completely renovated. It was a crying shame that all that hard work would have to be demolished.

Once the patients were relocated, my job was to make an inventory list. The nurses and medics boxed and labeled all the hospital equipment and medical supplies. The medics oversaw the demolition and the natives assisted. Most of the physicians were sent home and reassigned.

Major John and Doc Samuel stayed to the bitter end to help finish the final closing.

One afternoon, Major John and Doc Samuel came into the ward to see how everything was progressing.

Major John told Sam and me in private, "Don't repeat this but I know that one of the station hospitals in India packed every item up only to find that it was all dumped into the ocean because it was too expensive to ship back to the States."

"Oh, my Lord, that's tragic. Can't we give our supplies to the poor hospitals here, Major?" I asked.

Doc Samuel said, "I agree and I can't leave here until all our precious medical equipment is either shipped back or goes to a needy hospital, of which there are plenty as you well know."

Major John nodded. "I'll see what I can do."

"Major, I'll stay with you to make sure that happens," Doc Samuel spoke with conviction.

I felt satisfied that our best physicians would be the last to leave so they could take care of business. I knew the local hospitals in Burma, as well as India, would be thrilled to receive the desperately needed supplies.

The day before the nurses were scheduled to leave, Sam came by and whispered in my ear, "Do you have time for a date, Dottie?"

I gave a shy giggle. "With you, of course I'll make time!"

On our last rendezvous up the mountain, Sam asked, "Tell me, Chief, what are your plans when you return to the States?"

"I intend to take advantage of the GI Bill and continue my education to advance in the Army Nurse Corps. How about you?" I stopped and stared into his unusual, beautiful eyes and worried it might be the last time I would see him.

Sam put his arm around me. "I'm not sure."

We sat on our favorite bench, both of us silent, and took in the view of the jungle and the massive Himalayan Mountains for the last time. We fell into a long, endless kiss. We were both hungry for each other and moved into the remodeled dining room. Sam scooped me up and set me down on the table. Our lovemaking took me into another world as I remembered our romantic, slow dance together. Tears streamed down my face as we climaxed together.

Sam, alarmed, said, "Did I hurt you?"

"No, I'm just sad we'll have to leave each other."

"I know what you mean." He brushed a curl away from my face.

My heart pattered as he touched me.

A short time later, we walked down the mountain path back to the ward.

"We can write to each other, can't we?" I asked.

Sam took out a pen and small pad and wrote down his address in Pennsylvania. Then he tore off the page and handed it to me. I wrote my information for him and drew a tiny heart near my name.

As the ship left the dock, I touched the cool white railing. A soft, steady breeze blew on my face and I reflected on my life as an Army nurse. The past year in Burma had been such a challenge, and even a bit frightening at times, but it was a very rewarding experience. As a nurse, I learned an incredible amount in a short period of time and gained a whole new respect for all the different races of people there.

My 15 nurses and I gathered on the ship and exchanged our thoughts about the future. With sadness in my heart, we headed for New York. Once there, we hugged and said our goodbyes, then headed off in different directions.

Chapter Thirty-Five
Major Bea
Leyte, Philippines – San Francisco, CA
1945

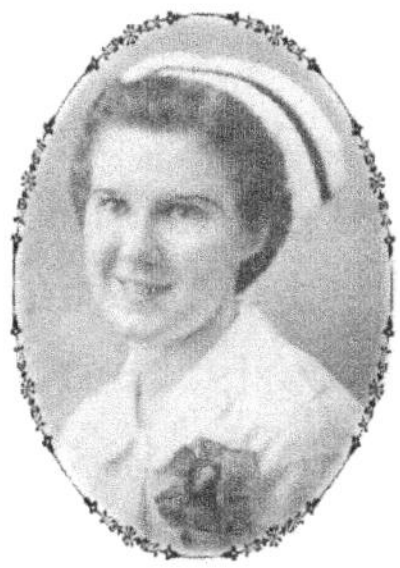

On February 19, 1945, we boarded two C-54 aircraft from Leyte, Philippines and flew to Hawaii, where we refueled at Hickam Field. When we got off the planes, we were greeted by a band that played "Star-Spangled Banner," which stirred pride in our hearts. On the layover, we were treated like royalty. Beauticians came in and gave us permanents, facials, and manicures plus a package of real silk stockings.

After we received our back pay, which averaged $6,500 each, the nurses went on a shopping spree at the post exchange and bought pens, wristwatches, jewelry, cigarette lighters, purses, and shoes. I purchased a new stylish pair of eyeglasses after an appointment with a U.S. Army optician.

Two days later, we took off for our beloved Mainland USA, Hamilton Field, San Francisco. During the flight, the thought of going to California made my heart flutter. *This is where Rob is from. Maybe he'll be at the ceremony when we arrive…* I thought hopefully. You'd think by now I would have given up on reuniting with him, but the thought of him always kept me in a positive state of mind.

Veronica, with full glamorous makeup on, looked out the window after we heard the announcement that we were about to land. "There it is! America! California! The good ol' USA!"

When the gals heard her say "California," they broke out into song. "California, here I come, right back where I started from!"

Shouts of exhilaration sprang from red-lipsticked smiles.

"We're home, we're really home!"

"Oh, gosh! America! I never thought I'd see you again!"

Several uniformed escorts boarded our plane after we landed and brought us down the stairs in our new ANC uniforms in the bright California sunshine. We stood on a section of the tarmac away from a crowd of over 1,500 people. A huge band played Sousa marches like the same music I heard when I first got off the ship in Manila in 1941. That seemed like many years ago instead of only three.

An Army public relations officer came over to us. "Get into formation, ladies."

We were joined by our nurses who had escaped to Australia from Corregidor. Many hugs and kisses were exchanged, and we felt a tremendous relief to be brought together at last.

The public relations officer commanded again, "The ceremony is about to begin. Please line up."

At that moment, I thought the government was keen to turn us into recruiting icons with this tremendous amount of publicity. Of course, the Army would lose 68 nurses and would need replacements since the war was not over yet. All the fanfare was meant to honor the nurses' sacrifices, but it was clear that our government wanted to present the nurses well-coiffed and in new, smart uniforms as a great recruitment method to obtain more signups.

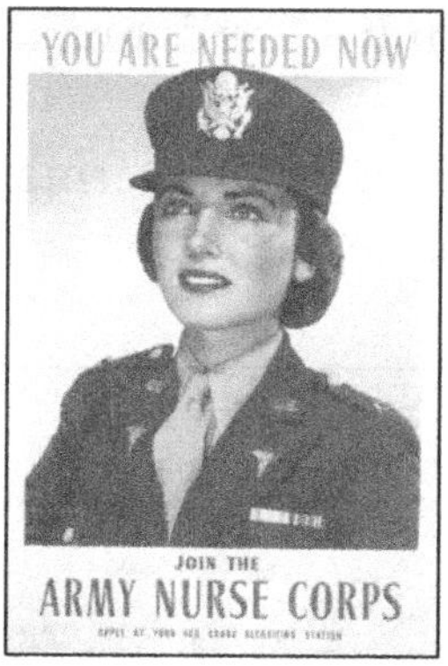

This had been a well-publicized event. The Army had rounded up as many relatives as possible for the ceremony. The public relations officer tried to keep the nurses in position, but it was a lost cause when Caroline shouted, "Mom! Sis!" and ran out of line toward them. Then the rest of the gals bolted and ran into the crowd to look for any family member who might be there.

I stayed where I was ordered and watched hungry grabs and embraces in the crowd. Annie got swung in the air by her father. The scene warmed my heart.

Officer Thomson glared at me. "Major, get your nurses back here. The Assistant Surgeon General of the United States has a speech to give."

The red-faced assistant surgeon general stood at the mike and tapped his fingers on the podium.

I went up to the microphone. "Nurses, time to come back for the ceremony."

The nurses returned and the speeches began. We stood tall as Brigadier General Raymond W. Bliss, Assistant Surgeon General of the Army, spoke. His long speech was peppered with the words *courage, self-sacrifice, and inspiration.*

The general ended with, "The nurses went above and beyond their expected role and we are grateful to the Almighty for your safe return."

Many officers, families, and my nurses had noticeable tears in their eyes.

At last, we were driven to Letterman General Hospital at the Presidio to recuperate.

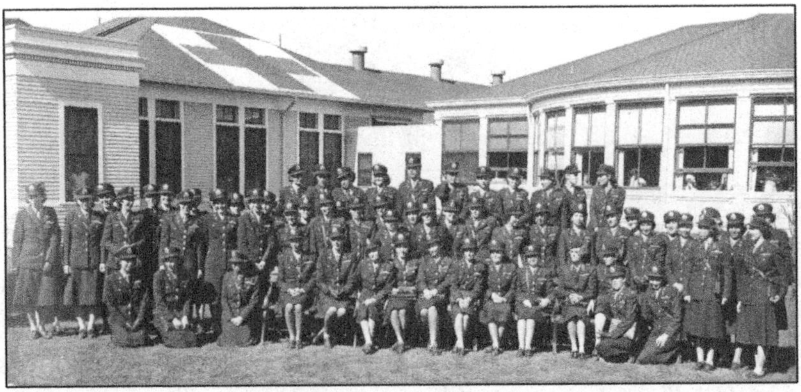

The former prisoner-of-war nurses at
Letterman General Hospital, 1945.

We were assigned to a ward with flower-filled vases, radios, boxes of candy, and Kleenex on a small table next to each bed. For several days, families and friends visited. It was a joy to hear the laughter of happiness even though there was no one there for me. I would take a train and see Mother in a few weeks.

We were given medical exams that were more thorough than at Leyte and included lab tests, chest x-rays, and eye exams. Most everyone had lost 10 or more pounds. Our lovely, vivacious Veronica lost 35. Annie had an enlarged liver and Molly had dysentery. Everyone had bad teeth from starvation. I still walked with a limp from beriberi and received high doses of thiamine. I was told I would get better soon. Yes, we all had health problems but were on the road to recovery, and a great feeling of hope prevailed.

The last ceremony was held at Letterman Hospital on the grounds and this facility was the most prestigious of all. The set-up was the best with the hospital in front of Presidio Park, and there were many photographers and news reporters. Hundreds of soldiers who had been wounded on the Bataan Death March were sent to Letterman Hospital to recover and watched the ceremony through the windows.

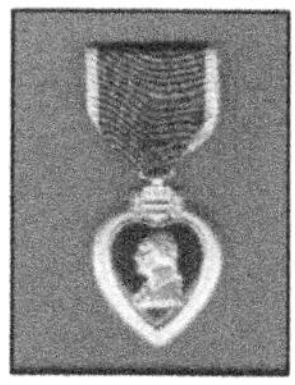

We were ecstatic when we heard Lieutenant Rosemary Hogan and Rita Palmer's names announced to come up to the podium to receive the Purple Heart for being wounded on Bataan. Both were promoted to a higher rank of first lieutenant.

Brigadier General Bliss pinned a medal on each woman's uniform and handed them both a letter from the White House, Washington, DC.

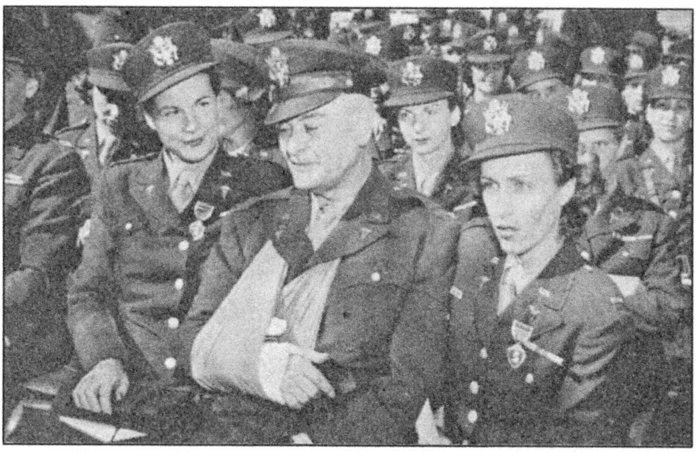

Colonel James W. Duckworth with two of the nurses who served under his command on Bataan, Lieutenants Rosemary Hogan and Rita Palmer.

Following the applause, each nurse was called and presented with an envelope with her name and serial number in the corner. I slid my finger over the embossed gold letters on the envelope and a shiver ran up my arm. Inside was a letter.

> *THE WHITE HOUSE*
>
> *WASHINGTON*
>
> *To MEMBERS OF THE ARMY NURSE CORPS BEING REPATRIATED FROM THE PHILIPPINES ON 23 FEBRUARY 1945:*
>
> *It gives me special pleasure to welcome you back to your native shores, and to express, on behalf of the people of the United States, the joy we feel at your deliverance from the hands of the enemy. It is a source of profound satisfaction that our efforts to accomplish your return have been successful.*
>
> *You have served valiantly in foreign lands and have suffered greatly. As your Commander in Chief, I take pride in your past accomplishments and express the thanks of a grateful Nation for your service in combat and your steadfastness while a prisoner of war.*
>
> *May God grant each of you happiness and an early return to health.*
>
> *Franklin D. Roosevelt*

It was an honor for all of us to receive a letter from the President of the United States—a valuable keepsake for all the nurses and their families to share and cherish.

General George C. Marshall, U.S. Army Chief of Staff, spoke from the podium. "These Angels of Bataan, the 68 Army nurses, will remain a beautiful legend of the Pacific War. The legend will fall short of what they stood for and what they did. Only those who were with them in their captivity can know the dread that must have haunted these nurses during three dragging years. Only those to who they ministered can know how they conquered fear and hardship and faithfully served the wounded and the sick under almost inconceivable difficulties. Their devotion to duty will be a continuing inspiration to all women, especially to those of the Armed Forces."

Epilogue
Major Dottie
1945

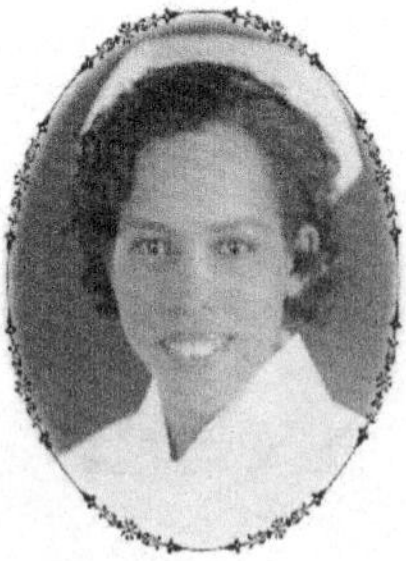

Molly and Charlie bought a small house right near where my mom lived, and I enjoyed visiting them both frequently. Clara wrote me from New York City, telling me that Major John had visited her often and they were going to marry. I had mixed feelings—I was happy for them but felt jealous because I had received only one letter from Sam. I wrote Clara back and wished them well.

Six months later, Clara wrote and told me she was pregnant, and that Major John had applied to law school in many states but was denied because none of them accepted Negro students. He passed the bar exam and started his own law school for Negroes.

Medic Stevie went to school on the GI Bill to study politics and religion, and became one of the most important civil rights men in Chicago. He also pastored a Black mega church.

Hilary continued in her nursing career and took up the long fight for civil rights. She attended the 1963 March on Washington, where a quarter of a million people rallied to demand an end to segregation, the need for fair wages, economic justice, voting rights, education, and long overdue civil rights protections.

I stayed in the Army Nurse Corps and was stationed to work post-war duty at the Birmingham General Army Hospital. It was an honor to care for the wounded soldiers who had returned from the war to the United States.

I wrote to Sam first, after a month of waiting to hear from him. I mentioned how much I missed him and told him about my work and school, and ended the letter with a little heart after my name. Sam wrote me a brief, impersonal letter and told me he had been happy to return home to his family and was taking a month off, then would resume his military career. He ended his letter with *Sincerely yours, Samuel Walker, MD*. I was devastated and scanned the letter over and over, searching for intimacy, but none was found. I wrote to Sam several times after that but never heard from him again. I was heartbroken and my disappointment led to a dreadful feeling of being used.

To ease the pain of losing my first love, I immersed myself in night school on the GI Bill and received my master's in nursing education.

On July 26, 1948, our wonderful president, Harry S. Truman, signed Executive Order 9981, banning segregation in the Armed Forces. The executive order stated, "It is hereby declared to be the policy of the President that there shall be equality of treatment and opportunity for all persons in the armed services without regard to race, color, religion, or national origin."

Several of the nurses who had served together had a party at a bar and grill and toasted the end of segregation. Unfortunately, the executive order may have ended segregation in the Armed Forces but in the South, it was painfully slow to occur.

I joined the National Association for the Advancement of Colored People, established in 1909, one of the largest

American civil rights groups. It focused on desegregating schools and universities. Whenever I had free time between work and school, I joined with the NAACP to protest segregation in sit-ins, boycotts, and marches, and proudly wore my WW II Army uniform.

When the war broke out in Korea in June 1950, I was called to serve in the Korean conflict. The Korean War was the first conflict in which Negro nurses participated not in segregated units but as integral members of the Army Nurse Corps. I was interested to see if it was truly possible to have a peaceful integration of the two races. I decided that I'd rather throw my heart into the service than worry about romance, though I did harbor a secret wish that perhaps Doc Sam might be there. I looked forward to working with White nurses in Korea now that the ANC was integrated. I knew I would do an excellent job, and would make my family proud of my continued nursing career.

Chapter Thirty-Six
Major Bea
San Francisco, CA – Atlanta, GA – San Francisco, CA 1945-1946

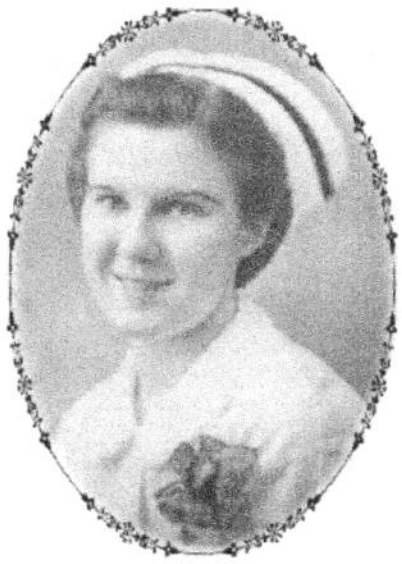

By the end of March, we were cleared to go home. Many of the nurses returned to their hometowns and were celebrated with parades in their honor. There were high school bands, Boy Scouts, Girl Scouts, and The American Legion.

Before I returned on leave to my hometown in Georgia, I searched the San Francisco phonebook for Robert L. Johnson. The listing was there—not junior but senior, Rob's father. I dialed the number with a nervous twitch in my finger.

An older woman answered the phone.

"Hello…" I stammered. "Is this Robert L. Johnson Junior's mother?"

She was quiet for a moment. "He is deceased," she said flatly. "Who is this?"

My heart dropped a beat when I heard her say "deceased."

I answered in a sad, quavering voice, "I met Rob at a dance at the officers' club in Manila, Philippines in 1941."

"Are you the nurse?" she asked.

"Yes, my name is Beatrice Harrington. I'm in the Army

Nurse Corps."

"I thought so. Rob wrote us a letter about you. He wanted us to meet you when the war was over. Did you know he was missing in action and the Army never recovered his body?" She blew her nose.

"I tried to find out about him after Manila was bombed, and in the hospital I asked every patient if they knew anything about him. Everywhere I was relocated, I inquired about him."

"Were you at the ceremony at Letterman Hospital for the Army nurses that I heard on the radio? Rob told us he wanted to marry you."

My heart sped up when she said *marry*. "Yes, I was the chief of our group."

"Are you still in California?"

"I am."

"My husband and I would be honored to meet you. Please come over for dinner."

I took a cab to Rob's parents' house and was warmly greeted. When we sat down for dinner, I kept my eye on the framed photograph of Rob in his Air Force uniform. We all shared our grief over his death after the bombing of his airbase.

After a wonderful homecooked meal with a homemade berry pie for dessert, I brought out Rob's watch to give to his parents. They were overcome with emotion to see it. When I told them how I had gotten the watch, it brought on a flood of memories. I clutched the watch in my hands and began to cry. We were all in tears as his mother held me on the couch. I presented the watch to Rob's father, who put it on his wrist and wore it with pride.

Before I left, his parents told me they would have loved to have had me as Rob's wife and part of their family. We all agreed on what a long, terrible, but necessary war it had been, then I left.

During the train ride home, I had time to think. I fell into a deep sorrow, but this time I had shared the reality of my beloved's death with his parents, and this eliminated my fantasies of finding him.

My mother met me at the train station. Our embrace had never been this emotionally charged. I had to lean over to hug her, and she suddenly seemed much shorter to me.

"Beatrice, praise the Lord you made it back," she whispered in my ear, then added, "Darling, you are too thin. And you have white hair now."

I blushed and thought, *You also look thin.* My mother appeared older with many more wrinkles on her face, and her gray hair was scant and wispy.

Mother remarked about my limp.

I said in a defensive voice, "It'll go away."

At first, I felt comforted to be home and savored the meals I had dreamed of during the years of my imprisonment. When I unpacked my musette bag, there in the bottom was the carved bamboo flower Manuel had given me in Baguio. I twirled the stem of the flower between my fingers and unexpected tears rolled down my face.

Occasionally, I shared what it was like to be a combat nurse with my mother, but she would brush my remarks aside and say things like, "Beatrice, you must put that all behind you. You're in the safety of America now."

Then after a month, I felt lost. I missed the camaraderie of my nurses, with whom I had shared hopes and dreams. I felt isolated and Mother's comments made me think that she didn't believe me or didn't want to know what I had been through.

I longed to see Rob's family again and accepted a job at the Veterans Administration at the Letterman Hospital in San Francisco. I was happy to obtain the status of corporal and thanks to the GI Bill, I earned a baccalaureate in nursing administration while I worked there. The war was coming to an end, and I felt needed caring for the influx of injured Army soldiers. I felt a closeness to the group of Bataan Death March soldiers who shared their nightmares freely with me, knowing that I had been a combat nurse in Bataan.

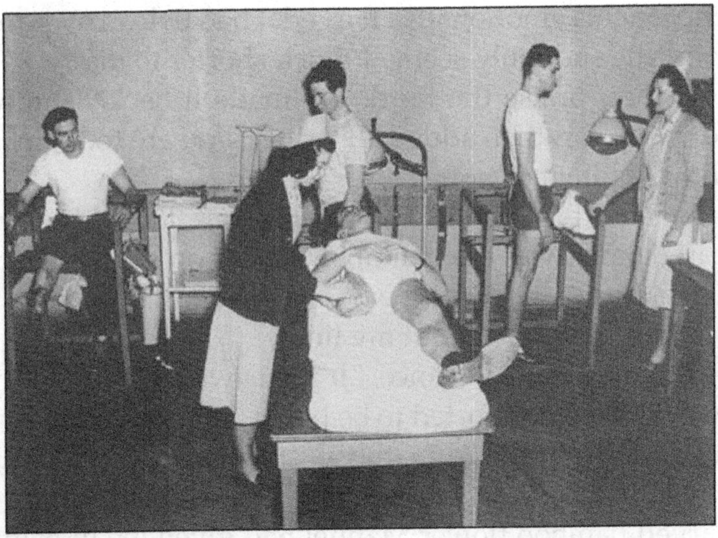

While I worked at Letterman Hospital, the muslin remembrance sheet of the imprisoned nurses on Corregidor was found. It was shown to me by an officer who framed it and hung it in the hospital. It threw me into a state of shock. Memories of being captured by the Japanese swirled through my mind. I was so taken aback, I had to leave work early that day.

It was awkward when I went shopping for items I needed. Clerks often asked, "Are you one of those Angels of Bataan?" After treating the Death March soldiers and knowing what they went through, plus what all the patients in the European concentration camps had experienced, I did not feel like I deserved the title of an angel.

I phoned Rob's parents, who were delighted that I had moved to the city. They invited me to dinner once a week. I embraced my new family. We were united by the love of a man who served and gave his life for his country.

In 1950, a war broke out in Korea, and I was assigned by the Army Nurse Corps to go.

Another adventure! I thought as I readied myself for the trip. I was honored to be called and I couldn't wait for the next chapter of my life to begin.

Epilogue
Major Bea
1945

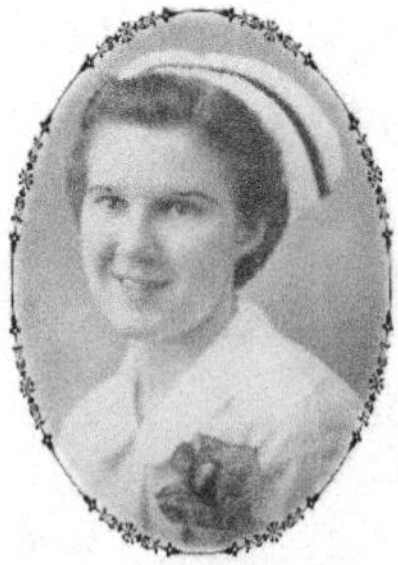

The 10 army nurses who escaped from Corregidor to Australia on an airplane arrived on May 1, 1942 in Port Darwin, Australia. It was a miracle flight of over 7,000 miles, which made it the longest rescue in US history. Late in May, they boarded a ship for San Francisco.

The 179 British and 21 Dutch captured at Santo Tomas Interment Camp were sent home to their countries via plane to Leyte, Philippines then by ship to Australia. A few of the former nurse prisoners of war stayed in the Army Nurse Corps and rose in rank.

Some of the Bataan Death March soldiers received compensation and others were denied. The captured physicians and medics on Baguio were taken to Camp O'Donnell in the Philippines and they brought their possessions with them, only to be looted by their captors. The Japanese took everything—razor blades, soap, rings, watches, and underwear. The compound at Camp O'Donnell was a mile square with 40,000 prisoners. The captives slept in 14 x 14 palm-roofed wooden huts. Ten men crowded into each one. Everyone had dysentery from contaminated water and the entire camp smelled like a sewer. Additionally, there were many dead bodies lying around waiting to be buried. The prisoners' diet was inadequate and did not meet the bodily requirements for protein and vitamins. The physicians and medics were there for 12 weeks after the surrender of Bataan. Many were sent on for work detail at nearby Cabanatuan Prison.

When the war was over, the city of Manila was left in shambles with many homeless children roaming the streets. A thousand Americans, 16,000 Japanese, and at least 100,000 unarmed Filipino civilians were killed. One in 10 Manila residents died at the hands of the Japanese army or U.S. artillery barrages in the war.

The city of Manila was rapidly rebuilt with U.S. aid. The United States granted the Philippines independence on July 4, 1946.

Lieutenant General Jonathan M. Wainwright, Commander of Allied Forces in the Philippines, after surrendering the island of Corregidor, was imprisoned in Camp Hsian, Manchuria, China in June 1942 for over three years. He was the highest-ranking American officer taken prisoner.

Our 68 nurses were the first members of the Army Nurse Corps to become prisoners of war. Because of the systematic starvation of the prisoners at Santo Tomas Internment Camp, most of the nurses lost 25 pounds, with the most lost being 40 pounds. Many also shrunk in height.

Symptoms that continued after the war included severe dental problems, wartime illness, and intestinal disorders. Several of the women lost all their teeth and had to get dentures, or had damaged roots, bleeding gums, or chronic gingivitis from starvation, poor nutrition, and a lack of calcium and vitamin D.

Agnes had severe hepatitis with a swollen liver, and stayed at Letterman General for a while before being discharged.

Susie had a decade-long struggle with amoebic dysentery and had a hemorrhoidectomy, which ended her symptoms.

Underweight Annie could not get rid of her symptoms of cramps and had a digestive disorder, which was later diagnosed as hookworms. When she recovered, she found a second "true love" and married.

Molly and Dr. Charlie had a fine marriage with six children.

One of the nurses had tuberculosis and a lung had to be removed.

Veronica surprised everyone by staying in the ANC and became the chief nurse of the 53rd Army Field Hospital in the European Theater of War after following General George Patton's Third Army into occupied Europe. She took care of the liberated patients from Buchenwald. Another one of our nurses married a Bataan Death March survivor. Sadly, many of the nurses developed dementia or what was called a deep melancholy and consequently had failed marriages.

Caroline was granted a 30% disability for arthritis. Some of the Bataan nurses applied to the Veterans Administration for compensation for their lasting injuries, like joints and limbs that ached from malaria and dengue fever.

A few of the "angels" did not have the stamina to work on post-war assignments. Exhaustion set in after having survived shootings, bombardments, famine, and disease.

Many reunions were held for the "Angels of Bataan" for those healthy enough to attend, where some of our original 68 women got to renew their close friendships.

At all of our nurse reunions, we reminisced about the good times, which helped erase memories of the bad times. One of the nurses stated that she never wanted to set foot in another hospital again.

Juanita Redgrave wrote in her diary about both hospitals in the jungle of Bataan and the Santo Tomas Internment Camp. She was the first person to coin the phrase "Angels of

Bataan" and published the 1943 book *I Served in Bataan*.

In 1980, Molly and I signed up for a special trip to the Philippines, arranged by an American veteran who fought there during the war. We visited Corregidor and navigated the old laterals of the Malinta Tunnel. She took her daughter, who realized that her mother had not been an ordinary housewife but a remarkable woman.

In March 1992, many of the surviving "Angels" traveled to Washington, DC to celebrate the 50th anniversary of their capture.

–The End–

About the Author

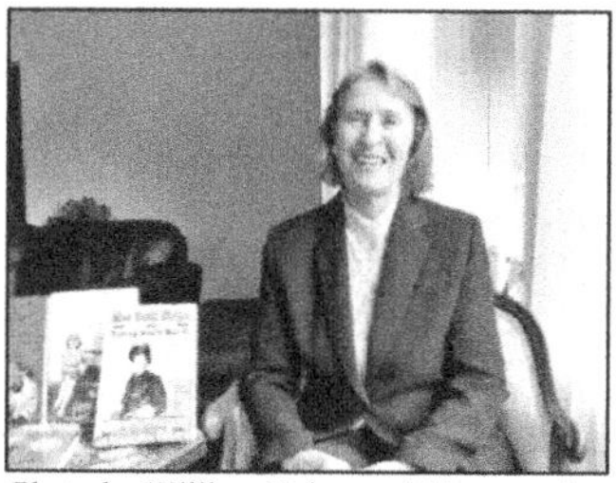

Photo by William Haigwood Photography

Jeane Slone is a member of the Pacific Coast Air Museum, Santa Rosa, CA and a 15-year member of Redwood Writers Club, a branch of the California Writer's Club. She received the Jack London award for service to the club. Ms. Slone has a Bachelor of Science degree in Health Education and a teaching certificate from Brockport State University, New York. She has taught several history classes at Sonoma State University's Osher Lifelong Learning Institute.

Ms. Slone has distributed local authors' books since 2010. She is also the owner of ESL Publishing, a dedicated company that prints quality textbooks for second-language learners. www.eslpublishing.com

Ms. Slone is the daughter of parents who both served in the Army during World War II. She has published five historical novels since 2007:

- *She Flew Bombers During WW II*, winner of the national 2012 Indie Book Award (also available as an audio book through audible.com).
- *She Built Ships During WW II*, which is also available in an ESL version with a workbook.
- *She Was an American Spy During WW II*
- *She Was a WW II Photographer Behind Enemy Lines,* finalist in the Indie Excellence Book Awards.
- *She Was an American Combat Nurse During WW II*

For more information, please visit the author's website:

www.jeaneslone.com

Resources & Additional Information

Copy of letter from the National Association of Colored Graduate Nurses, Inc. dated March 11, 1943.

National Association of Colored Graduate Nurses, Inc.

1790 BROADWAY NEW YORK CITY

Telephone
Circle 5-8000

Executive Secretary
Mrs. Mabel K. Staupers, R.N.

March 11, 1943

Dear Miss Lomax:

You may be assured that we are doing everything we can to remove the present discrimination which Negro nurses are facing in the Army.

Our Advisory Council, and the National Nursing Council for War Service, through Mrs. Biddle, are working on the matter and we hope very soon that you will be called for service.

I am turning your letter from the Service Command over to the National Nursing Council for War Service as another evidence of discrimination.

Kind personal regards,

Sincerely yours,

Mabel K. Staupers

mks/tsl

Mabel K. Staupers, R.N.
Executive Secretary

Miss Louise V. Lomax
1222 East Marshall Street
Richmond, Va.

History of Nursing and the Army Nurse Corps (Est. 1901)

Please note: ANC is the abbreviation for Army Nurse Corps. All references are to White nurses unless otherwise noted.

1818: Spelman College, Atlanta, GA established the first Negro student nurse school.

1836: National Association for Colored Graduate Nurses founded the Mary Mahoney Award in honor of Ms. Mahoney's achievements. This award is given to nurses or groups of nurses who promote integration within their field.

1850-1860: Harriet Tubman led 19 excursions into the hostile South to rescue 300 fugitive Negroes and nursed soldiers in hospitals.

1861-1865: During the Civil War, a small number of Negro nurses served both races.

1854: Florence Nightingale (May 12, 1820-August 13, 1910). She was a British woman who led a group of female nurses to Crimea in October of 1854 to deliver nursing service to British soldiers. Nightingale established the first nurse education programs in several British hospitals.

1862: United States Navy enlisted five Negro women to serve as nurses on the hospital ship *USS Red Rover*.

1873: Three White nursing educational programs—the New York Training School at Bellevue Hospital, the Connecticut Training School at the State Hospital, and the Boston Training School at Massachusetts General Hospital—began operations.

1879: Mary Eliza Mahoney (May 7, 1845 - January 4, 1926) was the first Negro nurse to become a professionally trained nurse in the United States. Mahoney was the first Negro to graduate from the New England Hospital School of Nursing and receive her nursing license.

1890: Two White professional organizations were established, The American Society of Superintendents of Training Schools for Nurses (later renamed the National League of Nursing Education) and the Associated Alumnae.

1893: Lillian Wald founded the Henry Street Settlement House, which provided nursing and other social services to impoverished populations in New York City (White nurse).

1896: The American Nursing Association was established to gain respect for the nursing profession. The ANA did not accept Negro nurses until 1964. The first Negro president was Barbara L. Nichols in 1978.

1900: Approximately 400-800 schools of nursing were established in the United States. The schools were either affiliated with or owned by a hospital. They were apprenticeship programs that used student nurses for their labor. The students received two to three years of training. At the end of the educational program, students received a diploma and were eligible to seek work as a trained nurse.

1901: Army Nurse Corps established.

1914-1918: During WW I, Negro nurses served in convalescent homes and U.S. government hospitals. None were allowed to remain following the period of demobilization.

1918: The influenza pandemic occurred and thousands of people died. A few Negro nurses attended to both Negro and White patients.

1920: Eighteen Negro nurses were assigned to duty in the ANC following the epidemic. Nine were assigned to Camp Grant, Illinois, and nine to Camp Sherman, Ohio. Their living quarters were separate but they were assigned to duties in an integrated hospital.

1930: There were 595 practicing Negro nurses *not* in the ANC.

1939: There were 672 White nurses who served in the ANC. Qualifications: 21-40 years old, unmarried, a graduate of a 3-year nursing training program, licensed in at least one state, a US citizen or a citizen of an Allied country, 5′0″-6′0,″ have a physician's certificate of health and a letter testifying to moral and professional excellence. Pregnancy was given an honorable discharge whether a woman was married or not.

October 1940: The surgeon general recommended that Negro nurses be admitted to ANC to care for Negro patients in segregated Army hospitals.

1940: There were 949 White nurses in the ANC. The demand for nurses increased and the available supply could not keep pace.

1941: New York City White nurses worked with Negro nurses.

1941: Only 14 nursing schools in the U.S. accepted Negroes, who were *not* given the same facilities as White students.

March 7, 1941: Surgeon General James C. Magee established a quota of 185 Negro nurses that would serve in hospitals or wards devoted exclusively to the treatment of Negro soldiers.

Until April 1941: The ANC only employed White nurses.

April 1941: Lt. Della Raney Jackson became the first Negro nurse to be commissioned in the U.S. Army. She was a graduate of Lincoln Hospital School of Nursing in Durham, NC. Lt. Della Raney was the first Negro Chief Nurse in the ANC at Tuskegee Airfield, AL.

1941: The Army had not met their quota of activating 185 Negro nurses. Only 22 Negro nurses were assigned to Fort Bragg, NC and Camp Livingston, LA.

1941: Racial segregation was policy. Mrs. Eleanor Roosevelt requested the Army surgeon general recruit Negro nurses in the ANC. This was before the attack on Pearl Harbor.

June 1941: The ANC authorized 6,894 Negro nurses with only 5,433 signing up. Most of the qualified Negro nurses were rebuffed.

March 1942: Julia O. Flikke was the first White ANC woman to hold the rank of full colonel.

June 1942: Six months after the Japanese bombed Pearl Harbor, there were 12,000 nurses on duty in the ANC.

October 1942: Married nurses were accepted into the ANC.

December 22, 1942: Congress authorized military nurses to receive pay equivalent to a man of the same rank without dependents. The nurses held the "relative" rank of 2nd Lieutenant and were admitted to officers' clubs and had the privilege of the salute.

1943: Twenty-eight nursing schools accepted Negro nurses.

1943: One hundred eighty-three Negro nurses were accepted in segregated hospital wards on Army bases located at Camp Livingston, LA and Fort Bragg, NC.

January 17, 1943: The first nurse to receive an Air Medal for meritorious service was White 2nd Lt. Elsie Ott. Lieutenant Ott served as a nurse for five patients who were being evacuated from India to Washington, D.C.

February 18, 1943: The first class of Army Nurse Corps flight nurses graduated by the School of Air Evacuation at Bowman Field, Kentucky.

February 18, 1943: Second Lt. Dorothy Shikoski was the second Army nurse to receive the Air Medal for risking her life trying to save a Marine navigator in a plane crash. Shikoski was the first American White woman in the first group of air evacuation women flight nurses to set foot on the island of New Georgia in the South Pacific. She was decorated for displaying heroism following a crash landing at sea during a severe storm in the South Pacific Theater. This was the first aerial evacuation flight in nursing history and the pioneer movement of transporting wounded soldiers by air over such a great distance (11,000 miles).

March 1943: Negro First Lt. Susan Freeman was chief of the 30 nurses of the 25th Station Hospital, Roberts Field, Liberia. Lieutenant Freeman was awarded the Ribbon of the Knight Official, Liberian Order of African Redemption.

July 1943 - September 1945: Approximately 27,330 newly inducted nurses graduated from 15 Army training centers.

January 1944: White Army nurses waded ashore on Anzio beachhead in Italy five days after troop landings on January 22,

1944. Six Army nurses lost their lives during enemy bombing attacks in early February.

June 6, 1944: Second Lt. Geraldine Dishroom received the first flight wings and was with the first air evacuation team to land on Omaha Beach after the Normandy invasion. She was a White nurse.

June 10, 1944: Four days after the Normandy invasion, White nurses of the 42nd and 45th Field Hospitals and the 91st and 128th Evacuation Hospitals arrived in Normandy.

June 22, 1944: Public Law 350, 78th Congress, granted Army nurses temporary commissions in the Army of the United States, with full pay and privileges of the grades from second lieutenant through colonel, for the duration of the emergency plus six months.

July 1944: Quota to accept Negro nurses lifted; however, only approximately 600 Negro women were accepted to serve in the entire Army Nurse Corps, even though 9,000 signed up.

1944: Approximately 2,000 Negro students enrolled in the Cadet Nurse Corps program and nursing schools for Negroes, and benefited from increased federal funding.

July 9, 1944: Gardiner General Hospital, Chicago, Illinois, was dedicated to the memory of 2nd Lt. Ruth M. Gardiner, the first White Army nurse to be killed in a theater of operations during World War II. Lieutenant Gardiner, a flight nurse, was killed in a plane crash near Naknek, Alaska, on July 27, 1943 while on an air evacuation mission.

September 27, 1944: Lt. Reba Z. Whittle of the 813th Medical Air Evacuation Transport Squadron became a prisoner of the Germans after the plane in which she was flying during an evacuation mission was shot down over Aachen.

October 21, 1944: Lieutenant Francis Slanger died of wounds caused by the shelling of her tented hospital area in Belgium.

December 1944: First Lt. Agnes B. Glass was the Chief Nurse of the 335th Station Hospital at Tagap, Burma (Negro nurse).

1945: There were 59,000 White nurses in the ANC.

January 6, 1945: Draft for nurses was proposed in a State of the Union Address, in which President Franklin D. Roosevelt stated that there was a critical shortage of Army nurses and that medical units in the European Theater were strained to the breaking point. He proposed that nurses be drafted. At the time, there were 9,000 applications from Negro nurses hoping to enlist in the Army Nurse Corps, but those nurses didn't count toward the goal. The House of Representatives passed a draft bill on 7 March 1945, but the Senate had not acted upon it because of the Victory in Europe on May 8, 1945.

January 1945: Army Nurse Corps opened to all qualified nurses regardless of race.

March 1945: Negro nurses first admitted into the Navy.

Apr 28, 1945: Six Army nurses and five Army medical officers were among some 29 people killed when the hospital ship *Comfort*, loaded to capacity with wounded being evacuated from Okinawa, was attacked by a Japanese "suicide" plane (all White).

May 8, 1945: The War Department notified the Senate on May 24, 1945 that a draft for nurses would not be necessary since there was an enrollment of over 10,000 nurses in the Army Nurse Corps.

May 8, 1945: Victory in Europe (V-E day). There were more than 52,000 Army nurses on active duty serving in 605 hospitals overseas and 454 hospitals in the United States.

September 1945: End of the war, approximately 500 Negro nurses held commissions compared to 59,000 White nurses, accounting for just 0.8% of the Army Nurse Corps. Negro nurses served in Africa, England, Liberia, China, Australia, Burma, New Guinea and the Southwest Pacific. There were nine Negro nurses in the grade of captain, 115 were first lieutenants, and 388 were second lieutenants.

1945: Five hospital ships and one general hospital used during the war were named after White Army nurses who lost their lives in service during World War II.

1945: End of the war, Army nurses were eligible for additional education under the G.I. Bill of Rights, which would enable them to pursue professional educational goals. World War II had forever changed the face of military nursing.

After the war: Nurses entered the ANC as second lieutenants, and the vast majority stayed at that rank. By the end of the war there were only 107 cases of nurse misconduct. During the first part of the war, Army nurses were not allowed to socialize with enlisted men.

1941-1945 During WW II, Army nurses served at station hospitals (military hospitals that give treatment to troops in the immediate area) and general hospitals throughout the continental United States. Overseas, they were assigned to hospital ships, flying ambulances, and hospital trains; clearing stations; and field, evacuation, and general hospitals. They served on beachheads from North Africa to Normandy and Anzio, in the Aleutians, Wales, Australia, Trinidad, India, Ireland, England, the Solomons, Newfoundland, Guam, Hawaii, New Guinea, New Caledonia, Puerto Rico, Panama, Iceland, Bataan, and Corregidor.

The nurses endured relentless bombing and strafing on land, torpedoing at sea, and anti-aircraft fire while evacuating the wounded by air.

In Europe, during the major battle offensives, Army nurses assisted in developing the concept of recovery wards for immediate postoperative nursing care of patients. The flight nurses helped to establish the incredible record of only five deaths in flight per 100,000 patients transported.

ANC nurses received 1,619 medals, citations, and commendations during the war. Sixteen medals were awarded posthumously to nurses who died as a result of enemy fire. In World War II, 201 Army nurses died, 16 as a result of enemy action. More than 1,600 nurses were decorated for meritorious service and bravery under fire. Decorations included the Distinguished Service Medal, Silver Star, Distinguished Flying Cross, Soldier's Medal, Bronze Star Medal, Air Medal, Legion of Merit, Army Commendation Medal, and the Purple Heart.

September 2, 1945: End of World War II, Army nurses became eligible for all veterans' benefits. Many former Army nurses attended colleges and universities in the post-war period under the Servicemen's Readjustment Act of 1944, commonly known as the G.I. Bill of Rights.

December 31, 1945: There were 27,850 Army nurses on active duty.

1946: During the occupation of Japan, Maj. Grace E. Alt organized a Nursing Education Council in Japan. White Army nurses offered refresher courses to the Japanese nurses.

September 30, 1946: A year after the end of World War II, approximately 85,000 nurses remained in the Army Nurse Corps.

July 26, 1948: President Truman signed Executive Order 9981, establishing the President's Committee on Equality of Treatment and Opportunity in the Armed Services, requiring the government to integrate the segregated military.

October 6, 1955: Second Lt. Edward T. Lyon became the very first White male nurse to be commissioned in the Army Nurse Corps in the US as a reserve officer.

July 15, 1964: Margaret E. Bailey became the first Negro promoted to lieutenant colonel in the Army Nurse Corps. In 1970, she was promoted to full colonel. She had a 27-year career in the ANC. In 1971, Bailey, after retiring, became a consultant to the surgeon general to promote increased participation by minority group members in the Army Nurse Corps.

Mabel Keaton Staupers, RN (1890-1989), Racial Integration Leader

1914: Graduated with honors from Freedman's Hospital School of Nursing, Washington, D.C.

1920: Established and became Director of Nursing in the first hospital in Harlem, NY—The Booker T. Washington Sanitarium—which helped treat Negroes with tuberculosis.

1921: Executive Secretary of the New York Tuberculosis and Health Association. Her research led to the founding of the Harlem Committee of the New York Tuberculosis and Health

Association. She became the organization's first executive secretary, a post she held for 12 years.

1934: Executive secretary of the National Association of Colored Graduate Nurses (NACGN), which helped Negro nurses gain unrestricted membership in state and national nursing organizations.

June 1941: Mabel Staupers wrote to the surgeon general to end segregation.

1944: Contacted First Lady Eleanor Roosevelt and organized a nationwide letter-writing campaign to convince President Franklin D. Roosevelt and other political leaders of the need to recognize Negro nurses.

January 1945: Worked to end discrimination in the Armed Forces Nurse Corps and achieved first full integration in the American Nurses Association by 1948.

1951: Staupers was awarded the Spingarn Gold Medal from the National Association for the Advancement of Colored People.

1961: Mabel Staupers published her autobiography, *No Time for Prejudice: A Story of the Integration of Negroes in Nursing in the United States.*

History of Fort Huachuca, Arizona

March 3, 1877: Fort Huachuca was built.

1913-1933: Negro Buffalo soldier unit established.

1942: 1,400 structures at Fort Huachuca were built to house the segregated Negro male and female personnel. There were 50,000 people posted at the base at this time, making it the third largest community in Arizona. The Mountain View Negro Officers Club, 17,000 square feet, featured celebrities such as Lena Horne and Louis Armstrong.

German Prisoners of War

From 1942 to 1946, there were 371,683 German POWs in more than 600 camps in the United States.

Interracial Marriage (Miscegenation Laws)

1751: Maryland banned interracial marriage.

1913-1948: Thirty out of the then 48 states enforced anti-miscegenation laws. Only Connecticut, New Hampshire, New York, New Jersey, Vermont, Wisconsin, Minnesota, Alaska, Hawaii, and Washington, D.C. never enacted them. As late as the 1950s, almost half of the states had miscegenation laws.

1921: The term "mulatto" (a person of White and Negro ancestry) was dropped from the federal census with the "one-drop rule" replacing it to stop Negroes from passing as Whites.

1924: Virginia passed a law that prohibited Whites from marrying anyone with "a single drop of Negro blood."

1924: Congress passed the Immigration Act, a series of strict anti-immigration laws calling for the severe restriction of "inferior" races from Southern and Eastern Europe.

1948: California was the first state to repeal its laws against interracial marriage.

January 31, 1967: Loving v. Virginia, 388 U.S. 1, was a landmark civil rights decision of the U.S. Supreme Court in which the Court ruled that laws banning interracial marriage violate the Equal Protection and Due Process Clauses of the Fourteenth Amendment to the U.S. A Netflix movie was made about this interracial couple during segregation.

1967: Alabama was the last state to repeal its laws against interracial marriage.

History of Skin Pigmentation

The one-drop blood rule or 1/16th rule

The one-drop rule was state and federally mandated to keep Negroes in their place and not mix with the White race. This law applied to American Negroes only. Nazi Germany had an Aryan blood policy. No other nations in the world had miscegenetic laws except U.S. and Nazi Germany.

1837: Jakob Henle, anatomist/pathologist, discovered the pigment melanin that produced cells in the skin called melanocytes. The origins of human skin color remained an enigma before the 19th century and generated a multitude of misconceptions.

Booker T. Washington (4/05/1856-11/14/1915) an American Negro educator, author, orator, and adviser to several presidents of the United States, said, *"It is a fact that, if a person is known to have one percent of African blood in his veins, he ceases to be a white man. The ninety-nine percent of Caucasian blood does not weigh by the side of the one percent of African blood. The white blood counts for nothing. The person is a Negro every time."*

1924: The Racial Integrity Act of Virginia ensured that all infants born in Virginia receive birth certificates that included their racial designation. The one-drop rule was applied.

1924: The term "White person" is only classified as such if they have no trace whatsoever of blood other than Caucasian. Laws were made at this time to stop racial passing.

The Virginia Racial Integrity Act of 1924 prohibited interracial marriage and essentially determined that if a White person had one drop of Negro blood they were classified as Negro, ensuring that all infants born in Virginia received birth certificates that included their racial designation.

1940: Terms "melanin" and "melanocyte" first reported. These cells are responsible for the pigment-producing cells in the hair, skin, and irises of the eyes in people and animals.

History of the American Red Cross

1941: Red Cross Blood Donor Program established.

1941-1945: 6.7 million volunteers donated over 13 million pints of blood at 35 fixed donor centers and 63 mobile units. There were more than 2,000 Red Cross chapters and branches. The Donor Service had 100,000 volunteer workers and hundreds of nurses. Plasma, serum, and whole blood were flown all around the world and transported to battlefield fronts on the backs of mules, on litters carried by natives, and planes dropped plasma by parachute.

1950: The Red Cross stopped requiring the segregation of Negro blood.

1969: Arkansas banned the segregation of Negro blood.
1972: Louisiana was the last state to ban the segregation of blood.

History of All-Black Hospitals

1942: The surgeon general was opposed to the integration of Negro doctors and nurses with White professionals. There was no other option but to establish all-Negro wards in some hospitals, such as Ft. Bragg, North Carolina and Camp Livingston, Louisiana. The Medical Department mostly employed its limited Negro staff in the Negro wards of White station hospitals, while the majority of Negro personnel either served in ambulance and sanitary companies, or in the medical detachments attached to segregated combat and support units.

1942-1945: Negro medical personnel were used on a non-segregated basis in four general hospitals, three regional hospitals, and nine station hospitals but were still under White command. Overseas, the 335th Station Hospital (CBI), the 268th Station Hospital (SWP), the 355th and 383rd Station Hospitals (CBI and Philippines), and the 25th Station Hospital (Liberia), as well as the 168th Station Hospital (England) had their complement of Negro nurses.

1945: Toward the end of the war, the Medical Department employed 342 Black officers and 19,587 enlisted men and women.

History of Grady Hospital, Atlanta, Georgia

1892: Grady Memorial Hospital opened with separate and *unequal* facilities.

1917: First Negro class graduated from the segregated nursing school.

1930: A fire occurred in the Negro section of Grady caused by rats chewing through the insulation; 125 patients and staff died. Negro Grady was called a disgrace with building and equipment being inadequate and no isolation wards for meningitis or measles, scarlet fever, chicken pox, or tuberculosis. The Negro dormitories were severely crowded.

1950: Negro physicians were able to visit and practice in the hospital's segregated Negro section.

June 1, 1965: Grady hospital became desegregated.

Liberia

1853-1903: Approximately 500 Negroes left the Chattahoochee Valley of Georgia and Alabama to start new lives in the West African Republic of Liberia. Most sought safety and escape from a white supremacist society. Liberia had available land and opportunities for prosperity more than the southern United States. Most emigrants were young families consisting of farmers, tradesmen, and clergymen.

Malaria

1942: 24,000 out of the 75,000 American and Filipino Armed Forces suffered from malaria during WW II.

1943: For every Allied soldier wounded in the struggle for Burma, 120 fell sick. The malarial rate that year was a staggering 84% of total manpower.

2021: Malaria vaccine became available.

History of the Term "Jim Crow"

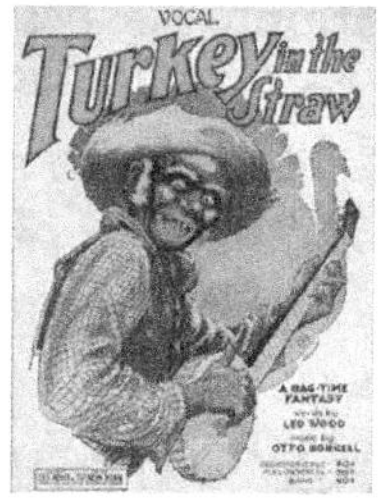

1830: Thomas Dartmouth Rice, a White man, performed a popular song-and-dance modeled after a slave he named Jim Crow. He darkened his face, acted like a clown, and spoke in exaggerated Negro vernacular. Many White performers imitated his acts.

1870-1960s: The term "Jim Crow" became used for laws, customs, and etiquette that segregated and demeaned Negroes.

History of the National Association of Colored Graduate Nurses (NACGN)

The trend in every section of the United States was toward complete segregation of the Negro. It was difficult for most Negro nurses to practice their profession and procure an education. Employment opportunities for a Negro nurse were mostly assigned to the care of Negro patients.

Despite the need for personnel, the Red Cross and the Army Nursing Corps had been refusing Negro nurses as volunteers. The NACGN aided Negro nurses to find employment amidst discrimination and segregation.

1908: NACGN was founded by RN Martha Minerva Franklin, a graduate of the school of nursing of the Women's Hospital of Philadelphia. The NACGN was established because the American Nursing Association denied Negro women jobs and membership.

1914-1918: NACGN got the Army to enlist Negro nurses during WW I and the flu epidemic.

1916: RN Adah Belle Samuels Thoms became the first president of the NACGN.

1941: WW II broke out and the NACGN urged all eligible nurses to enroll in the American Red Cross. The Red Cross did not accept Negro nurses and they registered through the NACGN. The Red Cross established a special membership category for these nurses:

National Association of Colored Graduate Nurses. The National Association of Colored Graduate Nurses (NACGN) – founded in 1908 for Negro registered nurses as an alternative to the ANA. With political pressure from civil rights groups and the Negro press, 56 black nurses were finally admitted into the U.S. Army Nurse Corps in 1941. Some went to Fort Livingston in Louisiana and others to Fort Bragg, in North Carolina, both segregated bases. The NACGN asked First Lady Eleanor Roosevelt for help and she gave her commitment to equal rights.

1951: NACGN dissolved.

History of Ledo Road

Multi-culture laborers worked day and night in the jungles of Burma, sometimes halfway up 10,000-foot mountains, drenched by 140 inches of rain in the five-month monsoon season. They went through raging rivers, pushed through swamps thick with bloodsucking leeches and swarms of biting mites and mosquitoes that spread typhus and malaria. Over 1,500 soldiers died during the construction of the Ledo/Stilwell Road. Some died from disease or fell to their deaths when construction equipment slid along soupy mud tracks and dropped off cliffs. Others drowned or were killed pulling double duty in combat against the Japanese.

December 16, 1942: U.S. Army engineers began construction of the highway to link the railheads of Ledo in Assam, India to Mogaung, Burma with 15,000 American troop members, 60 percent Negro. There were 35,000 soldiers consisting of Indian, Chinese, and Burmese nationals who assisted in the construction of the road. The goal was to have the road begin in Ledo, India, cross over the Patkai Mountains (where passes were as high as 4,500 feet) and end at Kunming, China.

1944: The road stretched 1,726 kilometers (1,072 miles), with 1,033 kilometers (642 miles) in Burma, 632 kilometers (393 miles) in China, and the remainder in India. It took over two years for the road to be completed from India to Burma to the western Chinese city of Kunming.

January 1945: U.S. spent almost $149 million to build the road and, at the request of Nationalist Chinese leader Chiang Kai-shek, it was named the Stilwell Road after U.S. Gen. Joseph "Vinegar Joe" Stilwell, Commander of Allied troops in the region.

May 20, 1945: Ledo/Stilwell Road officially opened.

September 13, 1945: Two atomic blasts finished the war with Japan, and a hard-won passage that soldiers called "the Big Snake" was abandoned to the rain forest. The road had cost 1,133 American lives—a man a mile.

1946-1990: Ledo/Stilwell road became difficult to travel on as the jungle encroached upon the road. Travel to this region was restricted by the Indian government. India imposed severe travel restrictions on Burma from 1962 until the mid-1990s, as fighting occurred between the Indian army and rebels who had taken refuge in Burma.

2005: India and China began to resurrect the overland trade route linking India to China again by mapping out plans to rebuild the road.

Reconstruction of the Ledo/Stilwell Road could cut 30% off the time to transport goods and increase trade and economy between China and India.

April 2008: The government of India considered a proposal to build 37 more roads along the India-China border.

2016: China called for restoration of Stilwell Road.

2022: Paved sections of roads from India to Myanmar (Burma) were constructed.

Interrogation of Alice M. Zwicker, 1st Lt., ANC, N-720222

To follow is the transcript of the interrogation of Alice M. Zwicker, 1st Lt., ANC, by the War Crimes Office in the matter of imprisonment of civilian internees and American prisoners of war under improper conditions at Santo Tomas Internment Camp, Manila, Philippines 1942 to 1945.

Mr. Rod Tenney, nephew of Alice M. Zwicker, and Mr. Walter M. Macdougall, author of *Angel of Bataan,* paid a researcher to find this war crimes interrogation in the National Archives in Washington, DC. Alice was one of the 68 nurses interned at Santo Tomas, Manila, Philippines by the Japanese. Rod wrote me and said, "This is important information that the majority of people have never seen. I'm glad that it is going to be included in your book."

The Process

I received quite a number of zip files from Rod Tenney (see acknowledgments) about the interrogation of his Aunt Alice, one of the 68 nurses interned at Santo Tomas. It was a daunting experience trying to read the 26 zip files as they were copies of microfilm on dark-gray paper. After an exhaustive process to get a clearer copy of the text, the resulting document displayed many anomalies, such as capitalization errors, etc. The files also had numerous Japanese and Korean characters dispersed throughout that were not seen in the zip files. I had them translated by two different translators and was told they were meaningless words or letters. Although this was a very time-consuming process, it was well worth it to add this recently declassified material to the book so readers could view an actual war crimes interrogation about the Santo Tomas Interment Camp.

The transcript is presented unedited and verbatim in its original form.

Interrogation of Alice M. Zwicker, 1st Lt., ANC, N-720222 by the War Crimes Office in the matter of imprisonment of civilian internees and American prisoners of war under improper conditions at Santo Tomas Internment Camp, Manila, Philippines 1942 to 1945.

CONFIDENTIAL
(stamped on every page)

For the WAR CRIMES OFFICE
Judge Advocate General's Department - War Department
United States of America

In the matter of Imprisonment of civilian internees and American prisoners of war under Improper conditions at Santo Tomas Internment Camp, Manila, P. I. 1942 to 1945
Perpetuation of the testimony of Alice M. Zwicker, 1st Lt., ANC, ASN N-720222.
Taken at: Conference Room, Base Headquarters, 138th AAF Base Unit, NAD, ATC, Presque Isle Army Air Field, Presque Isle, Maine. 24 July, 1945. In the presence of: Edward D. Flannagan, Agent, Santo Tomas Internment Camp, ASN 33064393. David W. Fuller, Agent, SIC, ASN 51146016. Reporter: Leger R. Morrison, Sgt., Squadron C, 1380th AAF BU, ASN 11097195. Questions by:
The Deponent was duly sworn by David W. Fuller, Notary Public.

Q. Will you state your name, rank, and Army Serial Number?

A. Alice May Zwicker, First Lieutenant, Army Nurse Corps, N-720222.

Q. What is your permanent home address?

A. 27 Pleasant Street, Brownsville, Maine.

Q. What is the name of your nearest relative living there?

A. James Zwicker, my father.

Q. When and where were you born?

A. Brownsville, Maine, August 6, 1916.

Q. When did you return to the United States from overseas?

A. February 24, 1945.

Q. Were you a prisoner of war?

A. Yes.

Q. By whom were you captured?

A. By the Japanese Army.

Q. In what places were you held prisoner, and for about what periods of time?

A. I was held at Fort Mills on Corregidor from 7 May 1942; then I was interned at Santa Catalina, Manila, from 2 July 1942 until 28 August 1942; then I was held at Santo Tomas, Manila, from the 28th of August 1942 until the 3rd day of February 1945, at which time I was liberated.

Q. In what schools or colleges where you educated?

A. Brownville High School, Brownville, Maine, and the Eastern Maine General Hospital School of General Nursing in Bangor, Maine.

Q. Are you a registered nurse in this State?

A. Yes.

Q. Are you a registered nurse for any other State?

A. Yes, New York.

Q. When did you enlist in the Army Nurse Corps?

A. April 20, 1941.

Q. At what places did you serve while you were in the Army Nurse Corps?

A. Camp Edwards, Massachusetts from April to September 1941, then I went overseas, and I spent all the rest of the time there. I went to Fort McKinley, Risal, in the Philippines, and stayed there until the war broke out.

Q. Can you tell us something about your employment before you enlisted in the Army Nurse Corps?

A I did both private duty and Institutional nursing.

Q. Did you specialize in any particular type of nursing before you entered the Army?

A. Surgery mostly surgical patients and surgery operating rooms.

Q. Did you specialize in any particular type when in the Army before you were captured?

A. No, just general nursing general duty.

Q. What types of nursing did you do after you were captured by the Japanese?

A. General duty looking after all the patients.

Q. In other words, you had an opportunity to observe patients who were injured in different ways and patients who were sick from different diseases?

A. That is correct.

Q. Did you experience or observe any particular mistreatment of military prisoners of war or civilian internee while you were at Corregidor or Santa Catalina?

A. No.

Q. Can you tell about how large a camp Santo Tomas was and where it was located? Do you have any idea of the acreage?

A. The area was about sixty acres.

Q. Was it located in Manila?

A. On the outskirts, it was right in the city proper; It was on the out-skirts, and at the same time it was thickly populated. It wasn't out away from anything.

Q. What classes of people were interned there?

A. Civilians and Army Nurse Corps personnel. There were a few military personnel, very few, in the beginnings then they were taken out.

Q. About how many people were held there when you first went there yourself?

A. I should say about two thousand; fifteen hundred or two thousand, approximately.

Q. What was the largest number you remember having

there?

A. About four thousand.

Q. About how many were there when you were liberated?

A. About three thousand.

Q. Was there any turnover of prisoners, or were the same ones there all the time?

A. There was a turnover.

Q. During the first year or so that you were at Santo Tomas who had charge of this camp for the Japanese.

A. The Japanese civilian administration.

Q. Do you know the names of these authorities?

A. Mr. Kodaki and Mr. Koroda

Q. What were their capacities?

A. Kodaki had charge of the various camps, because he wasn't there all the time, and he came in at intervals and looked the place over. Koroda was in all the time. He stayed right in the camp; he was actually the head of the camp.

Q. From the middle of 1944 to February 1945, who had charge for the Japanese?

A. The Japanese Military Administration.

Q. Do you know the names of any Japanese connected with the camp during that period of time?

A. There were Abiko, Horosi, Honda, and Ohasi. They were officers, but I don't know what their ranks were.

Q. Do you know what has become of any of these Japanese since?

A• Horosi, Honda, and Ohashi surrendered when the American troops came in, and they were taken prisoner. Abiko was killed when our troops came in.

Q. Did the first three try to treat the prisoners decently?

A. They did, definitely.

Q. What sort of management did the Internees have to govern themselves?

A. We had committees and sub-committees, central committees, and subordinate committees. The central committee was the main committee, where we could take our problems to.

Q. Could the central committee handle negotiations with the Japanese if any were necessary?

A. Yes.

Q. Can you give the names of any members of that committee and their home addresses If you know them, and whether or not they were liberated?

A. I know only a couple, C. G. Grinnell; he represented General Electric. He wasn't liberated, he was killed by the Japanese. There was Mr. Earl Carroll, and he was liberated. I believe he's back in the States. I believe he lives in Los Angeles, California.

Q. How did Carroll get along with the Japanese?

A. He got along very well with the Japanese. He was all American, but he wasn't a "yes man", The Japanese made a statement that Carroll was probably the best man we had.

Q. What were your own duties?

A. Hospital duties as a nurse; just general ward duty. We didn't have space to have wards for the various things.

Q. Who was in charge of the hospital?

A. Dr. Fletcher.

Q. Do you know what his home address was?

A. I really do not know.

Q. Was he liberated?

A. Yes.

Q. Do you know the names of any other medical men at the camp?

A. Dr. Theodore Stevenson, Dr. Waters, Dr. Baldwin.

Q. Do you have any ideas what cities these people came from?

A. Dr. Waters and Dr. Fletcher were in the Islands quite a while before the war. I don't know where Dr.

Stevenson's home is.

Q. Do you recall any other names?

A. Lee Gardiner was head of the hospital. Dr. Fletcher was medical advisor and was head of the hospital from a medical standpoint.

Lee Gardiner was head of the hospital as far as supplies were concerned. Dr, Gardiner was connected with either General Electric or Standard Oil.

Q. Do you know his position with this company?

A. No, I don't.

Q. What, in general, would you say of living conditions during the period while the Japanese Military authorities had control of Santo Tomas?

A. I would say they were very good, all things considered.

Q. Good, for internment?

A. That is right.

Q. In general, what would you say as to living conditions during the period while the Japanese military authorities had control?

A. They went from bad to worse. The principal criticisms were lack of food and lack of medical supplies.

Q. Can you tell us what type of food was issued by the Japanese for these of the internees?

A. In the beginning, we had enough meat. It was rationed, and we had enough food with what we supplemented in the beginning by buying our own things. Then rice was the main rations, a few camotes (that is a form of sweet potato)and a few native greens and ground corn.

Q. Would you have any idea, during that period, how many calories per day per person were issued by the Japanese?

A. I think at first our diet as adequate so far as food and vitamins are concerned. About the beginning of the internment, we had about fourteen hundred calories per day per person. During the last six months, we had about hundred calories a day per person.

Q. For how many months did you get six hundred calories per day per person?

A. About six or eight months.

Q. What measures did you take to supplement the camp diet while you were under the Japanese military authorities?

A. We were able to get money through various sources while in camp, and we bought food when we could. After the Japanese military took over, the markets stood open a little longer and we bought what food we could. There wasn't much to buy and the prices were exorbitant.

Q. Did the Japanese control the market?

A. I don't think they did at first, I think it was the Filipinos. The Japanese came in, and later on the Filipinos left, and the Americans would sell the food in the market. They made nothing, and turned over what little they collected to the Japanese, and prices were high.

Q. That was during that period of six months?

A. It was about May 1944, and that we had about a month after that and no supplemental rations.

Q. Was this the situation, that the Japanese civilian authorities had control of this camp and you were allowed to go out yourselves?

A. No, we were allowed to send a representative out to purchase food or to arrange contact with these Filipinos for them to come into the camp so that we could purchase food from them.

Q. Was the closing of the markets to the Internees a punishment for breaking rules or regulations for that camp?

A. No, it wasn't for that purpose that the Japanese closed them.

Q. What was the reason?

A. Slow starvation, I guess. To starve the internees.

Q. Was there available food for the internees during the period from 1943 on until your liberation, and for the Japanese as well as the internees?

A. It was available, but towards the end the Japanese wouldn't permit food to come into camp.

Q. What food was available for the internees?

A. All native fruits and vegetables were available. I think the meat supply was rather low. We didn't expect too much of that, but all fruits and vegetables you can grow around there, and they could have been plucked from the trees. Sugar, we didn't get much but it was easy to obtain for the Japanese, but we didn't have much.

Q. You could have continued to procure most types of food from the Filipinos at no expense to the Japanese if they had been willing for you to do so that is if the Japanese had been willing?

A. That is right, if they had kept prices down too, because I think that is important. They charged $3.50 for a coconut, and bananas were about fifty cents apiece, bananas you can pick from a tree. The prices were so high that it was almost impossible to buy anything.

Q. Who raised the prices, Captain? Was it the Japanese military management?

A. I think it must have been. The first two years the prices were approximately the same, although perhaps a little higher, but not too much. Then they assigned Americans in camp to sell the food. The Japanese arranged to have it brought in, and various people in camp sold it. At first you could buy as much as you wanted; then in 1944 it was rationed.

In late 1944 when the Japanese military took over the camp from the Executive Committee, we still had the market for approximately two months, Then, that was out entirely, and there was no more contact with the outside. I think from having talked to the Filipinos after liberation, that in the beginning, what profit they made was their own. The Filipinos would raise the stuff and when it was ready to harvest, it was confiscated, or they got only a small percentage of the harvest.

Q. After the Japanese military took over, did they allow food to come in or were representatives of the internees allowed to go out?

A. After the military took over, a representative was sent out. Before, we could buy as much food as we wanted. If you wished, at first, you bought ten papayas then, all you could buy was one papaya for ten people. Then we had ration cards to get food.

Q. While you were a prisoner, did you receive Red Cross food boxes?

A. We received them once in December 1943 that 1s all. We were given individual food kits, bulk medical supplies, bulk clothing, in that package.

Q. How many people were these for?

A. Each person in the camp received a kit and there were extras. There were about four thousand kits, maybe more.

Q. When you received these kits did it affect the quantity of food you received from the Japanese?

A. No.

Q. Do you have any knowledge of whether or not Filipinos who had food for the American prisoners were excluded from this camp by the Japanese? In 1944-45.

A. Yes, I was told by both our elected guards and by Filipinos that Filipinos came to the gates of the camp with food and that the Japanese would not let them bring it in.

Q. Do you have any knowledge of Red Cross boxes that were received by the Japanese, but weren't delivered to the internees?

A. Yes, we got word from those on work details that were sent out to assist the Japanese. They were sent out of camp to help the Japanese in emptying their food bodegas (big warehouses), and around there, there were some remnants of kits, that is food kits.

Q. What was the condition of these kits as described to you by men of these work details?

A. The cartons and the cans looked new. It certainly didn't look anything that had been left over for a year.

Q. These cans contained food?

A. That is right.

Q. There were food cans both empty and filled which resembled the ones which had been received in your Red Cross packages received in December 1943?

A. Correct.

Q. Do you know the names of any men on these work details who saw these Red Cross cans and cartons?

A. No. As in an ordinary community of that size, one comes in contact with people and know their faces, but I don’t recall their names.

Q. Do you feel that there is a reasonable possibility that these last packages and cans may have been from Red Cross supplies delivered to other camps in the vicinity by the Japanese?

A. No, I don't. The only other prison camp in Manila was Bilibid, and those men were not allowed out who were there. So, in the first place, If they received the cans, there would be no reason why food should be out there near those bodegas; and in the second place, the civilians were treated much better than military prisoners, and I felt sure that we didn't get Red Cross supplies, they didn't either, After our liberation, I talked to prisoners of Bilibid prison camp, and they said they received kits once.

Q. Do you have any knowledge of other Red Cross supplies which were received by the Japanese but were not delivered to the internees?

A. Yes, in December 1944, I saw a newspaper which was smuggled in over the wall.

Q. What newspaper was it?

A. It was edited by the Japanese and printed in Manila ~- a small newspaper. It said that a Red Cross ship had landed in Tokoyo. We have reason to believe that if it had gotten that far, the Japanese could have gotten supplies to us if they had wanted to.

Q. What was the effect upon you of the diet at the prison camp of Santo Tomas?

A. I had beriberi and general fatigue from lack of proper diet.

Q. Did you lose weight?

A. About thirty-five pounds.

Q. How much did you originally weigh, and how much did you lose!

A. I weighed one hundred thirty-five pounds when I went into camp, and I weighed one hundred pounds when I was liberated.

Q. Were you sick in bed with beriberi?

A. I was in bed for a while after that I took vitamin shots and continued to work.

Q. Did you feel weak as a result of this diet?

A. Toward the last, it was just about all one could do to get out of bed for four hours duty and then go back to bed.

Q. Can you tell us something about the effect of the diet on the other internees as you observed it.

Q. The other internees, the majority of them, probably suffered a lot more from vitamin deficiency than I did. Those who were hit the hardest were the old men. I don't know why it seemed to hit them the hardest, but it did and most of it was just caused from improper diet, and toward the last, they were complete bed patients. We had many deaths which were definitely caused from just starvation and although my loss of weight was only thirty-five pounds, many of the men lost as much as one hundred thirty-five pounds.

Q. You were in a position to observe this yourself?

A. That is right.

Q. About how many of the internees died from various causes?

A. Well, in the early days of internment it was not very high that is the death rate. We had deaths of course, but I don't think any more than you would find for a similar number of people in a community of that size. They were deaths from natural causes, and I honestly don't feel that those people would have been saved had they been on the outside. I feel that in the majority of those cases, it was not due to internment. But from the middle of 1944, I think patients could have been saved in some cases had they been able to get proper treatment and medical supplies from the outside. We were limited because we had only what was in the Islands to begin with and nothing was coming in.

Q. How many months was that for?

A. That probably covers the last six months.

Q. You could really put your finger on it as starvation being the cause of death?

A. Yes. The last six months of camp our mortality rate increased with an average of 12-15 deaths a day and they were definitely due to starvation and nothing else.

Q. Can you tell us something about the medical supplies available for the internees at Santo Tomas?

A. In the beginning, representatives were sent out of camp to arrange for the purchasing of medical supplies for the camp from places in Manila.

Q. How long did they do that?

A. About a year and a half after internment.

Q. After the Japanese military came in, what about it?

A. After the Japanese military took over from the executive committee they stopped It.

Q. Did the Japanese ever issue medical supplies for the use of the internees at the camp?

A. No.

Q. Do you know whether they had medical supplies they should have issued to the camp?

A. I don't know whether they did or not, but they had control of the whole south Pacific.

Q. After the Japanese military authorities took control could you obtain Medical supplies from any sources?

A. No.

Q. Not even the Red Cross?

A. These supplies we received from the Red Cross is in the last part of 1943 were the only ones we received from them.

Q. After December 1944, you didn't get any medical supplies at all until you were liberated?

A. That is right.

Q. During the last few months you were allowed to purchase medical supplies, were the prices raised in the same manner as the prices of food?

A. Yes.

Q. Do you remember any instances where any of your medical supplies for the camp were confiscated or stolen by the Japanese?

A. No.

Q. What diseases were prevalent among the internees which required medical supplies for treatment?

A. Almost any of the diseases, including malaria, beriberi, amebic dysentery, basilary dysentery, and the ordinary things which you find anywhere.

It was very difficult to diagnose, because we had no X-Ray and not very much to work with. You just hoped the patient wasn't telling a wrong story.

Q. Any pneumonia or influenza or others?

A. There were several cases of diphtheria and several cases of infantile paralysis. There were cases of pneumonia, influenza, and a lot of dengue. In the beginning because of the unsanitary conditions, they didn't clean up the pools of rainwater both outside and inside of the camp until we got the camp and organized it in order to house that many people.

Q. There is no doubt in your mind that the absence of medical supplies tributed materially to the death rate.

A. That is correct.

Q. Was it the practice at this camp to keep medical records covering the causes of death and the types of diseases?

A. Yes.

Q. Do you know whether or not these records were still at the camp when you were liberated?

A. I do not know whether they were or not. The Japanese had to sign or see the death certificates, and whether they kept them I do not know.

Q. Who made the diagnosis if the cause of death was

beri-beri?

A. Our doctors in camp. The doctors we had at the hospital.

Q. These are the same ones whose names we already have?

A. That is right.

Q. About how many patients did you have in the hospital during the latter part of your imprisonment?

A. About three hundred.

Q. What was the condition of these patients?

A. Very poor. The majority of them were not ambulatory. The majority would not have been able to get out of bed, The beriberi was taking such a toll, and it was hitting the lower part of the body. Most of the patients were so emaciated and yet so edematous from the bottom of their legs up that they would not have been able to get away.

Q. And it was the diagnosis of these medical men that part of the deaths of the internees or prisoners was caused by starvation and part of them by these various diseases?

A. Yes.

Q. Were the doctors in the camp allowed to diagnose the cause of death and enter it in the records?

A. In the beginning, yes. As far as I knew, there was never any comment on any death certificate that they signed. About two weeks before liberation, Dr. Stevenson signed a death certificate as "starvation". and the Japanese wanted him to sign it "malnutrition". They called him in and wanted him to change the diagnosis to "malnutrition". He refused because malnutrition is not the same as starvation. In malnutrition, one has enough food but is not getting the proper vitamins. Because he refused to sign the statement to read "malnutrition" instead of "starvation", he was put in jail for about ten days on a bread and water diet, only he didn't get any bread. Then the American troops came into Manila. I think Dr. Stevenson lost fifteen pounds in those ten days.

Q. How did you know this?

A. I was told by Dr. Stevenson when I saw him after he got out of jail.

Q. While you were in the hospital at Santo Tomas, did you have occasion to see civilian internees who showed evidence of physical abuse?

A. Yes, although the patents never talked; never said anything, I don't know whether they had been cautioned by the Japanese or whether they were just afraid to say anything. Anyway, they didn't talk, but we saw evidence so far as malnutrition and starvation were concerned, and bruises on their bodies, and even some wounds when they were brought in the camp and taken out for some reason or taken to Fort Santiago before they were brought in (picked up in Manila for some reason or other) Although they didn't say anything. it was obvious they had been mistreated.

Q. Had they obviously been beaten in some cases?

A. Yes.

Q. What was Fort Santiago, as you understand it?

A. Fort Santiago was a walled city, an old jail, very seldom used to my knowledge. When the Japanese got it, they used it for headquarters for people who didn't tow the mark.

Q. Can you give us the names of any persons imprisoned who would be able to give additional information?

A. Yes, First Lieutenant Rita G. Palmer, Army Nurse Corps, Hampton, New Hampshire. She was a casualty. I believe she is now in Cushing General Hospital in Framingham, Massachusetts

I, Alice M. Zwicker being duly sworn on oath, state that I have read the foregoing transcript of my interrogation and all answers contained therein are true to the best of my knowledge and belief.

____

Alice M. Zwicker,1st Lieutenant, ANC

Subscribed and sworn to before me on this 17 day of September, 1945.

I, David W. Fuller, Agent, SIC, ASN 31146016, certify that Alice M. Zwicker 1st Lieutenant, ANC personally appeared before me on 24 July 1945 and testified concerning war crimes and that the forgoing is an accurate transcription of the answers given by him to the several questions set forth.

I, Roy Rutland, Jr., Agent, Security Intelligence Corps, Eight Service Command certify that on 17 September 1945 personally appeared before me Alice M. Zwicker, Capt., ANC, ASN N-720222, who, after having read the transcription of the foregoing

questions propounded by David W. Fuller, Agent, Security Intelligence Corps, First Service Command, ASF, at Presque Isle Army Air Field, Presque Isle, Maine on 24 July, 1945, acknowledged them to be true and correct to the best of her knowledge and belief, and affixed her signature thereto in my presence.

Place: San Antonio, Texas, 17 September 1945.

Date: 17 September 1945

WAR CRIMES OFFICE, 16 April 1945

AT WHAT ENEMY CAMPS AND HOSPITALS WERE YOU CONFINED AND WHEN WERE YOU AT EACH? (If never a prisoner of war or internee, then state principal places you have been from time to time while overseas.)

Corregidor 7 May 1942 to 2 July 1942, Santa Catalina 2 July 1942 to 28 August 1942, Santo Tomas 28 August 1942 to Liberation (Feb. 3, 1945)

DO YOU HAVE ANY INFORMATION ABOUT ANY ATROCITIES AGAINST, OR MISTREATMENT OF AMERICANS, PRISONERS OF WAR, CIVILIAN INTERNEES, OR THE CIVILIAN POPULATION FOR WHICH YOU THINK THE PERPETRATORS SHOULD BE PUNISHED? (Answer by stating YES or NO in the spaces provided below).

1 Killings or executions -----------------------NO

2 Torture, beatings or other cruelties

Imprisonment under improper conditions----------NO

3 Massacres, wholesale looting or burning of towns--------------------NO

4. Use of prisoners of war on enemy military works or Operations---------------NO

5. Exposure of prisoners of war to danger of gunfire, bombing, torpedoing, or other hazards of war YES SEE OTHER SIDE

6. Transportation of prisoners of war under improper conditions-----------NO

5. Public exhibition or exposure to ridicule of prisoners of war----------NO

6. Failure to provide prisoners of war with proper medical care, food or quarters YES

7. Collective punishment of a group for offense of others-------------NO

8. Any other atrocities not specifically mentioned above for which you think the guilty persons should be punished--------------NO

IF ANY QUESTION IS ANSWERED YES, THEN STATE THE FACTS BRIEFLY ON REVERSE SIDE OF THIS SHEET. YOU MAY ANTICIPATE AN EXTENSIVE INTERVIEW AT A LATER DATE

CONFIDENTIAL

DECLASSIFIED: AUTHORITY: NND 735027

THIS FOLLOWS THE YES, NO

DETAILS OF ATROCITIES

STATE: KIND OF CRIME, WHERE IT OCCURRED, WHO WAS THE VICTIM, STATE IF YOU SAW IT YOURSELF OR IF YOU DID NOT SEE IT WHO TOLD YOU ABOUT IT.

1. Approximately one year prior to liberation, the Japanese turned the cantonment itself into a motor pool and supply base - where military supplies (Ammunition, gasoline, etc.) were stored. Innumerable drums of gasoline were buried within 100 ft. of the hospital - where American prisoners of war were confined as patients.

1. The American Medical Units were charged with the responsibility of caring for their own. During the first year and one half of captivity, the camps were under the administration of civil authorities and treatment was as good as could have been expected. If

a patient became seriously ill, it was permissible to have him transferred to one Manila's larger hospitals where more adequate services and treatment were available. However, sometime during the latter part of 1943 the Japanese Military assumed administrative control and conditions changed abruptly. From then on, the seriously ill were not allowed to be removed. With reference to medical supplies, we were allowed to purchase them from the Philippine Drug House but the price became exorbitant and some items became unattainable. During all of 1944, we were dependent on almost wholly, Red Cross supplies. I never saw any medical supplies which were placed at our disposal by our captors.
I estimate a daily average of 12 deaths just prior to liberation - ten of which were due either directly or indirectly to malnutrition and insufficient diet.

Q. Did the Japanese ever make use of the compound at Santo Tomas which was occupied by the internees or prisoners?

A. Yes. Barracks were put up as housing for Japanese soldiers eventually in the compound. They built a high fence so that we couldn't actually see the barracks, but they were still there. Originally the space used the far the building of the barracks as a part of Santo Tomas.

Q. Was this apace inside the cement wall?

A. Yes, it was.

Q. Did the Japanese ever make any other use of this? Was this apace inside the cement wall?

A. Yes, it was.

Q. Did the Japanese ever have any other use of this compound?

A. Yes, approximately a year before the liberation, the Japanese set up machine guns in the camp. They had the guns on top of the buildings, and they had then in various corners within the four walls they also had them set up directly behind the hospital within the compound.

Q. Did it appear to you that they were set up to prevent the internees from escaping, or was It for some other purpose?

Have you any idea what that purpose was?

A. Nobody wanted to get any place, because we would have been picked up by the Japanese outside. We all felt that they were getting ready for things when they started to happen. They dug fox holes in the compound too. They were getting ready for the invasion of Manila.

Q. They were really getting ready to use the compound as a fortification?

A. Definitely.

Q. Did the Japanese use the compound in any other way?

A. They used it as a place of storage for military supplies, Of course, a lot of the stuff was crated, but marked on the outside in Japanese, and our interpreters told us it was ammunition. Then the Japanese stored gasoline not more than fifty feet from the hospital, drums of gasoline.

Q. Has anything else used by the Japanese placed inside the compound walls?

1. Yes. Trucks were inside the compound wall and something that looked very much like big guns, of course they were crated, and most of these supplies, the Japanese brought in at night, transported them at night and usually tried to keep them covered, that is camouflaged with bamboo or palm or something like that. The drums of gasoline were buried under the ground. The Japanese dug something like trenches and put the drums in them.

Q. By whom was this done?

A. By Japanese soldiers.

Q. How was the ammunition stored? In what building?

A. It was just piled up on the outside on the front lawn of the camp.

Q. It was camouflaged?

A. That's right.

Q. Did the Japanese try to evacuate the hospital or the rest of the compound before storing these materials there?

A. No.

Q. Did the camp officials in your central committee make any complaint?

A. I don't recall if they did. But knowing the camp officials at this time, I know they must have registered a complaint. I feel sure it was a waste of breath.

Q. Did you ever hear any of the Japanese military authorities in charge of Santo Tomas make any statement about the Geneva Convention?

A. Yes they said they didn't sign the Geneva Treaty, and so there was so reason why they should live up to it.

Q. What was the Japanese attitude toward the rights of prisoners of war?

A. They said we didn't have any rights as prisoners of war. We first complained about housing. We were just jammed in there after a while, the Japanese said we had no rights as prisoners of war. I heard that myself.

Q. Do you recall the name of the individual who said that?

A. Korada, he was the civilian administrator. He treated us reasonably well, but the Japanese said they had not signed the Geneva Treaty, and we knew that there was no point in dwelling on it. If they said "No", they meant "No". At times we did assert ourselves, but that was once where they were holding the whip in hand, and so no one said anything.

Q. Could the Internees have moved the hospital away from the military supplies?

A. Not without the consent of the Japanese, and even so, we had no place to move It. Were you given any reason by anyone as to why these military supplies were stored where they were?

A. We weren't given any definite reason. The Japanese just didn't feel we were entitled to any reason. Naturally, our Air Force certainly knew where the camp was, while prisoners there, we knew we would not be bombed, and we felt the Japanese knew that too. Knowing the Americans, the Japanese knew they wouldn't bomb the camp with the American prisoners in there. So the Japanese knew it was an excellent spot to put something they didn't want touched.

Q. Did the storage of these military supplies in the compound at Santo Tomas take place at about the time of the invasion of the

Philippines by the United States forces?

A. Yes. On September 21, 1944, we saw our first American planes. That we had our first bombing a beautiful sight, I must say.

Q. What was bombed?

A. The Port Area that is a military objective. The Port Area in Manilas airfields, Nichols Field and Grace Park.

Q. Were there other bombings of Manila and the vicinity before the United States forces eventually landed?

A. Yes, we were bombed from the 1st of September until

Liberation Day, February 3rd, 1945.

Q. Do you have any ideas about how many times or how frequently?

1. Until about January 6th, 1945, approximately three or four times per week, I mean three or four days out of the week. Some days it would last four- or five-hours other days, all day long from early morning to night. And after January 6th, it was about every day.

Q. That was about the time of the invasion of Linayen (correct)Gulf. Did any shells, shrapnel, or bomb fragments drop in the compound?

A. Yes. Probably more of it was from anti-aircraft fire than from actual bombs. The Japanese had guns set up outside, and all around the place, so when the planes would fly over the camp, the Japanese shot at them, and shrapnel came down.

Q. When shrapnel would fall in the camp like that, could it have set off the ammunition or gasoline?

A. I don't imagine It would have. However, some shells were found in the camp, and were found to be duds. Others were found to have exploded in the camp, but nobody was hurt.

Q. Do you have any idea of the area of this camp at Santo Tones?

A. About 60 acres.

Q. It was located near Manila?

A. On the outskirts of Manila, but not out away from anything.

Q. What classes of people were interned there?

A. Civilians and Army military Corps personnel. A few military personnel, very few were there in the beginning; then they were taken out.

Q. About how many were there when you were liberated?

A. About three thousand.

Q. About how many patients did you have in the hospital while this army aircraft fire was going on?

A. About three hundred.

Q. And the storage of military supplies?

A. 300

Q. What was the condition of the patients?

A. Very poor. The majority of them were not ambulatory.

Q. They would not have been able to get out of bed?

A. The beriberi was taking a toll and it was hitting the lower part of the body. Most of the patients were so emaciated yet so edematous from the bottom of the their legs up, that they would not have been able to get away.

Q. Was there any apparent reason why the Japanese had to store their materials where they did?

A. I wouldn't say there was any reason for it except the one I Just gave. They stored their ammunition and war supplies, military supplies, in churches and schools and places which the Americans wouldn't ordinarily hit. You saw this yourself?

A. I saw the Japanese store military supplies, in churches. Santo Domingo in Manila was one of the churches.

Q. Do you know of any protests being made about the

storing of the Japanese military supplies in Santo Tomas?

A. I do not.

Q. Do you know who was the Japanese commanding officer during the time they were using the compound at Santo Tomas to store military supplies as you have described?

A. I don't know who was in command when they started. We changed commandments about every six months in that camp.

Their superiors would come in and say that they weren't harsh enough. During the last six months, Abiko was in command.

Q. Would you care to add anything else on this matter of the

storage of military supplies?

A. When they first started bringing in these military supplies, for sone reason which I don't know, they (the Japanese) were bringing them in one day and perhaps taking them out the next day. But there were usually some in the compound at all times, although there was a turnover, they were using the compound as a supply depot more than anything else.

State of Texas. County of Bexar:

I, Alice M. Zwicker, being duly sworn on oath, state that I have read the foregoing transcription of my interrogations and all answers contained therein are true to the best of my knowledge and belief.

Subscribed and sworn to before me this 17 day of September, 1945. C.M. Koss, Lt. Col., MD, AAFSAN, Randolph Field, Texas

SUMMARY COURT (stamped)

CERTIFICATE

I, David W. Fuller, Agent, SIC, ASN 31146016, certify that ALICE M. ZWICKER, 1st Lt., ANC personally appeared before me on 24 July 1945 and testified concerning war crimes; and that the foregoing is an accurate transcription of the answers given by him to the several questions set forth.

Signed: David W. Fuller, Agent, SIC

I Roy Rutland, Jr., Agent, Security Intelligence Corps, Eighth Service Command ASF, certify that on 17 September 1945 personally appeared before me Alice M. Zwicker, Capt. ANC, ASN N-720222, who, after having read the transcription of the foregoing questions propounded by David W Fuller, Agent, Security Intelligence Corps, First Service Command, ASF at Presque Isle Army Air Field, Presque Isle, on 24 July 1945, acknowledged then to be true and correct to the best of her knowledge and belief and affixed her signature thereto in my presence. Place: San Antonio, Texas Dates: 17 September 1945

(stamped) DECLASSIFIED

CONFIDENTIAL (stamped)

HEADQUARTERS, ARMY SERVICE FORCES

Office of The Judge Advocate General

Washington 25, D. C.

10 May 1945

SUBJECT: Request for interview and interrogation of

Alice May Zwicker

TO: Director, Intelligence Division, Army Service Forces ATTENTION: Major Tucker, Room 3-E-572, The Pentagon

1. Reference is made to ASF letter, 14 March 1945.

2. Attached hereto is War Crimes Questionnaire of: Alice May Zwicker

Name: Alice May Zwicker

Rank: lst. Lt. Serial No.: N720222 ANC

Home Address: Brownville, Maine

It is requested that she be interviewed and any testimony pertinent.

CONFIDENTIAL

Army Service Forces, Office of the Commanding General, Washington D. C.

To: Commanding General Service Command

(Attn: Director, Security and Intelligence Div.)

Forwarded for compliance with request set forth in basic

letter. In the event the individual referred to in basic letter has departed from your jurisdiction, this request should be forwarded for compliance to the Headquarters of the Service Command in which he is located, directed to the attention of the Director of Security and Intelligence Division.

BY COMMAND OF GENERAL SOMERVILLE: CHARLES T. TUCKER, Major,

Chief, Domestic & Branch Intelligence Division.

Interview and Interrogation of Alice May Zwicker, 1st Lt., ANC, ASN N-720222

Headquarters First Service Command, Boston 15, Massachusetts, 4 September 1945.

To: Commanding General, Eighth Service Command, Santa Fe Building, Dallas, Texas.

ATT: Director, Security and Intelligence Division.

1. Ist Lt. Alice M. Zwicker, ANC, ASN N-720222, was interviewed on 24 July 1945 and her testimony subsequently transcribed in deposition form. Prior to obtaining her signature, Lieutenant Zwicker was transferred to the School of Aviation Nursing, Randolph Field, Texas.

2. It is requested that Lieutenant Zwicker's sworn signatures be obtained for the attached three depositions and the Enclosed memoranda, to the Director, War Crimes Office, Munitions Building, Washington 25, D.C. FOR THE COMMANDING GENERAL.

1945 WAR CRIMES OFFICE

6 August 1945, SUBJECT: War Crimes. Death of Mr. C. C. Grinnell, a civilian interned by the Japanese at Santo Tomas, and believed to be an American citizen.

The following information was obtained from 1st Lt. Alice May Zwicker ANC,N-720222, Brownville, Maine who is now stationed at the Presque Isle, Maine AAP Base. Lt. Zwicker was prisoned by the Japanese at Santo Tomas.

She stated that management of the internment camp and negotiations with the Japanese authorities were handled through a so-called Central Committee and various sub-committees chosen by the internees and prisoners.

A member of the Central committee was a Mr. C. C. Grinnell who had been a representative of General Electric Corporation, He was put in jail by the Japanese about one month before the American forces arrived and liberated the prisoners. Then two weeks before the Americans arrived, he was taken out of the "jail" at Santo Tomas and removed from the camp.

Lt. Zwicker says that it was common knowledge that after the arrival of the American troops, Grinnell's body was found full of bullet holes. Further details are unknown, but Lt. Zwicker believes this man was imprisoned at Santiago after his removal from Santo Tomas, Santiago being the place where prisoners of war and internees who had incurred the displeasure of the Japanese were taken.

David W. Fuller, Agent, SIC, (Santo Tomas internment camp).

This interrogation was stamped unclassified twelve years after the last interview.

Photo Credits

All photographs and images in this book are from the following sources:

Airforce Medical Service
Army/Military Photos
Army Nurse Corps Border Institute
Centers for Disease Control and Prevention
GGNRA Park Archives, Golden Gate National Recreation Area
iStock Photos
Library of Congress
National Archives
National Institute of Health
National Library of Medicine, Medical History Section, Bethesda, MD.
National Park Service Public Domain
US Army Signal Corps
US Army Center of Military History
US Militia Forum
Wikipedia
WW2 US Medical Research Center

Special Attribution by Chapter

Chapter photograph of Bea credited to Rod Tenney of his Aunt Alice M. Zwicker, 1st Lt., ANC, N-720222, 1941-1947

Chapter photograph of Dottie credited to Mary Robertson of her Aunt Olive Lucas, 1st Lt. ANC, 1942-1945

Chapter Two: Poster of nurse at Grady Hospital, Atlanta, GA, University of Library News, Georgia State University.

Chapter Ten: Map of Liberia, the Office of the Geographer and Global Issues.

Chapter Ten: Ambassador Lester A. Walton, Dale Genius Collection, Louisiana History Museum, Alexandria, LA.

Chapter Twelve: Camp Livingston, Dale Genius Collection, Louisiana History Museum, Alexandria, LA.

Chapter Thirty-Five: The former prisoner of war nurses at Letterman General Hospital, 1945. Golden gate National Recreation Archives.

Chapter Thirty-Five: Colonel James W. Duckworth with the wounded nurses, Lieutenants Rosemary Hogan and Rita Palmer who served in his command on Bataan, GGNRA Park Archives.

Bibliography

BOOKS

Adams-Ender, Clara. *My Rise to The Stars*. Cape Associates, Inc. Lake Ridge, VA.

Farrell, Mary Cronk. *Pure Grit.* Abrams Books, New York 2014.

Fessler, Diane Burke. *No Time for Fear.* Michigan University Press, East Lansing, Michigan 1996.

Grady Memorial Hospital, School of Nursing history book. Georgia State University, Atlanta, Georgia 1962.

Hartendorp, A.V. H. *Santo Tomas Internment Camp*. McGraw-Hill Book Company 1964.

How to Shoot the U.S. Army Rifle. The Infantry Journal, Inc. Washington, D.C.

Jackson, Kathi. *They Called Them Angels.* University of Nebraska, Lincoln, Nebraska 2000.

Kaplan, Carla. *Passing Nella Larsen*. W.W. Norton & Company, Inc. New York, N.Y. 2007.

Movie on Netflix 2021 based on the book.

Macdougall, Walter M. *Angel of Bataan.* Down East Books. Lanham, Maryland 2015.

Monahan, Evelyn M. & Heidel-Greenlee, Rosemary. *All This Hell.* University Press of Kentucky, Lexington, Kentucky 2000.

Monahan, Evelyn M. & Heidel-Greenlee Rosemary. *And if I Perish: Frontline U.S. Army Nurses in World War II.* Random House, Inc. New York 2003.

Mullenbach, Cheryl. *Double Victory.* Chicago Review Press 2017.

Norman, Elizabeth M. *We Band of Angels*. Pocket Books, New York, N.Y. 1999.

Powell, Patricia Hruby. *Loving vs. Virginia: A Documentary Novel of the Landmark Civil Rights Case.* Chronicle Books, San Francisco, CA.

1/31/17.

Redmond, Juanita. *I served on Bataan.* J. B. Lippincott Company 1943.

Sarnecky, Mary T. *A History of the U.S. Army Nurse Corps*. Henry M. Jackson Foundation 1999.

Staupers, Mabel Keaton. *No Time for Prejudice: a Story of the Integration of Negroes in Nursing in the United States.* The Macmillan Company, NY 1961.

Tomblin, Barbara Brooks. *G.I. Nightingales*. University Press of Kentucky, Lexington, Kentucky 1996.

Webster, Donovan. *The Burma Road.* Farrar, Straus, Giroux, New York 2003.

Weinstein, Alfred A. M.D. *Barbed-Wire Surgeon.* Deeds Publishing, Marietta, GA 1948. (Poem in Ch. 9)

Whitcomb, Edgar Doud. *Escape From Corregidor*. Arcadia Press, Mt. Pleasant, SC 1958.

SONG LYRICS

Song of the Army Nurse Corp
Official Anthem of the Army Nurse Corps
1944, Leeds Music Corporation
Words by Pvt. Hy Zaret, Music by Lou Singer

WEB SITES

Academic Accelerator. "Ledo Road." https://academic-accelerator.com/encyclopedia/ledo-road

African American Registry. "The Lee Street Riot Occurs." 2023. https://aaregistry.org/story/the-lee-street-riot-occurs/

American Nursing Association. "The History of the American Nursing Association." https://www.nursingworld.org/ana/about-ana/history/

Arcado, Nickii Wantakan. "Recognizing African American Efforts in Building the Ledo Road" Pacific Atrocities. 2/23/2011. http://www.pacificatrocities.org/blog/black-history-month-recognizing-african-american-efforts-in-building-the-ledo-road .

2/23/19.

BBC News. "Will the famous Indian WWII Stilwell Road reopen?" 2/8/2011. https://www.bbc.com/news/world-south-asia-12269095

"The Army Nurse Corps." U.S. Army Center of Military History. https://history.army.mil/books/wwii/72-14/72-14.HTM

"Camp Livingston, Louisiana, WWII Army Camp." 2023. https://www.alexandria-louisiana.com/camp-livingston-louisiana.htm

Caparas, Kheem. "Intramuros: The Historic Past Inside the Walled City." 8/01/13. Vitattintourism. https://www.vigattintourism.com/index.php?/tourism/articles/Intramuros-The-Historic-Past-Inside-the-Walled-City

Centers For Disease Control and Prevention. "The History of Malaria an Ancient Disease." https://www.cdc.gov/malaria/about/history/index.html

City of Alexandria, Louisiana. 2/26/20. https://www.cityofalexandriala.com/press-release/city-erects-marker-recognizing-lee-street-riot-1942

Clark, Alexis "The Army's First Black Nurses Were Relegated to Caring for Nazi Prisoners of War." 5/15/18. Smithsonian Magazine. https://www.smithsonianmag.com/history/armys-first-black-nurses-had-tend-to-german-prisoners-war-180969069/

Conde, Mavic. "The History of Manila's Walled City of Intramuros" 12/24/19.

CULTURE TRIP. https://theculturetrip.com/asia/philippines/articles/the-history-of-manilas-walled-city-of-intramuros/.

Dash, Dipak K. "Government mulling proposal to build 37 more roads worth Rs 13,000 crore along India-China /Border." 3/27/2023. Published by The Times of India. http://timesofindia.indiatimes.com/articleshow/99018344.cms?from=mdr&utm_source=contentofinterest&utm_medium=text&utm_campaign=cppst

Davis, James F. "Who is Black? One Nations Definition." 1995-2014. PBS Frontline, WGBH educational foundation. https://www.pbs.org/wgbh/pages/frontline/shows/jefferson/mixed/onedrop.html

Feller, Carolyn M. Lieutenant Colonel, ANC, USAR and Moore, Constance l. Major, ANC. "Highlights in the history of the Army Nurse Corps." U.S. Army Center Military History. Washington, D.C. 1995. https://history.army.mil/html/books/085/85-1/CMH_Pub_85-1.pdf

Georgetown Washington University, Washington, DC. "Mabel Keaton Staupers: Nurse, Advocate, Changemaker." 3/8/2021. https://blogs.gwu.edu/himmelfarb/2021/03/08/mabel-keaton-staupers-nurse-advocate-changemaker/

Gillespie, James O. Army Medical Department, Office of Medical History. "Malaria in World War II." Army Heritage Foundation. 2023. https://www.armyheritage.org/soldier-stories-information/malaria-in-world-war-ii/

Guglielmo, Thomas A. "Desegregating Blood: A Civil Rights Struggle to Remember." 2/4/18. KQED PBS News Hour.. https://www.pbs.org/newshour/science/desegregating-blood-a-civil-rights-struggle-to-Remember#:~:text=Officially%2C%20at%20least%2C%20the%20distinction,and%20Louisiana%20overturned%20si

Guglielmo, Thomas A. "Red Cross, Double Cross": Race and America's World War II-Era Blood Donor Service." The Journal of American History volume 97 issue 1. 2010. https://academic.oup.com/jah/article-abstract/97/1/63/719496?redirectedFrom=fulltext.

Hinda, Radhe Director (IT) and DIO "Stilwell Road (Ledo Road)." Compiled by: District Administration, Changlang District, Arunachal Pradesh, Developed by National Informatics Centre. https://changlang.nic.in/stilwell-road-ledo-road/

Hinton, Capt. Dr. Clarence David Army MS. The 335th Station Hospital. https://335thstationhospital.org.

History.com editors. "Jim Crow Laws." 8/11/23 https://www.history.com/topics/early-20th-century-us/jim-crow-laws#jim-crow-in-the-north

Hollinger, David A. "One Drop & One Hate." American Academy of Arts & Sciences, Cambridge, MA. https://www.amacad.org/publication/one-drop-one-hate

Infectious Disease: Superbugs, Science, & Society, A High School Course in Biology. "A Brief History of Malaria and Its Treatment." https://sites.duke.edu/superbugs/module-3/malaria-scourge-of-the-developing-world/a-brief-history-of-malaria-and-its-treatment/

The Jackson Sun Big Rapids, Michigan. "1876-1965 Examples of Jim Crow Laws- Oct. 1960-Civil Rights." 2001 https://jimcrowmuseum.ferris.edu/links/misclink/examples.htm

Jones, Philip H. "African American 'First' Key to Army History." 2/5/09. https://www.army.mil/article/16455/african_american_firsts_key_to_army_history

Ferris State University, Big Rapids, Michigan "Laws that Banned Mixed Marriages." May 2010. https://jimcrowmuseum.ferris.edu/question/2010/may.htm

Los Angeles Times Staff Writer. "Burma's Stilwell Road: A Backbreaking WW II Project." 12/30/2008. https://www.latimes.com/world/la-fg-road30-2008dec30-story.html

Lovasik, Brendan P., M.D., Priya, R. Rajdev, M.D. "The Living Monument": The Desegregation of Grady Memorial Hospital and the Changing South." The American Surgeon. 3/1/2020. Vol. 86, issue 3. https://pubmed.ncbi.nlm.nih.gov/32223800/

National Museum of African American History and Culture. "Victory at Home and Abroad African American Army nurses in World War II." https://nmaahc.si.edu/explore/stories/nurses-WWII

National Nurses United Blog. "Celebrating the pioneering National Association of Colored Graduate Nurses." 2/10/2023. https://www.nationalnursesunited.org/blog/celebrating-the-pioneering-national-association-of-colored-graduate-nurses

Office of the Historian, Foreign Service Institute *United States Department of State*. "Founding of Liberia." *https://history.state.gov/milestones/1830-1860/liberia*

Pilgrim, Dr. David Professor of Sociology Ferris State University. "The Tragic Mulatto Myth." 11/2000. The Jim Crow Museum. https://www.ferris.edu/HTMLS/news/jimcrow/mulatto/homepage.htm

Pistininz, Michael. "America's African Colony: A History of Liberia." 2/24/21. https://www.ourcityforest.org/blog/2021/2/23/americas-african-colony-a-history-of-liberia

Robinson, Greg. Université du Québec À Montréal. "Camp Livingston (detention facility).” https://encyclopedia.densho.org/Camp_Livingston_(detention_facility)

Robertson, Mary. “The story of Olive Lucas” The Talbot Spy. Five part series in The Talbot Spy. https://talbotspy.org/?s=The+Story++of+Olive+Lucas+by+ 7/19/2019, 8/8/2019, 8/31/2019, 9/27/2019,11/10/2019.

Jhonnyespanadique's Blog. Runners of Tomorrow “History of Santo Tomas Manila.” 11/12/2010. https://jhonnyespanadique.wordpress.com/2010/11/12/history-university-of-santo-thomas-manila/

Saikia, Jaideep. “Opinion | Stilwell Road Holds the Key to India’s ‘Act East’ Policy.” 2/18/2023. CNN News 18. https://www.news18.com

Shanks, Dennis G. “Historical Review: Problematic Malaria Prophylaxis with Quinine.” 2/22/20. National Library of Medicine https://www.ncbi.nlm.nih.gov/pmc/articles/PMC4973170/

Smilie, Jim. “City Erects Marker Recognizing Lee Street Riot of 1942.” . 2/26/2021. City of Alexandria, Louisiana. https://www.cityofalexandriala.com/press-release/city-erects-marker-recognizing-lee-street-riot-1942#:~:text=(February%2026%2C%202021)%20%E2%80%94,at%20the%20Randolph%20Riverfront%20Center

Spring, Kelly A. M.D. “Mary Elizabeth Mahoney (1865-1926).” 2017. National Women’s History Museum. https://www.womenshistory.org/education-resources/biographies/mary-mahoney

Stroock, William. “Final Battle For Burma, 1945.” Warfare History Network. https://warfarehistorynetwork.com/article/final-battle-for-burma-1945/#:~:text=In%20February-March%201945%2C%20the

Sundin, Sarah. “Army Nursing in World War II – Nursing Uniforms.” 10/15/18. https://www.sarahsundin.com/army-nursing-in-world-war-ii-uniforms/

Sundin, Sarah. “Army Nursing in World War II-Who Could Serve.” Blog. 10/1/2018. https://www.sarahsundin.com/army-nursing-in-world-war-ii-requirements/#:~:text=To%20serve%20in%20the%20Army, of%20an%20Allied%20country%2C%205

Tisdale, David. "USM Professor Organizes Formal Discussion of Rumored Mass Grave for African Americans Killed in 1942 Riot." 10/01/20. The University of Southern Mississippi. Camp Livingston, Lee Street. https://www.usm.edu/news/2020/release/formal-discussion-rumored-mass-grave.php.

Tucson Historic Preservation Foundation. "Mountain View Black Officers Club." 2023. https://preservetucson.org/stories/mountain-view-black-officers-club/

University of Houston, Texas. "To Bear Fruit for our Race." 2023. https://uh.edu/class/ctr-public-history/tobearfruit/story_1927-1954_section06.html

US Medical Research Center. "Venereal Disease and Treatment During WW2." https://www.med-dept.com/articles/venereal-disease-and-treatment-during-ww2/

Weidenburner, Carl Warren. "The Hoverfly in CBI. First helicopter used in CBI in 1944. First medivac rescue." 2/4/22. http://www.cbi-theater.com/hoverfly/hoverfly.html

Weidenburner, Carl Warren. "Stilwell Road Story of The Ledo Lifeline." 2008. https://www.cbi-theater.com/ledoroad/first_convoy/firstconvoy.html

Westerhof, Wiete. "The discovery of the human melanocyte." Published by Researchgate. https://www.google.com/search?q=%E2%80%9CThe+discovery+of+the+human+melanocyte.%E2%80%9D+Published+by+Researchgate&rlz=1C5CHFA_enUS849US858&oq=%E2%80%9CThe+discovery+of+the+human+melanocyte.%E2%80%9D+Published+by+Researchgate&gs_lcrp=EgZjaHJvbWUyBggAEEUYOdIBCjM2MzI4ajBqMTWoAgCwAgA&sourceid=chrome&ie=UTF-8

WGBH | PBS Online. "People and Events American Colonization Society 1816 – 1865." https://www.pbs.org/wgbh/aia/part3/3p1521.html

Whelan, Jean C. Adjunct Assistant Professor of Nursing. "American Nursing: An Introduction to the Past." University of Pennsylvania School of Nursing. https://www.nursing.upenn.edu/nhhc/american-nursing-an-introduction-to-the-past/

WW2 Medical Research Center. "Venereal Disease Treatment During WW2." https://www.med-dept.com/articles/venereal-disease-and-treatment-during-ww2/

Made in the USA
Monee, IL
13 November 2023

46453895R00246